Psychosocial & Behavioral Aspects of Medicine

Psychosocial & Behavioral Aspects of Medicine

HANNO W. KIRK, PhD, LICSW

JO WEISBROD, MA, LPC, ADTR

KAY ERICSON, PA-C

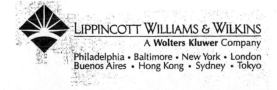
LIPPINCOTT WILLIAMS & WILKINS
A **Wolters Kluwer** Company
Philadelphia • Baltimore • New York • London
Buenos Aires • Hong Kong • Sydney • Tokyo

Editor: Neil Marquardt
Managing Editor: Jacqui Merrell
Marketing Manager: Scott Lavine
Art Director: Doug Smock
Printer: Data Reproductions Corp.

351 West Camden Street
Baltimore, Maryland 21201-2436 USA

530 Walnut Street
Philadelphia, Pennsylvania 19106-3621 USA

The publisher is not responsible (as a matter of product liability, negligence, or otherwise) for any injury resulting from any material contained herein. This publication contains information relating to general principles of medical care which should not be construed as specific instructions for individual patients. Manufacturers' product information and package inserts should be reviewed for current information, including contraindications, dosages, and precautions.

Printed in the United States of America

Library of Congress Cataloging-in-Publication Data
Kirk, Hanno W.
   Psychosocial and behavioral aspects of medicine / Hanno W. Kirk, Jo Weisbrod, Kay Ericson.
     p. cm
   Includes bibliographical references and index.
   ISBN 0-7817-2700-6
    1. Clinical health psychology. 2. Social medicine. 3. Medicine and psychology.
  I. Weisbrod, Jo. II. Ericson, Kay. III. Title.

R726.7 .K56 2002
616'.001'9--dc21

2002028647

The publishers have made every effort to trace the copyright holders for borrowed material. If they have inadvertently overlooked any, they will be pleased to make the necessary arrangements at the first opportunity.

To purchase additional copies of this book call our customer service department at (800) 638-3030 or fax orders to (301) 824-7390. International customers should call (301) 714-2324.

Visit Lippincott Williams & Wilkins on the Internet: http://www.lww.com. Lippincott Williams & Wilkins customer service representatives are available from 8:30 am to 6:00 pm, EST, Monday through Friday, for telephone access.

02 03 04 05
1 2 3 4 5 6 7 8 9 10

Authors

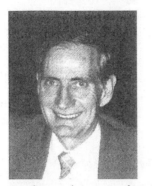

Hanno W. Kirk, PhD, LICSW, has been a trainer/educator for the past 30 years. His diverse experience in the subjects of addictions, corporate cross-cultural skills, domestic violence, ethics, gerontology, medical social work, and guided imagery for cancer patients made him uniquely qualified to develop the curriculum for a course *Psychosocial Aspects of Medicine,* which he and Jo Weisbrod taught for the Physician Assistant Program at Mountain State University in Beckley, WV. Seeing that there was no textbook for such a course, Hanno Kirk, Jo Weisbrod, and Kay Ericson (the director of the PA program) wrote this textbook. His current activities include lecturing at the West Virginia School of Osteopathic Medicine on the topics discussed in this book; teaching sociology, social psychology, and abnormal psychology at Bluefield State College; conducting regional workshops for health care workers and child social service workers; and maintaining a private practice in psychotherapy.

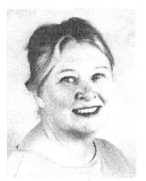

Jo Weisbrod, MA, LPC, ADTR, is a licensed professional counselor, a creative arts therapist, and a hypnotherapist. She brings a total of 37 years of mental health experience to this book. She has worked at St. Elizabeth's Federal Mental Hospital in Washington, DC and has taught creative arts therapy in the Department of Psychiatry at George Washington University and dance at the University of Maryland. Jo Weisbrod jointly taught *Psychosocial Aspects of Medicine* with Hanno Kirk in the PA program at Mountain State University; they are copresenting selected topics from this text at the West Virginia School of Osteopathic Medicine, Lewisburg, WV. She is an instructor in psychology and creative arts therapies at Bluefield State-Greenbrier Community College Center; conducts regional and national workshops; and has an active private practice in mental health counseling. She lives with her husband, Hanno Kirk, in Lewisburg, WV.

Kay Ericson, an NCCPA certified physician assistant for 25 years, has extensive experience in medical and physician assistant education as well as practicing in pediatric primary care. She was Assistant Professor in the department of family medicine at the Southeastern College of Osteopathic Medicine and a faculty member in the Physician Assistant Program at the Medical College of Georgia. She held the administrative position of Program Director for the new Physician Assistant Program at Nova Southeastern University and later became the Program Director for the new Physician Assistant Program at The College of West Virginia (now Mountain State University). Kay is currently Assistant Professor and Academic Coordinator of the Physician Assistant Program at the University of Findlay in Findlay, Ohio.

Acknowledgments

This book covers a wide range of topics. It is the product of a team effort going beyond the three authors. We want to thank the professional team at Lippincott, Williams and Wilkins who shared our vision that a book on psychosocial and behavioral aspects of medicine would fulfill a need in the training for a wide range of health care professionals. We want to express our special thanks to Jacqui Merrell, our development editor whose enthusiasm and patient prodding kept us on task. We also want to thank Mary Frances Bodemuller, the Librarian at the West Virginia School of Osteopathic Medicine who put all the resources of the library at our disposal, including two able assistants Valeria Barfield and Amber Cobb. We owe a debt of gratitude to Trudy Laurensen, the Director of the Lewisburg Family Refuge Center who gave us sage advice on the chapters on domestic violence and child maltreatment. Leslie Bakker who teaches nursing at the University of Charleston (WV), gave us valuable feedback on technical and medical terminology. Paul Rose deserves a special thanks for contributing his research on the role that key neurotransmitters play in ADD/ADHD, and in chemical and behavioral addictions, as well for proof reading. Thanks to Ritchie Shoemaker who shared his discovery of a simple test for diagnosing signs and symptoms caused by neurotoxins and thus differentiate them from somatization complaints. We appreciate the generosity of Gregory Carroll, Director of the Bayer Institute for Health Care Communication, who put the Institute's considerable training materials at our disposal. Similarly we want to thank Professor Benjamin Sadock for permission to use tables and materials from his books. We want to thank our clients and patients from whom we learned how to treat and manage individuals with a variety of issues from a wide spectrum of backgrounds. We are grateful for our supportive families and community of friends who stood by us through the writing of this book.

Preface

Educators and students often teach and learn in a pressurized atmosphere. The demand to keep up with the latest medical advances may lead to a relative neglect of the other part of the equation of being a good health care provider: The ability to relate to patients. This human element includes the ability to understand how psychosocial factors in the patient's environment influence health and disease, how the patient responds to the care provider, and the impact of that response on compliance with treatment. Students entering the clinical part of their training indicate that they often feel unprepared to address the psychosocial and behavioral needs of patients.

PURPOSE

A major goal of this book is to raise health care providers' level of self-awareness and to offer them insights and skills that enable them to look beyond physical symptoms and explore the psychosocial factors that could be affecting a patient's presenting condition. The book rests on the following assumptions:

- Psychosocial factors play a crucial role in the etiology and maintenance of wellness and disease. These factors can facilitate or hinder communication and treatment outcomes.

- In numerous physical and behavioral dysfunctions or pathologies, psychosocial factors may outweigh organic factors or are of major importance in the etiology and maintenance of a patient's complaint or disorder.

- Health care providers must be aware of their own psychosocial factors that they bring to the examination room. Core beliefs, hidden assumptions, and prejudices, as well as issues of transference and counter transference can affect how providers relate to patients, and how providers perceive and process information they receive from patients.

- Establishing good communication with patients is the key to effective assessment, patient participation, and treatment. Communication skills also are essential to a health care provider's career satisfaction.

- Health care providers need to stay informed about social, economic, and political developments and how they may impact the way they practice their profession.

ORGANIZATION

Part I of *Psychosocial and Behavioral Aspects of Medicine* provides the conceptual framework for the elements of the psychosocial perspective, including communication skills and self care guidelines. In Part II, these elements provide the basis for effective recognition and treatment of specific patient populations. It also explores the special management problems presented by some types of challenging patients including those with Somatoform Disorder, Pain Disorders, Factitious and Malingering Disorders, Borderline Personality Disorders, and drug seeking patients. Part III examines how complementary and alternative medicine, as well as contemporary social, political, and ethical issues affect the practice of health care.

FEATURES

The following features reinforce the goals for this book:

- Each chapter begins with an **introductory paragraph** that summarizes the goals and general concepts presented in the chapter.
- **Key terms** are highlighted throughout the text to reinforce essential elements.
- **Patient Profiles*** provide assessment interviews based on real cases that illustrate teaching goals in each chapter. Each profile contains a brief description of the practice setting, a dialogue between the provider and patient, and concludes with the feature Points to Consider to go over critical elements in the interviewing process. The profiles include a wide range of practice settings that encompass the varied environments in which health care providers work. The dialogue portion of the profiles contains both expressed and internal dialogue to clarify underlying psychosocial and behavioral issues that may affect participants.
- **Sidebars** present additional information and definitions of common terms or concepts.
- **Boxes, tables, and figures** support and expand upon concepts in the text.
- **Extensive reference lists** offer resources for readers who want to learn more about a particular topic.

SUMMARY

Psychosocial and Behavioral Aspects of Medicine provides a much-needed bridge between what traditionally has been considered a divide between "medical" and "non-medical" elements in the provision of health care. More attention given to the psychosocial and behavioral elements in health care will improve provider-patient communication, enhance health care, and create more satisfaction for both provider and patient.

---

*DISCLAIMER: The Patient Profiles are based on actual patient cases. All identifying information has been changed to preserve patient confidentiality.

Contents

Preface ix

Introduction xiii

PART I
Foundations of Treatment: The Psychosocial Perspective

CHAPTER 1
What is the Psychosocial Perspective? 1

CHAPTER 2
Multiculturalism and Treatment 13

CHAPTER 3
Life Span and Human Development 35

CHAPTER 4
Basic Counseling and Communication Skills 59

CHAPTER 5
Sensitization to Prejudice and Discrimination 79

CHAPTER 6
Stress Management and Self Care for the Healer 93

PART II
Addressing Specific Psychosocial Issues in Practice

CHAPTER 7
Human Sexuality 111

CHAPTER 8
Care Giving and End of Life Issues 131

CHAPTER 9
Chemical and Behavioral Addictions 155

CHAPTER 10
Domestic Violence 183

CHAPTER 11
Child Maltreatment: Abuse and Neglect 205

CHAPTER 12
Mental Disorders 221

CHAPTER 13
Challenging Patients 243

PART III
Current Practice Concerns

CHAPTER 14
Sociopolitical and Ethical Issues 265

Index 287

Introduction

Health Care Today

The pace of discoveries and advances in the medical field has led to a virtual explosion of knowledge. The Human Genome Project has revealed the possibility of identifying individual and combinations of genes involved in specific pathologies. Research in genetics has pushed the frontiers of treatment in diseases previously considered incurable. Genetic engineering, which is tailored to specific disease conditions or even to individuals, is creating a new pharmacology. At the same time, neuropsychopharmacology has made advances that render conditions such as schizophrenia, depression, and bipolar disorders more treatable with a prognosis for a better outcome. Various mechanical devices, replacement joints, and prostheses have opened new dimensions in geriatric medicine and life extension. Animals are now being trained to use their special senses to assist persons with conditions such as diabetes, epilepsy, or Parkinson's disorder.

Educators face the dilemma of how to fit this rapidly growing store of biomedical information into an already-crowded curriculum. Until recently, academic committees have generally opted to route new information into the core curriculum to increase the empirical knowledge base. However, the struggle facing most schools that train health care providers is unless the period of the academic training is increased, addition of any new material quickly becomes a game of zero-sum choices, a question of what to delete to make room for the additions.

In many schools, psychosocial and behavioral aspects of health care are discussed in various core subjects. Coverage often depends on an instructor's level of comfort with these topics, or whether an instructor believes discussing these topics will "take away" from the core subject they teach. As a result, fragments of psychological and behavioral components are addressed in discussions on the physical system in which primary symptoms rest: sexual problems during discussions about the urogenital system, stress during cardiovascular coverage, or addictions during discussions about the nervous system. The thrust of this book, however, is that psychosocial and behavioral aspects form a common thread that transcends these individual core subjects, and therefore needs an integrated approach.

The authors acknowledge that an empirical approach to teaching health care will always be necessary. Students will continue to have to memorize facts from a wide variety of core curriculum subjects. In the clinical component of their training, they must apply the knowledge gained in the classroom to patient care while getting supervised, hands-on practice. Students will be expected to use deductive reasoning, or apply diagnostic algorithms to correlate symptoms with specific causes. Being able to evaluate a patient, make an accurate assessment, and then develop a treatment plan is good science, and it is good medicine.

The concern of the authors and other observers is that a strictly empirical approach places too much emphasis on physical symptoms. For example, it may be simple to diagnose irritable bowel syndrome. But pharmacological alleviation of unpleasant symptoms does not identify or address the underlying stressful conditions in the patient's life that may have caused the patient's peristaltic movements to go out of balance.

The traditional model of practitioner-patient interaction casts the health care provider as the "expert" and the patient as passively receiving and carrying out instructions. However, evidence in the research literature about the mind-body connection reinforces the concept that successful treatment depends as much on the patient as it does on the health care provider. The holistic treatment paradigm calls for a partnership between health care provider and patient. This approach encourages the practitioner to engage their patients as active participants in the assessment process and the treatment regimen. Providers must also educate patients about their role in achieving long lasting or permanent relief. Once a practitioner and patient reach a common understanding of the patient's psychosocial environment, and how this environment either supports or adversely affects the patient's health and treatment, they can reach an agreement as to what behavioral or lifestyle changes the patient needs to make to assure that medical treatment can be effective.

Health care providers may object to such a comprehensive and holistic approach as beyond the scope of their training. They may feel it is not part of their job to attempt to understand a patient's thoughts and feelings because it is not "real medicine." Providers may be concerned that in today's volume-oriented health care system, there is not enough time to consider psychosocial concerns. The authors acknowledge these concerns and provide guidance on how to navigate these barriers through focused, empathic interviewing, the use of self-administered patient questionnaires, and through teamwork with specialists, social workers, and other mental health professionals. The authors trust that adopting such a holistic approach will allow you to efficiently provide personalized health care that will be appreciated by your patients as well as by those whose concern is third party reimbursements. Moreover, the authors believe that this holistic approach to managing a situation through organized teamwork will reduce the stress of working with emotionally difficult patient issues, such as domestic violence, child maltreatment, or mental disorders.

Book Overview

Part I of *Psychosocial and Behavioral Aspects of Medicine* forms the foundation for the engagement process. Chapter 1, *The Psychosocial Perspective,* explains how the belief systems and values of the health care provider and patient, as well as factors in the psychosocial environment, can enhance or interfere with the personal interactions between them. Chapter 2, *Multiculturalism and Treatment,* explores how family and cultural traditions influence how a patient reacts to the health care system, the individual health care provider, and treatment recommendations. Chapter 3, *Lifespan and Human Development,* discusses how patients negotiate stage-appropriate tasks in the life cycle in the face of expected or unexpected events, and how shock or trauma can affect their physical and psychological well-being. Chapter 4, *Basic Counseling and Communication Skills,* presents proven techniques for developing crucial skills for effectively engaging, educating, and enlisting the patient in the biomedical task of finding and fixing the "problem." Chapter 5, *Sensitization to Prejudice and Discrimination*, discusses and gives guidance on recognizing and countering the ways in which prejudice and discrimination can distort health care. Because health care is stressful as well as satisfying, Chapter 6, *Stress Management and Self Care for the Healer,* addresses what the authors consider a serious training gap for health care providers. This last chapter in Part I discusses a variety of internal and external reasons for stress, and outlines effective strategies on how providers can reduce or manage it.

Part II focuses on applying the psychosocial approach to specific patient populations or to types of presenting problems. Chapter 7, *Human Sexuality*, addresses overcoming barriers to objective discussion of health problems related to sexuality, and also discusses the range of human sexual behaviors. Chapter 8, *Care Giving and End of Life Issues*, has a two-fold purpose: First, it examines how culturally conditioned attitudes affect how patients at various stages of development react to impending death, and how they prepare for death. This chapter also looks at the special problems of treating older patients and the ethical issues surrounding comfort or terminal care. In Chapter 9, *Chemical and Behavioral Addictions*, providers are guided to recognize and effectively work with patients who have developed pathological addiction patterns. Chapter 10, *Domestic Violence*, provides details about how to pierce the veil of secrecy and shame surrounding this issue, explains the psychophysiological progression of domestic violence, and details how to assist the victims of such violence. Chapter 11, *Child Maltreatment: Abuse and Neglect*, informs providers how to recognize victimized children, set up protocols for interviewing and recording information, and alleviate the emotional stress of working with such children. Chapter 12, *Mental Disorders*, examines how to get past the barriers of fear, stigma, and denial about mental illness. This chapter augments standard psychiatric information with the psychosocial and behavioral perspective, and gives guidance for using auto-mated patient assessment instruments. In Chapter 13, *Challenging Patients*, the health care provider is given information and precautions concerning several types of patients that may require special handling, including those with factitious disorders, malingerers, disability-seeking and drug-seeking patients, and those with borderline personality disorder.

Each of these chapters is designed to provide enough information to reduce your personal doubts and discomfort so that in your role as health care provider you *will* ask necessary and sometimes difficult questions about what is going on within the patient's family or psychosocial environment. In addition to guidelines provided about how to recognize issues facing the patient, each chapter also gives practical suggestions on how to *manage* the situation through organized teamwork, such as appropriate consultation with, or referrals to, medical specialists or mental health professionals.

Part III, the final section in *Psychosocial and Behavioral Aspects of Medicine*, looks at practice concerns created by social, economic and political developments in the larger societal context. Legal and policy decisions impact the way health care providers practice their profession. Chapter 14, *Sociopolitical and Ethical Issues*, discusses managed care, complementary and alternative medicine, reproductive issues, right-to-die, eugenics, the ethics of genetic engineering in health care, and encourages the reader to stay abreast of the psychosocial and behavioral issues in medicine.

CHAPTER 1

What Is the Psychosocial Perspective?

The psychosocial approach looks at the reciprocal pattern of transactions and interplay of the person and four elements:

1. The Individual and their belief system
2. The Family as a system
3. The Community as a context
4. The Culture as the wider context

This chapter examines the first three elements. The purpose of looking at these elements is to help you identify at which level the patient's stress is occurring, and how it interferes with assessment and treatment compliance.

What Is the Psychosocial Approach?

The word **psychosocial** first achieved wide usage in the field of social work and was developed in part to emphasize the impact of the sociocultural context on human development and behavior. Earlier theories, like Freud's psychodynamic approach, had asserted that our personality and behavior were the results primarily of internal mechanisms. Psychosocial theories emphasize the interaction between the individual and their social environment, which makes demands or exerts social pressure in the form of social expectations, norms and values. The social environment includes not only the family, but also the neighborhood or community, and the culture.[1]

INDIVIDUALS AND THEIR BELIEF SYSTEM

Each of us has an individual and idiosyncratic belief system. To a large extent, our beliefs are shaped by our family, our community, and our culture. Our interactions at a very early age begin to form our beliefs, our character and how they may be modified later in life. Most **core beliefs** are learned at an early age. These very deeply held beliefs are about the nature of the Self, others, the world and God. On a basic level, they reflect our beliefs whether our needs are going to be met, or at least attended to; whether the world is safe, whether others can be trusted, whether the self is worthy or not and other meaning-of-life questions. These core beliefs are held as deeply embedded internal messages that rarely change, and if they do, it is under the impact of great trauma, stress, or insight (Box 1-1). For example, if you grew up believing the world to be a relatively safe place, and one night you are awakened from a deep sleep and are facing a robber or a rapist at gunpoint in your home, the belief in a safe world may be shattered forever. Such a harrowing experience might also change your values and priorities about what else is important in your life. In a cascade of subsequent changes, you might adopt new attitudes on such issues as gun control, the legal system, and even the death penalty.[2] Another perplexing example of a deeply ingrained, unchanging belief comes from the nursing home industry. It was found that some elderly residents would sneak food from the dining room and hoard it in their beds or closets, thus, presenting a hygiene hazard. Although one might assume the residents were responding to a lack of food, they were not. Rather almost all of these residents had lived through severe deprivation or hunger during the Great Depression. Being in a nursing

---

Box 1-1 Personal Belief Structure

Each person holds beliefs, values and attitudes on a number of major issues. Core beliefs are those most deeply held internal messages. Values are about everyday living and behavior and institutions. Attitudes usually come out of our core beliefs and values. The sample of dichotomies below should be viewed as a continuum. Most people fall somewhere in between the extremes listed. This list is by no means exhaustive.

CORE BELIEFS

- World: safe vs unsafe.
- Nature of self: self-sufficient (internal locus of control) vs dependent (external locus); I am good, adequate, worthy of love vs bad, inadequate, unworthy or not measuring up.
- Nature of others: loving vs hurtful; honest vs dishonest; trustworthy vs untrustworthy; all human beings equally worthy vs some less equal or less worthy.
- Purpose of life: spiritual journey vs struggle for survival & suffering; service to others vs quest for power and success.
- Nature of God: loving and forgiving and a source of solace and strength vs judging and punishing and a source of fear, guilt or shame.
- Family: source of love, nurturance and strength vs source of struggle, tension and pain.

VALUES

- Work: work to live and serve vs work to make money and survive.
- Education: valuable and desirable for self improvement and its own sake vs something you have to endure to get ahead.
- Conduct of relations with others: being "nice" (getting along at any price) vs honest communications including expressions of disagreement or anger.
- Emotions: OK to enjoy or express vs sign of irrationality, loss of control or weakness; take risks by expressing love and affection vs take no risks by being "safe" cool, detached.
- Honesty: best policy in relations with others vs lying is OK.
- Religion: structured belief in God and fellowship vs waste of time.
- Prejudice and discrimination: always wrong vs some groups should be restricted.

ATTITUDES

- TV viewing: way to relax vs harmful or a waste of time.
- Abortion: sometimes a solution to unwanted pregnancy vs always wrong.
- Welfare: a safety net for the deserving poor vs a program for the idle and undeserving.
- Politics: the way to get things done (including compromise) vs unpleasant and dishonest activity in which principles are compromised.

---

home, often in a state of slight or moderate dementia, brought up primitive survival fears stemming from old core beliefs about this being a world of scarcity and hunger.

Similarly, people's spiritual beliefs can directly affect their reaction to disease. For example, people who see themselves as "unworthy" in the sight of God, may regard cancer, or having a disabled child as a "punishment from God" for being "bad." Other patients do not believe in "earthly" remedies or medical procedures, but instead place their faith in a "healing from God." You may also treat patients who have positive regard for themselves and their spirituality who will find it appropriate to complement the treatment you prescribe with spiritual practices.[3-6]

Religious beliefs are but one example of how core beliefs shape your patients' responses to health care in general. The important point to remember is that core beliefs may influence patients' reactions to you in the role of the health care provider. In addition *your* core beliefs will influence how the patient interacts with you as the health care provider. Knowing your core beliefs is as important as understanding the patient's core beliefs. The student exercise on

What are my beliefs

Take a blank piece of paper (or a notebook) and a pen. Review each of the Beliefs, Values and Attitudes of the Personal Belief Structure in Box 1-1 on the previous page. Reflect for a moment where along the continuum of each sample dichotomy your inner assumptions appear to be. Formulate your own version of each belief, value, and attitude (add any that are relevant to you) and record them on paper. You might reflect further on the events or forces that shaped specific beliefs, values and attitudes. If you feel inclined, you may wish to share and discuss this student exercise with a trusted friend.

the next page will help you identify core beliefs and values that may influence the relationship between you and your patients.

THE FAMILY

From almost any perspective, the family is seen as the basic community subsystem in which each of us exists and acts most of our lives. In the **systems approach** to analyzing families, emphasis is placed on **patterns, interconnectedness, and reciprocal influences.** (See Figure 1-1, and 1-2).[6,7]

An image often used to represent the family systems approach is that of a mobile. When one part of the hanging mobile is "disturbed," all the finely balanced parts will bounce up and down and the whole mobile will sway and rotate. After a while when the source of the disturbance is no longer agitating the "system", the mobile settles into balance again. This tendency to return to homeostasis or balance is a central assumption of family systems theory. This return to balance occurs regardless of whether the family is "healthy" or "unhealthy". Some changes, like the birth of a child, grown children leaving home, or death of aged parents, are an inevitable part of the life course of any family. However, some shocks — a divorce or a sudden death — can be so great that the family needs to rearrange itself into a new constellation of interdependent parts.

How a family weathers such shocks and makes the transition to the next life stage are often determined by its resilience and ability to handle change in an orderly and accepting manner. The ability to change and for the system to evolve depends on how **functional** or **dysfunctional** a family is. (Chapter 3 "Life Span and Human Development" details the **life course stages** of families and the tasks and difficulties that mark each stage.)

Functional families tend to display consistent caring and love for its members as well as mutual respect for each other's boundaries and roles. What is important for the health care provider is that members of functional families tend to be consumers of health care who communicate their problems relatively openly with their health care provider, and either follow treatment regimens, or else let their health care provider know why they are not following them. In contrast, **dysfunctional families** tend not to display the consistent caring, love and mutual respect for the boundaries and roles of its members. Members of dysfunctional families may be noted for their tendency to be poor communicators, for manipulative behaviors, and for non-compliance with treatment regimens. However, because dysfunctional families may outwardly present the "right" or ideal pattern of a nuclear or extended family, such families may look "normal" to you. The type of family household recognized by the 2000 US Census has grown past the traditional nuclear family to include a wide constellation of permanent or semi-permanent living arrangements. Some healthcare providers may have difficulty in seeing certain arrangements as "family."

CAUSES OF DYSFUNCTION

Although we may be quick to blame certain family structures — such as the single parent household — we need to remember that families are dysfunctional due to multiple psychosocial factors. For example, poverty produces stress. The struggle to cover basic survival needs, the lack of transportation, if combined with low education and poor self-esteem, can produce

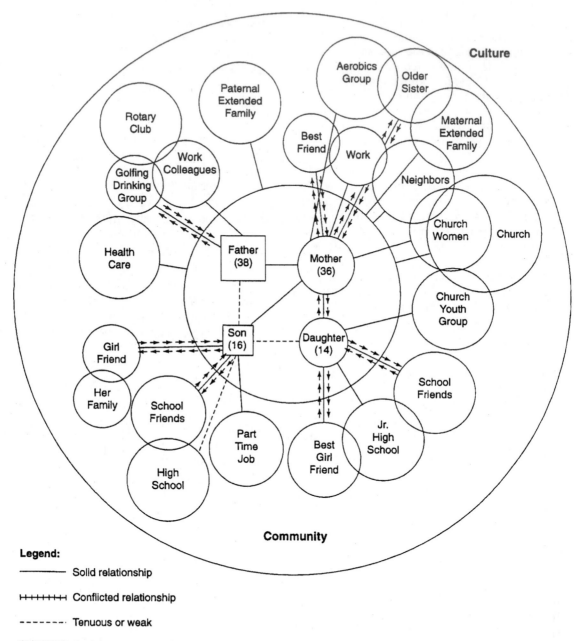

Legend:

———— Solid relationship

+++++++ Conflicted relationship

- - - - - Tenuous or weak

⩬⩬⩬⩬ Social support or positive energy flow

Figure 1-1 Functional family system tied into the community. Note multiple overlapping ties into community and friends. Adapted from Hartman A. Diagrammatic Assessment of Family Relationships. Social Casework 1978;59:465-476.

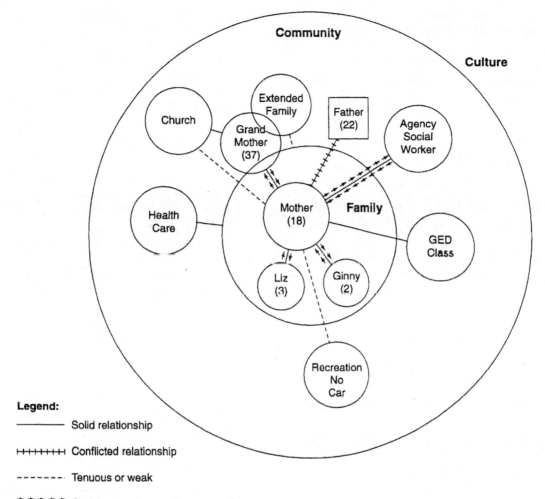

Figure 1-2 Single parent family system with few community ties. Note the few social connections, partly due to poverty and the lack of transportation. Adapted from Hartman A. Diagrammatic Assessment of Family Relationships. Social Casework 1978;59:465-476.

inadequate communication skills within families and isolation, as contrasted with the extensive social support network that functional families are tied into, as illustrated in Figure 1-2. Intergenerational poverty and low self-esteem often produce feelings of hopelessness, helplessness and severe depression. The lack of social skills in dealing with the "outside" world leads to frustration and alienation and a sense of powerlessness. Family members may compensate for this by exercising rigid control and power over other members of the family. Indeed the dominant members may become emotionally or physically abusive to one or more family members. (However, abuse is not restricted to poor people. It occurs in all social strata. See more detail on domestic violence in Chapter 10.)

Chemical or behavioral addictions play a major part, both in creating and maintaining, dysfunctional family patterns. In general, addic-

---

Box 1-2 Characteristics of Functional Family

1. Provides safety, warmth and nurturance
2. Provides love and belonging needs
3. Provides need for autonomy and separateness
4. Promotes self-esteem or sense of worth
5. Members mistakes are tolerated
6. Members can have fun
7. Members individuate and grow spiritually

CHARACTERISTICS OF DYSFUNCTIONAL FAMILY[12]

1. Physical, emotional, or sexual abuse and/or neglect
2. Rigid rules, life styles and/or belief systems, and shame-based enforcement
3. Keeping "family secrets"
4. Inability to identify and/or express feelings (except destructively)
5. Intolerance for mistakes (perfectionism)
6. Triangulation or using one person as an intermediary to communicate messages to another
7. Double messages/double binds (whatever you do, you can't win)
8. High tolerance for inappropriate behavior/pain (substance abuse, physical or sexual abuse)
9. Enmeshment (no one has an identity of their own)

THE DYSFUNCTIONAL FAMILY "RULES" [13]

1. Control - Always be in control of all interactions, feelings, and personal behavior. Control is the major defense strategy to deal with shame.
2. Perfectionism - Always be right. The members live according to an externalized image. No one ever measures up.
3. Don't make mistakes. Mistakes reveal the flawed, vulnerable self. Cover up your own mistakes (denial). If someone else makes a mistake, shame him or her.
4. Blame-Whenever things don't turn out as planned, blame yourself or others.
5. Don't express your own reality. You should think, feel, desire, perceive or imagine only the way the perfectionist ideal demands.
6. The "no talk rule". Families should hide their true feelings, needs and wants, and never reveal them to outsiders.
7. Don't trust anyone and you will never be disappointed.

---

tions — whether chemical like alcoholism, or behavioral like gambling — disrupt or inhibit the normal development of the family. They take a heavy toll of its members, both psychically and physically. Life in families with addictions is often marked by unpredictability, chaos, and frequently high levels of violence and abuse. You need to be aware that patients and their family members will tend to minimize or deny the addiction problem(s) within the family, thus maintaining the family as a closed system.

FAMILY SECRET RULE

One of the characteristics as well as one of the cardinal rules of most dysfunctional families is the **family secret** rule. This is when members of the family, either because of threat, shame or embarrassment, agree not to reveal to outsiders what goes on within the family. When this rule is in effect, the family tends to be a **closed** system. The family secret rule is a serious impediment for the health care provider who is trying to make sense out of presenting symptoms — such as a strange pattern of physical bruises or injuries — when those are explained away either by the patient or by an accompanying family member as the result of a household accident as illustrated by the Family Rules in Box 1-2. Because most health care providers in the past lacked specific training or practical experience in treating family violence, certain key symptoms ranging from psychosomatized complaints, to bruises, bleeding from orifices, fecal incontinence, functional encopresis, burns, or broken

---

Box 1-3 Diversity of "Family" Patterns[14]

1. Nuclear family consisting of one couple, and their offspring living together surrounded by a fringe of relatives in the vicinity as illustrated in Figure 1-1).
2. Multi-generational extended family consisting of spouses, their children, living together surrounded by a fringe of relatives.
3. Single parent usually a mother and her children living with her parent(s). Often grandmother takes care of the children while mother finishes her education or works (Figure 1-2).
4. Single parent and her children surrounded by other sources of support (friends).
5. Multi-generational group consisting of grandparent(s), parents, and a returned adult child with or without young offspring living together. This can be caused by death, divorce, bankruptcy, job loss, and out-of-reach housing costs in urban areas.
6. Blended family consisting of one or two adults who bring children from previous unions into the household (his, hers, theirs, adopted).

7. Same gender couple living together and raising children.
8. Two single persons living together without children. The union can either be heterosexual or homosexual.
9. Several single persons of either or both genders living together in the same household as friends, but sharing care burdens of housekeeping like a family.

FAMILY CONSTELLATION AND FUNCTIONALITY

None of these different family constellations is either inherently functional or dysfunctional. Stable family patterns are a crucial element in setting the beliefs, values and behaviors of children. How family members relate to each other and especially how much support and caring and love they express for each other is an important factor of stability affecting child development.

---

bones — all too often have gone unrecognized as signs of child abuse, domestic violence or sexual abuse. The "family secret" rule is usually also operative in families with addiction problems. Members from such families will rarely know or volunteer to their health care provider that their anxiety, depression, aches and pains or physical illnesses might be related to the stress of living in a household with an alcoholic or other type of addict. Special sensitivity and interview skills are required to penetrate the wall of secrecy and denial of patients from dysfunctional families. Later chapters focus on those skills.

INAPPROPRIATE BOUNDARIES

Closed families are often marked by either too much distance or too much closeness, i.e., **emotional distancing or enmeshment.** These terms are used to describe problems of respecting the individual private space of other family members and are known as **boundary** problems. Emotional distancing usually comes out of emotional neglect. The inability to provide consistent care, love, and emotional nurturance interferes

with the capacity of both child and parent to bond and to form strong attachments. This emotional insufficiency pattern may be intergenerational with poor modeling within the family going back several generations. Relations within a family of emotional distance are characterized as cold and disengaged. Persons from disengaged families may present with monotone voices, blunted affect, poor communication, and inadequate social skills. Alternatively they may be full of resentment and suspicion, quick to take offense and misinterpret simple requests for information in the health history. Often they relate to the "system", i.e., health care system, school system, social service agencies, or even their employer in a passive-aggressive manner. It may be hard for you to establish rapport with patients from this background.

When families are too close, we call it **enmeshment.**[8] Enmeshment is an unhealthy sense of dependency among family members. It is characterized by a lack of respect for the boundaries of the members within the families. When parents are overprotective and controlling, children fail to individuate or separate from their parents. They become dependent appendages within the "family system". They have trouble functioning separately from their families and as they become adults, the roles of parent and child may be reversed, with the adult child taking care of the parent.[9] In both enmeshed and disengaged families, the lack of respect for boundaries can lead to either emotional or sexual incest and physical abuse as dominant members need to exert their control and display their power by taking advantage of younger, weaker members of the family.[10] Health care providers should be aware that members of dysfunctional families may define their family situation as "normal", especially if the pattern has been present for generations.

In health care settings, patients from an enmeshed or poorly socialized rural family can be recognized because often the whole family will show up at the appointment for one family member. (See next chapter.) If the other family members are not in the waiting room, they may be outside waiting in the car. Knowing this can be an advantage. For example, if you are unable to get key information from a patient, you can ask the patient if it is acceptable for another family member who may be with them to come into the examining room to "help" you understand.[11] This communication technique usually works, unless the enmeshed family enforces the *secrecy rule* to appear "normal" to the outside. However, if you have honed your skills in listening and observation, you will be able to make sense of puzzling symptoms that may not match the verbal explanations of the patient or family members. (See Chapter 3 for more detail on communication skills.)

Health Effects of Dysfunction

Any one or a combination of the above mentioned patterns of dysfunctional families produce high levels of stress for its members, especially those who are victimized by more dominant members. This stress corrodes good physical and emotional health. On the physical level, you may see psychosomatized symptoms such as pain in the head, chest, or abdomen, or suicide attempts, severe anxiety or panic attacks, post traumatic stress disorder, selective mutism, or dissociative identity disorder, to name a few. Anxiety-related symptoms can include irritable bowel syndrome, tachycardia or brachycardia. In extreme cases of psychosomatization, you may observe conversion disorders (e.g., patient inexplicably loses function of an arm, leg, or vision). As we discuss in greater detail in Chapter 12, when you encounter such symptoms, utilizing diagnostic procedures to identify the "physical" cause may prove frustrating, fruitless and costly. With many of these symptoms, you are challenged to correctly identify and connect the symptoms with the psychosocial situation. Then you must integrate your knowledge of the consequences of the dysfunction within the psychosocial context of your patient and follow up with appropriate communication and interviewing techniques. Later chapters are designed to give you the specific knowledge for the different special situations you are likely to encounter. A major goal of this book is to give you the eyes to see, and the skills to delve below the surface of the psychosocial factors operative within the family context and the larger community context.

The Community As Context

The community is both the place in which you as the health care provider practice your profession, and also the context in which your patients live their lives. Being aware of how a community shapes the values and behaviors of its members, what its structure is, and what kind of resources it offers, will directly affect your personal and professional performance and sense of accomplishment. Printouts available from state health departments, or even the US Census Bureau on the socioeconomic and demographic profile of the community can give you answers to the following questions:

- What is the average income?
- What percentage is employed?

- Who are the major employers?
- What is the rate of families who receive benefits from the government?
- What is the adolescent pregnancy rate?
- What percentage is on disability and for what reasons (black lung, brown lung, asbestosis, etc.)?
- What is the level of health care coverage, i.e., employer insurance, Medicare or Medicaid?

For example, uninsured or underinsured persons tend not to get routine health care checkups, or to see a health care provider for minor ailments. Instead, they visit emergency rooms in hospitals with serious, sometimes fatal problems that could have been cured if treated earlier. Knowing these figures gives you an idea not only on the kind of health care consumer you are likely to encounter, but what type of medicine you will be practicing, such as preventive, palliative, or crisis-oriented.

Opportunities for Social Interaction

A community is also shaped by its layout. Are there places where the members can exchange information and socialize? Driving to away-from-home games, sitting together, cheering, and the shared pride in their local high school team becomes a bonding experience for a community. In rural areas, a general store (now a convenience store) or a post office may serve as a community-gathering place. In urban or suburban areas, community centers, malls, recreational facilities (movie theaters, video game arcades, outdoor playgrounds), college cafeterias, bars, restaurants, pool halls, coffee houses or even parking lots of fast food places can serve as places where adolescents and young adults congregate, socialize and exchange information. In addition, senior adults in some areas may form physical exercise clubs and use the safety of indoor malls for early morning walks. Others may gather at senior nutrition sites. Older men may gather for fellowship in an American Legion Hall, a union hall, or the various secret lodge organizations from Freemasons (and its associated orders) to Elks, Goodfellows, or Moose.

Many women participate in less formally structured activities. For mothers these are centered around their children's activities, from birth preparation classes, meeting at the park or playground, to planning car pools, overnights, with mothers of their children's friends. Some may be class mothers, or be active in parent teacher organizations, and church circles. In urban areas, women without children may also meet at the local gym, workout center, health spa, or fitness center. Alternatively they may participate in professional associations, volunteering, or even in book discussion groups. All these activities provide opportunities for social networking. A community without such opportunities is also likely to be less open, and possibly less friendly. In your practice, you will probably notice a distinct difference in the level of social and communication skills between those who are well connected with their community and those who do not participate in social activities.

Religion As a Social Force Shaping Community

Depending on the geographic area or subculture, churches, temples, and mosques may be the dominant social element as well as a political force in a community. For example, often in African-American communities, religion is the cement of the social fabric. Churches function as centers for community action, and their ministers frequently also became prominent political leaders in the community. Socially active religious institutions often become community centers providing space for meetings of various civic groups, senior citizen activities, health care screenings, day care, head start, prenatal and parenting classes, various support groups, as well as providing food and clothing for poor and homeless persons. Such exemplary centers often supplement other social support institutions. They create a sense of community and pride through participation in a meaningful effort.

Availability of Health and Social Services

As a health care provider, you need to know not only what is available, but also how accessible services are, and for whom. Answers to the following questions will give you a picture of how well the community functions to provide needed social services:

- What is the adequacy of the local or nearest hospital and what kinds of specialized services can be provided there?*
- Are there home health agencies?
- How active is the Committee on Aging in providing Meals on Wheels and personal care services to elderly home-bound persons?
- Are there retired persons who serve in various volunteer capacities?
- How accessible is the nearest office of the state Health and Human Services Department (often known as the welfare office)?
- How available and adequate are community mental health services and facilities?
- Is competent outpatient counseling available?
- What inpatient psychiatric services are there? How can they be accessed?
- What services exist for developmentally delayed and physically disabled persons?
- What kind of self help groups, such as the various Twelve Step programs are available and do they meet regularly?
- Are there informal networks of "natural helpers," students, or adults who often supplement the community health and mental health services by being good listeners for teens or adults in crisis?†

---

*If some services such as mammography, cholesterol and blood testing and other health screenings are not easily available in the community, do mobile units come into the community periodically to offer them?

†Some public high schools train "natural helpers" in basic counseling and crisis skills, listening and empathy, to act as a first line of defense against adolescent misinformation, depression and suicide. Some churches and temples also provide similar training for adults for outreach into the community.

For example, if a community does not support mental health services, is this an indication that these problems, including developmental disabilities, are taboo subjects? When you hear your patients using euphemisms like "nerve pills" for prescription mood drugs, or "slow learners" for even severely developmentally delayed relatives, you realize that they are trying to avoid the stigma of being labeled "crazy."

Educational Opportunities

Another major indicator of a community's health is its involvement in, and the resources it is willing to invest in education. In addition to the K-12 public education, what other educational resources are available? Is there access to adult continuing education and vocational training? Aside from the public schools, do institutions like churches, temples, community centers or mental health centers offer classes in self improvement, childbirth preparation and parenting, to name a few? Are there cultural offerings for children and adults in the arts — from painting and crafts to music, dance and theater? Is there access to higher education through a community college or other tertiary educational institution? The attitude of the community towards learning can give you an indication of how open your patients may be to learning from you about their health habits.

Community Spirit or Ethos

The various institutions and services named above contribute to a community's **ethos** or spirit. This is the feeling that its members have about themselves as a collective entity. It is akin to how families function and how the individual members feel about themselves. Where there is a strong sense of connection and mutual support, the spirit of community pride, optimism or even ebullience is expressed spontaneously by many of its members. Where this sense of connectedness and mutual support is missing, indifference, pessimism, resignation or shame may be expressed more often which in large part is due to how well the above factors work together.

Summary

This chapter has provided an overview of the elements that comprise the psychosocial perspective. Several of these elements will be discussed in more detail in subsequent chapters. For example, your personal belief system, as well as amount and type of exposure to persons of different cultures or different belief systems, will affect how you relate to such persons as patients. That is why the next chapter is on the role of culture. It examines the specific influences of the major subcultures within America. The significance of this examination for you as a health care provider is that patients you treat may hold widely differing beliefs about sickness, health and health care providers, depending on the regional, ethnic, religious or racial culture from which they originate. Building on that examination, Chapter 5 looks at prejudice and discrimination in the health care system. Chapter 3, Life Span and Human Development, enlarges on this chapter's brief discussion of the family. It discusses how a patient's adjustment of a specific phase of life can directly influence how they view their body, how they feel and behave, and how they react to illness and the health care system.

REFERENCES

1. National Association of Social Workers (1987). *Encyclopedia of Social Work* (18th Ed). Bethesda, MD. NASW Press.

2. Koss MP (1993). Rape: Scope, impact, intervention, and public policy responses. *American Psychologist,* 48: 1062-1069.

3. Achterberg J (1985). *Imagery in Healing: Shamanism and Modern Medicine.* Boston: New Science Library.

4. Achterberg J, et al (1994). *Rituals of Healing: Using Imagery for Health and Wellness.* New York: Bantam.

5. Dossey L (1997). *Healing Words: The Power of Prayer and the Practice of Medicine.* New York: Harper Mass Market Paperbacks.

6. Bowen M (1978). *Family Therapy in Clinical Practice.* New York: Jason Aronson.

7. Minuchin S (1974). *Families and Family Therapy.* Cambridge, Mass: Harvard University Press.

8. Germain CB (1991). *Human Behavior in the Social Environment: An Ecological View.* New York: Columbia University Press. p 125.

9. Love P (1991). *Emotional Incest Syndrome: What To Do when a Parent's Love Rules Your Life.* New York: Bantam Doubleday.

10. Briggs R (1999). *Transforming Anxiety, Transcending Shame.* Deerfield Beach, FL: Health Communications.

11. Korsch BM, Harding C (1997). *The Intelligent Patient's Guide to the Doctor-Patient Relationship: Learning How to Talk so Your Doctor Will Listen.* New York: Oxford University Press.

12. Fossum MA, Mason MJ (1989). *Facing Shame: Families in Recovery.* New York: WW Norton & Co. p. 86.

13. Bradshaw J (1988). *Healing the Shame that Binds.* Deerfield Beach, FL: Health Communications.

14. US Census (2000). "Households by Type" in Profile of General Demographic Characteristics US Census Press Release, May 15, 2001.

CHAPTER 2

Multiculturalism and Treatment

This chapter surveys how cultural differences in beliefs and values about health and health care affect provider-patient interactions. We call your attention to differences in verbal and nonverbal communication patterns, attitudes toward the health care system, and how such differences can affect treatment planning and patient compliance. We highlight the salient differences of the major cultural minorities in North America, as well as those between urban and rural dwellers.

If current populations trends continue, by the year 2020, White European Americans will be a minority in the United States. (US Census Interim Report, September 1999)

Terminology

To understand multiculturalism and its role in health care delivery, you need to familiarize yourself with certain terms. **Culture** is a collection of beliefs, values, ideals, and customs handed down in history and commonly accepted either by a society or a large group within that society, which we call a subculture. **Norms** are the rules of behavior generally accepted in a culture or subculture. They are justified by the **values** held by culture or subculture. **Ethnic groups** exist on the basis of "sentiments that bind individuals into solidarity groups on some cultural basis."[1] **Race** is a classification for a group with distinct observable biological features, such as skin color, hair texture and eyelid shape. **Prejudice** arises when those visual differences are assigned negative cultural meanings by the dominant culture.[2]

An Historical Perspective

The roots of "American" culture are for the most part Judeo-Christian, Western European traditions, which were molded by the unique conditions and historical experience of our society. Although the American population comprises many ethnic and cultural sources, in reality, the norms and values of our society, its politics and legal system have been those of the dominant White majority. Other ethnic and racial groups were expected to conform to this value system.[3] While new immigrant groups that were considered White, generally assimilated into the dominant culture by the second or third generation, those with visible differences, such as African-Americans, as well Asian-Americans, faced barriers of prejudice and discrimination that largely prevented them from blending into the American culture.[4] (See chapter on prejudice and discrimination for further details.) Historically, such minorities were forced to live segregated from the majority population of Whites until the Civil Rights laws of the 1960s brought about changes. However, ethnic and racial groups still tend to be concentrated in large enclaves in major cities in America as well as in rural areas in the South, Southeast, and parts of the Midwest and Southwest. Some of these are recent immigrant refugee groups from places as diverse as Southeast Asia, Central America, Haiti, the Balkans, or the Middle East.[5] If the second generation members of these subcultures continue to live in ethnic enclaves, their values are likely to still be influenced to a greater or lesser extent by their familial culture. In many locales in America, especially in some large cities and in the Southwest, non-Whites now outnumber English speaking Whites.[6] As this trend continues, you are likely to provide health care in locales where the value system, norms for behavior, and language of many or most of your patients will *not* be the same as that of the traditional American culture.

Cultural Differences and Their Effect on Provider-Patient Interactions

VERBAL AND NONVERBAL COMMUNICATION

One of the difficulties you may face is **language** differences. Culture is expressed as well as transmitted through language, which structures meaning *and* determines perception.[7] You, as the health care provider, will interact with patients who not only speak a different language, but for whom standard English medical terms or definitions of disease and wellness may have dramatically different meanings. Even if they speak English, you may have difficulty understanding them because pitch, volume, rhythm, inflection, speed, and hesitations might be unfamiliar to your ears. For example, even if listening intently, you may miss that a Cambodian-Montagnard woman is trying to communicate to you about some "female problems" — a taboo subject in her culture — by using some vague terms. A person from rural Appalachia may tell you that they are taking "a water pill," which turns out to be for hypertension. Nonverbal communication, which makes up a large part of communication, often differs from culture to culture. For example, most Asian cultures believe that direct eye contact with a person in "authority" is insolent, or disrespectful. Similarly, smiling, which we tend to take as a sign of being kind, friendly, and warm, may be regarded by Japanese or Koreans as "inappropriate" or frivolous in a "serious" situation, such as a health care interview. At other times in those cultures, smiling can be a mask for hiding "unacceptable" emotions, such as fear, terror or even pain.[8]

ATTITUDES TOWARD HEALTH CARE

You may also be challenged by patients' different attitudes toward health care and toward you as a health care provider. You may encounter "home remedies" that are based on ancient cultural traditions and indigenous methods of healing. These remedies may work surprisingly well, despite not being rooted in the Western scientific tradition and possibly sounding risky.[9,10] You may also encounter practices based on magical beliefs embedded in their culture that may stretch your credulity or that may revolt you by their seeming harshness. Health care providers have been known to call child protective services because they assumed that a child was being physically abused, when in fact the parents had simply used a healing method accepted in their culture for treating an illness.*

In working with different ethnic groups, you may encounter negative attitudes toward you as the health care provider. These negative attitudes may be based on a patient's fear of you as the "expert" or "authority". This fear may come out of a cultural heritage of feelings of inferiority vis-a-vis the ethnic group to which you as the healthcare provider belong.† For example, persons classified as "illegal aliens" may have contact with the health care system only in extreme or life-threatening situations because they fear being reported to the immigration authorities and being deported.

---

*One such case was Cambodian Montagnard parents who placed heated pennies on the back of their child to draw out a disease. When that did not bring about the cure, the parents took the child to a clinic. The HCP, observing the "burn" marks on the child's skin, immediately alerted Child Protective Services. The bewildered parents were charged with child abuse. The charges were dropped only after an interpreter explained to the court that this was a culturally based healing practice.

†Persons with low self esteem of any race or culture may exhibit similar behavior.

Historical Hostility

Some of the negative feelings directed toward you may be a result of **historical hostility**. Historical hostility arises whenever one group sees itself as having been exploited, or oppressed over time by the privileged "in-group."[11] Such hostility is evident around the world in societies split by long standing divisions of hostility along racial, tribal, or religious lines. In the United States, people of color often feel that they have to suppress their cultural values to gain social acceptance in the dominant culture. Health care providers who are part of the dominant American culture may find it hard to understand the almost daily struggle of persons who are not part of the "privileged class" to adapt and overcome barriers to personal, social, and economic acceptance. Health care providers belonging to a cultural minority in America may be able to apply their experience, perceptions, and insight to working through issues of historical hostility.

Historical hostility has several implications for the health care provider: Persons of color, ethnic minorities, and even many rural patients may feel insecure in many standard health care settings because of the cultural gaps in language, communication styles, education, and economic status. Such patients doubting their abilities to behave appropriately in the formal medical setting, may self-consciously focus more attention on not "making fools of themselves" than on communicating clearly about their health problems. Patients from a historically "exploited" minority group (e.g., Native Americans and African-Americans) may feel ambivalent towards health care providers that are White European Americans. By the same token, a White American patient meeting a provider from a minority culture may also experience an ambivalence based on prejudices they hold about that culture.

Medical need may dictate that a patient place themselves in your care, but the patient may have negative feelings toward the health care provider based on various personal or cultural reasons. You, as the health care provider, may experience some of these unconscious attitudes as passive resistance, sullen non-cooperation, and non-compliance. You may be frustrated by such ambivalent behavior. You may interpret their resistance to supplying needed clinical information as deliberate non-cooperation. Chapter 4, Basic Counseling and Communication Skills, provides specific guidelines on how to reach past this ambivalence, establish good rapport, and listen and communicate effectively.

IMPLICATIONS OF CULTURAL DIFFERENCES

The frustration with cross-cultural communications affecting both patients and health care providers can create serious barriers to effective health care for minority groups. Major surveys have shown wide disparities in the level of health care services between ethnic minorities and Whites. For example, it has been shown that ethnic minorities had higher *excess death* rates‡ in six health status categories: 1) cancer, 2) cardiovascular disease and stroke, 3) chemical dependency, 4) diabetes, 5) homicide and accidental injuries, and 6) infant mortality.[12] In analyzing these disparities, most studies point to limited access to health care by minority populations.[13,14,15] Several factors were cited: 1) low income, 2) lack of community health services, 3) high cost of health insurance, and 4) absence of "culturally competent service providers."[16] The following section will highlight the challenges you may encounter when working with patients who have different health care values and behaviors and how these challenges may affect your goal of creating good patient relations and providing good health care.

American Subcultures

We have chosen four ethnic minorities based in part on their ranking in numbers according to US Census data (African-Americans, Hispanics),

---

‡Excess deaths were defined operationally as the number of deaths that would not have taken place if the rates of minority populations had been equal to those of white Americans.

and in part based on the special problems they may present to the health care provider (Native Americans and Asians). Because there is a divide in values and norms between urban and rural dwellers, we also include a section on Rural Americans. One note of caution: generalizations are used in this chapter that describe *tendencies* for persons from specific subcultures to have certain beliefs, values, and attitudes and to behave in culturally specific ways. These are based on composite cultural data from a variety of sources.[17] However, you, as the health care provider, *must* be aware that patients are individuals. You will encounter a high degree of individual variability based on several factors: 1) the patient's level of separation from, or assimilation into the cultural values of the dominant White culture, i.e., how much they have internalized their cultural group's commonly accepted beliefs, values, attitudes, and behaviors, vs. how much they have internalized the values of the dominant culture; 2) the amount of education; and 3) previous contact with Western health care. Some individuals have bicultural competence, i.e., they carry some of the beliefs and norms of their ancestral culture, while at the same time being able to accept and operate successfully within the norms of the dominant American culture.[18] How readily you will see any of the culture specific characteristics in any given patient depends on your sensitivity and your willingness to recognize these various factors.

AFRICAN-AMERICANS

African-Americans or Blacks have been the largest non-assimilated minority in the United States. Historical hostility, based on skin color, has been one major reason why assimilation has not been open to African-Americans, as it has been for other White immigrant subcultures. One cause is the historical meaning of the color black. As one scholar points out, "The values embedded in the English language affirm White superiority — on our way to heaven we are bathed in a white light or on our way to hell, it

will be a black day."[19] This way of thinking based on semantics predated contact with African slaves, but anti-black stereotypes were applied with ferocity to the "heathens" who replaced white slaves from the 16th century on.[§] Researchers will tell you that the automatic (as contrasted with "conscious") acceptance of this belief may predispose persons to believe in the superiority of white over non-white persons.[20] Race relations in the United States also need to be seen from the perspective of oppression. African slaves comprised the largest group of "forced residents" in the history of the United States. Perhaps more importantly, the dehumanizing nature of the institution of slavery has left an historic imprint of inequality between Black Americans and the dominant White majority[‖].[21] Gunnar Myrdal, a Swedish sociologist, in his monumental analysis of American race relations called the contradiction between democratic ideals and racist practices "the American Dilemma."[22] Struggling against many ingrained societal beliefs has made the struggle by Black Americans to achieve equality with the dominant White culture very difficult.[23] The Civil Rights Act of 1965 outlawed overt prejudice and discrimination against African-Americans. Research, however, indicates that covert prejudice — prejudice based on subconscious fears aroused by blackness and stereotypes handed down within families — is still widespread and continues to represent a barrier to assimilation for Black Americans.[24] Health care providers

---

§The word *slave* comes from the Slavs of Eastern Europe, who for centuries were the traditional target of raids for servants in European and Islamic nations. Sowell T (1994). *Race and Culture: A World View.* New York: Basic Books.

‖The institution of slavery and the contacts between master and slave enabled Whites to see slaves as unequal. African American slaves were required to behave as if they were not fully human: They were traded and sold like prize livestock; they were required to be subservient and behave in a child-like manner; they were denied experience, knowledge, and literacy, thus keeping them ignorant.

need to be alert to stress-related diseases in Black Americans that may be caused by the difficulty in adapting to dominant cultural values as well as perceived prejudice, discrimination and hostility of not only Whites but also persons from other ethnic minority groups. For example, Black professionals often feel themselves held to higher standards in the work place than their White coworkers and thus have a higher frequency of some psychologically based health problems, such as hypertension. Those who have internalized oppression or have accepted the negative labels applied to them by Whites can have related self-defeating or high-risk behaviors and health problems. Seen in that context, the following prevalence rates may not seem surprising. Fifty-two percent of the persons infected with HIV are Black Americans;[25,26] the prevalence of HIV infection among gay Black men is 30%;[27,28] while young Black women have a high incidence of drug addiction, suicide, and anorexia.[29]

Black Cultural Values

The forced social isolation or segregation of Black Americans has led to a high level of retention of cultural values, speech patterns, and behaviors dating back to African origins. These retained patterns are often barriers to communications. One such barrier may be **Black English** dialect, which has its roots in Africa.[30] Generally, Black patients who use this dialect have grown up in or lived in segregated ghetto neighborhoods or in isolated rural areas. A health care provider accustomed to standard English, may regard a patient speaking Black English, with its simplified grammar, as uneducated or lacking in intelligence. In addition, some words or phrases in the Black English dialect or in street slang may have different meanings for the speaker and for the listener, as illustrated in Patient Profile 2-1. With such a person, you have to be careful not to assume a common understanding when you communicate using standard scientific terms for parts of anatomy, or for physiological processes and medical treatment. Misunderstandings about such assumptions could have adverse con-

sequences for the assessment and treatment of the patient. (The chapter on Basic Counseling and Communication Skills will discuss effective ways to prevent such misinterpretations.)

● ●

PATIENT PROFILE 2-1

FELL OUT

SETTING: Ms. Logan brings her 2-year-old son, Jerome, to the ER of a large urban hospital. The PA to see them is Melissa, who has been working the evening shift for 4 months now.

Melissa: Hello Ms. Logan. How can I help you and Jerome today?

Ms. Logan: My baby was playing and just fell out ...

Melissa: Fell out? Fell out of what?"

Ms. Logan: Like I said, he just fell out! You know fell out!

Melissa: Humm, I guess I don't know, Ms. Logan. Perhaps it is best to describe to me what you saw happen.

While Melissa and Ms. Logan are discussing what happened with Jerome, they both glance over at Jerome who is playing quietly with some toys.

Ms. Logan: OK...Jerome was standing next to his play table, leaning against it like he does. He was banging away on his xylophone and then just fell out.

Melissa: Ah-ha...So he was standing there one minute and suddenly he fell to the floor?

Ms. Logan: Yes! That's it...playing one minute and on the floor the next. It was very frightening. I ran over to him, he was shaking, but not crying, and no bleeding. I thought maybe he was having a spell.

Melissa: A spell?

Ms. Logan: Yes. It reminded me of my brother. He had spells when he was a little boy.

Melissa: So tell me more about Jerome. How long was he lying on the floor shaking?

Ms. Logan: Oh, for about a minute. Although it seemed to be forever. I was so scared. You know, Jerome is our first child and we just love him so much. My husband's family just think he's the greatest kid on earth. I hope you can tell me everything is OK. He has been fine, his usual self, since that first horrible minute an hour ago.

Melissa: You were right to bring Jerome in to us. I understand how frightening something like that can be. Let's talk more about what happened, as I need more details to help determine what caused Jerome to fall to the floor. Then I will examine Jerome and talk to my supervising physician about him. If need be, he will also take a look at Jerome and maybe even ask you some of the same questions.

Ms. Logan: That sounds just fine with me. What else do you need to know?

POINTS TO CONSIDER:

- Melissa realized there was a communication problem and acknowledged that to the mother.

- The understanding of the language expressed by the mother was critical for an accurate history and diagnosis and Melissa pursued that understanding.

- Reassuring the mother that she has made the correct decision is comforting to the mother.

- Explaining what will happen assures the mother that her concerns will be answered and Jerome will receive the attention he needs.

• •

The health care provider also needs to be aware that some beliefs about illness, held by African-American patients, may include ancestral healing practices that may look illogical. Health care providers must be careful not to dismiss, ridicule, or belittle such beliefs but instead endeavor to help their patient to integrate these beliefs into the framework of standard medical treatment procedures. Properly harnessed, the power of positive cultural or religious beliefs may enhance the healing process.[31] You also need to be aware that Black culture is permeated by a strong sense of communalism. Powerful kinship

ties extending beyond the nuclear family unit are a common phenomenon.[32] It is not unusual for Black children to be parented by a grandmother or female aunt.[33] When conducting a medical interview, keep in mind that relevant members of the extended family may have better historical information than the patient or their attending parent. Because time may be measured in terms of social events rather than chronologically, specific dates for previous medical procedures may be difficult to identify. Similarly, when informed consent is required, the rules of biological order may not apply. For example, when consent is required to perform a medical procedure on a child, it will probably be more effective to get the oral or written approval of the person doing the actual parenting, possibly an aunt or a grandmother, than the possibly less knowledgeable biological parent. In end-of-life situations, a communal decision may be made by some of the older female relatives.

NATIVE AMERICANS

The history of relations between the original inhabitants of the North American continent and immigrant Europeans is filled with instances of extreme clashes of cultural values. One of the first clashes was when the European settlers, imbued with Lockean ideals of property rights, wanted to protect their newly established farms.[34] The settlers believed that their property rights were being "violated" by the nomadic Native Americans, who in turn believed that land could not be owned, but was for all to share and enjoy. The Protestant work ethic that included concepts of hard work, frugality, and piety[35] clashed with Native American tradition of sharing for strengthening social bonds.[36] These different world views led to early violent efforts to keep Native Americans from trespassing on the settlers' homesteads. Within a short time, the mainly English-speaking settlers took the collective position that the Native Americans were indolent uncivilized savages who interfered in what they believed was the God-given rights of

European immigrants to settle the North American continent. The dominant culture thus attached a label of "subhuman" to Native Americans, making it easy to justify extreme denials of human rights with the official weight of government action. As described by the Assistant Secretary of Indian Affairs in a belated apology to Native Americans in September 2000,[37] "The US Government engaged in ethnic cleansing, deliberate spread of disease, the decimation of the mighty bison herds, the use of the poison alcohol to destroy mind and body, and the cowardly killing of women and children [which] made for tragedy on a scale so ghastly that it cannot be dismissed as merely the inevitable consequence of the clash of competing ways of life."

"This agency forbade the speaking of Indian languages, prohibited the conduct of traditional religious activities, outlawed traditional government, and made Indian people ashamed of themselves. Worst of all, the Bureau of Indian Affairs committed these acts against the children entrusted to its boarding schools, brutalizing them emotionally, psychologically, physically, and spiritually."

By conservative estimates at least two thirds of the indigenous population was wiped out between the arrival of White settlers in North American and the end of the 19th century.[38] As one writer put it: "Trauma experienced by generations of Native Americans has led to unresolved grief in many cases" carried forward to the present time.[39]

Cultural Values Affecting Health Care

This history of trauma has several implications for the health care provider. Suspicion and distrust are natural consequences against a health care system that was implicated in some of the mistreatment of Native Americans. Add to this a fundamentally different philosophical approach to the concept of health or health care, and it is understandable that many Native Americans might be suspicious of Western medicine.[40] Most Native American cultures have a holistic concept of health that integrates traditional spiritual beliefs with mind and body,[41] whereas Western health care tends to focus on removing obstacles (such as pathogens) or repairing physical damage to restore optimal body functioning. For example, if you had been trained in Western medicine, you would consider having achieved a "cure" for a broken leg if, after following the appropriate procedure for realigning and setting the bones and placing the leg in a cast, the bones had healed and the leg had been restored to full functioning. For a Native American, however, the cure might be incomplete unless they also address the lack of balance or harmony that allowed the injury to occur. This may involve the medicine man or healing woman, as well as the family, or even tribal elders to assist the patient to mobilize resources from both the patient's inner world, his tribe, as well as from the spirit world to overcome the barriers to harmony and balance that produced the injury or illness. Sometimes when a seriously ill member of a Native American tribe is in the hospital, the whole family and/or the medicine man may remain in the room with them for hours. They also may chant incantations and burn "smudge sticks" to keep away evil spirits, or bring ritual objects with them and place them in the room.[¶]

Although there is great diversity among Native American tribes, most tribal belief structures adhere to four basic cultural elements: medicine, harmony, relation, and vision.[42] The concept of *medicine* in Native American belief systems is defined as the deeply felt experience of everything being alive. *Medicine* could be translated as healing, and healing is everywhere. *Medicine* can include natural elements (wind, earth), animals, or even a certain place. *Harmony* is a concept that allows for acceptance of living in balance in one's world. *Relation* concerns

---

¶Smudge sticks are usually made of dried sage and other herbs and are burned like incense to cleanse a room and to create a sacred space. In some instances, the wise healing woman or shaman may sprinkle corn meal in a circle on the floor around the perimeter of the patient's bed.

being connected into one's world. *Vision* is the honoring of one's nature, life's gifts, and one's purpose. As with other subcultures, the extent to which a patient with Native American heritage holds to the traditions and beliefs of his or her culture depends largely on the degree of his or her assimilation into the majority culture.

Points for Effective Communication

For purposes of identification, the research literature places Native Americans on a cultural continuum that focuses on four styles of living: *traditional, marginal, middle class, and pan-Indian.*[43] The health care provider's approach to a patient may be determined by which style of living the patient has developed in their life. For those living in a traditional style, the family may need to be brought in as a supportive and protective unit, and Western healing efforts will need to address the interplay between physical healing and restoring social and spiritual harmony. To accommodate the more fluid sense of time of "traditional" Native Americans, you may need to adopt flexible scheduling for appointments.

When working with either "marginal" or "middle class" Native Americans, it is important to identify how comfortable they are with Western medicine. Harwood[44] proposed the following indicators to help identify patients with a relatively high level of acculturation: 1) at least some college education; 2) several generations since leaving the reservation; 3) a low degree of encapsulation within the traditional extended family network; 4) limited contact and few visits to the reservation; and 5) previous experiences with Western health care in the immediate family. However, even persons who fit all the above criteria (i.e., are either assimilated or at least comfortable with White cultural values) may occasionally have physical or psychiatric problems that relate back to their Native American heritage. Those who are living "marginal" or "middle-class" lifestyles are often caught between their traditional roots and the values and behaviors of White society. The tension of trying to balance or combine the values of both cultures, often leaves these persons feeling not accepted by either culture. This puts them at great risk for stress-related diseases.

"Pan-Indians" are those who having lived in White society — often for generations — struggle to return to elements of a lifestyle that embraces traditional Native American values and behaviors. Usually they come from families who had some Native American heritage or "blood", but had suppressed knowledge of that connection out of shame, fear of prejudice, or lack of awareness. Native American activism brought about a change in the 2000 Census forms allowing persons to list more than one ethnicity. Many of those who had previously hidden their ancestry, listed their Native American ancestry. Thousands of "Pan-Indians" are seeking fulfillment of identity by joining modern multi-tribal groups.# Some attend cultural gatherings (Pow-Wows) and try to blend Western traditions with Native American spirituality. These persons may try Native American healing techniques but will mostly rely on Western medicine in emergencies. Other "Pan-Indians" become purists, who oppose wholesale exploitation of traditional Native American names, rituals, or shamanic objects (like "dream catchers") for New Age commercial use. "Pan-Indians" who have an extreme ideological position tend to be disdainful of Western medicine and are less likely to use Western health or mental agencies.[45]

In order to effectively treat the various "types" of Native Americans according to their

---

#During the persecutions of the 19th Century many Native Americans, escaped into the remote hills and hollows of Appalachia, or mountain areas in the Southwest, went into hiding, or tried to pass themselves off as Whites or Mexicans. In the late 1980s and 90s there were several movements to bring about greater recognition and pride in having Native American heritage. For example, in 1995, one of the author's (Kirk) graduate students, who was half Cherokee himself, took on a social work research project to find out about West Virginians with Native American heritage. As a result of his work many people, who had previously hidden their Indian heritage became proud members of the West Virginia Indian Tribes, a vibrant organization of over 5,000 members by the end of 2001.

self-identified relationship to their culture, you need to be alert, respectful, and curious. If you are practicing in an area with persons of Native American heritage, you need to be sure to inquire about possible Native American ancestry during the first meeting with a patient. If appropriate, you should support the patient in their identity as Native American or member of a specific Indian "nation." You might also take a little longer to establish rapport with such patients by encouraging them to discuss their heritage and ties to Native American culture. These discussions are likely to reveal where the patient belongs on the continuum of identification with cultural heritage. An added bit of alert listening will give the health care provider clues about how much Western medicine the patient will accept, thus influencing the treatment plan and how much allowance the health care provider will need to make for traditional practices, such as including family or others in the process or concurrent spiritual healing treatment.

. . . .

PATIENT PROFILE 2-2

Wanna Make Something of It?

SETTING: Bet, a 13-year-old adolescent, has come to a Family Planning Clinic in Kentucky. Her Nurse Practitioner, Lucy, is treating her for her second infection with an STD. She had chlamydia last spring and now gonorrhea.

Lucy: *(I am concerned that she's heading for a pregnancy, PID, or AIDS. How can I get her to value her body? Her self? Have some self-esteem?)* So, girl to girl, let's talk about what you're doing to yourself.

Bet is silent and thinks: *(What does she know about my life? Who does she think she is? She thinks she can get me talking with that "girl to girl" crap.)*

Lucy is silent also and thinks: *(There she goes with those defensive eyes, her gaze averted. Zilch with the girl to girl stuff. How can I develop some rapport with her? She is so young and so vulnerable but acts so tough. Her cheekbones are high —*

look at that dark, rich hair — she has a soft tannish hue to her skin — could she have some Native American ancestry? I'll chance it.)

Lucy: Do you have Native American background? *(There's that wary "Am-I-gone-be-put-down-by-Miss-know-it-all-doctor" look. Is that a subtle shift in her expression?)*
Bet: Quarter Cherokee.

Bet juts out her chin as if to say "wanna make something of it?"

Lucy: Wow, cool. *(Bingo! Her voice tone was soft and a little shy sounding. Here is a possible bridge to self esteem. There's that chin. I wonder if she's been teased at school about being Cherokee.)* Bet, I don't know much about the Cherokee Nation, maybe you could tell me something about your background.

Bet's face perks up and she smiles.

Bet: Sure, what do you want to know?
Lucy: Because the Whites mistreated and killed so many Cherokee out on The Trail of Tears, some Native Americans used to be ashamed of their heritage. But now I know you can be proud of it. How do you feel about being quarter Cherokee?

POINTS TO CONSIDER:

- Lucy's perception that Bet's sexual and reproductive health might be compromised leads Lucy to wonder about Bet's self-esteem and how to get to the possible fundamental issues underlying her high risk behavior.

- Lucy's initial attempt to develop rapport was unsuccessful so she extended her observational skills to examine Bet's physiognomy and her nonverbal communication.

- Sometimes taking a chance on one's intuitiveness yields useful results. Lucy knows she can treat the infection but needs to discuss the risk factors in order to fully help Bet.

- When Lucy shares some of her knowledge about the Cherokee Nation, she offers Bet a familiar topic to open communications and improve their rapport.

. . . .

HISPANIC AMERICANS

The Hispanic population in the US has grown by 35% between 1990 and 2000. By 2004 Hispanics will be largest minority.[46]

The terms **Hispanic** and **Latino** are often used interchangeably to refer to persons whose primary language is Spanish or Portuguese. They are generally persons who came to the United States from South America, Central America, or the Caribbean. Many are refugees from political strife or civil wars (e.g., Guatemala, Nicaragua, Honduras, Columbia). But by far the largest number of Hispanic Americans immigrate to the United States to escape the poverty in their country of origin and to seek economic well being for themselves and their families. Many of these immigrants have come either from Mexico, or have moved through Mexico to come to this country. They have congregated most heavily in the southwestern and southeastern United States. In addition, large Spanish-speaking communities are found in most large American cities. In urban areas, these communities often reside in low income inner city sections referred to as *barrios.*[47] Although some Hispanic Americans, such as highly skilled middle-class Cuban Americans in Florida, have prospered economically, other Hispanic Americans who immigrated with less marketable skills have not escaped the poverty cycle. The poor first generation families hampered by language barrier, lack of education, or illegal or pending legal immigration status represent a collective concern in the health care community because they have high rates of dropping out of school, alcoholism, drug abuse, HIV/AIDS, and neonatal complications caused by lack of prenatal care.[48] Health care for Hispanic Americans is complicated by the reluctance of "illegal" immigrants to seek medical care because they fear that any contact with an official institution, like a hospital, will lead to their being deported. Thus, as with other populations living in poverty, the health problems of Hispanic Americans tend to be extreme when these patients present to a health care provider, usually in the Emergency Room.

A language barrier also complicates their health problems. Most large city public hospitals and those in the southwest United States, schedule Spanish speaking nurses, doctors or staff to be on hand 24 hours a day to manage the flow of Hispanics into their ERs. However, smaller private hospitals or clinics that do not specifically serve a significant Hispanic patient population, usually do not have such coverage. In such hospitals, the personnel or human resources department should maintain a current list of who among the nurse aides, maintenance, and service personnel in the clinic or hospital speaks Spanish, so you can call on them for interpreter duty,** when needed. The names of local Spanish speaking priests also need to be handy for times when you cannot reach anyone else, or when a dying patient needs the "last rites" of the Catholic religion performed. Given the strong tradition of the extended family, it is likely that a bilingual relative might accompany the patient and they may be able to act as an interpreter. If no bilingual relative is available, you may need to find a bilingual person in the community. Of course, if you are going to practice in an area with a large Hispanic patient population, and your own Spanish proficiency is poor, a good option would be for you to learn Spanish.

Hispanic Values

As with other immigrant groups, Hispanics tend to assimilate into the American mainstream by the second generation. At the same time, certain cultural attitudes and beliefs about health and health care may persist, especially if the patient still lives in a primarily Hispanic community. Despite the considerable cultural as well as racial diversity among Hispanic Americans, there are some values and behaviors that are characteristic of "Hispanic culture." Family and extended family is very important, and decisions are often made as a unit. A Hispanic patient will

---

**Often these low paying jobs, low skill jobs attract recent immigrants. Indeed in any hospital, the personnel department should create a list of all the languages spoken by all employees.

likely want to consult with their family before responding to a treatment recommendation made either by you or a social worker. Hispanic societies also tend to have an emphasis on respect for family and for not questioning the authority of the older generation, especially males. The cultural tradition of Latino *machismo* is demonstrated by the show of virility, courage and manliness. This often translates into denial of health problems by men, until the health concerns are so serious that they cannot be ignored. Because of the "double standard" in sexuality, (i.e. women are supposed to be virgins before marriage, but men can "fool around"), men are likely to have higher rates of STDs, and AIDS, which unfortunately are being transmitted to an increasing number of women.[49]

Another common denominator, aside from the Spanish language, is religion. Upward of 95% of Hispanic Americans are Roman Catholics. Some combine the teachings of the Catholic Church with some folk beliefs from their own country dating back to pre-Columbian times. For example, the tradition of the *santeria* or belief in healing saints is a mixture of Catholic beliefs superimposed on a whole host of pre-Columbian pagan spirits. Some patients will wear miniature statues of their personal *santero*, or insist on having it in the hospital room.[50] The Church also tends to occupy a central role in the social and spiritual life of many Hispanics. This needs to be factored into the assessment of the social support system of a patient. At the same time, the prohibitions of the Church on family planning, contraception, and abortion can be a complicating factor when these issues arise. For example, you will need to explore with some sensitivity your female patient's personal degree of acceptance or disagreement with Church dogma before you discuss family planning and contraception.[††] When broaching medical

issues, you will also need to be aware of another cultural value, the reluctance to disagree. This is reinforced by the belief that relationships are hierarchical, and so your patient may be submissive and may outwardly defer to your authority, but privately not follow treatment regimens. However, if you have established good rapport, and your patient regards you as *simpatico*, i.e., agreeable and trustworthy, it may be easier for them to share their personal views with you.

Generally Hispanics tend to be a population needing health care provider's special attention. Just as other cultural minorities, they tend to be underserved in health care. They may also have stress related health problems from the effort to live in two cultures simultaneously.[51] Serving them effectively may require special collaborative outreach programs for prenatal and neonatal care, child vaccinations, and routine health checkups.[52]

ASIAN AMERICANS AND PACIFIC ISLANDERS

The official US census label of **Asian Americans and Pacific Islanders (API)** encompasses more than 30 distinct cultural and linguistic groups. The sudden influx of refugees in 1975 after the Vietnam conflict and the genocide in Cambodia in the 1980s, increased the Asian American and Pacific Islander population by almost 40% between 1990 and 1998. Census projections predict that this group will reach almost 20 million or 6.1% of the US total population by the year 2020.[53] The largest Asian American groups are Japanese, Chinese, Filipino, Korean, and East Indian. Some are from Southeast Asia, mainly Vietnam, Cambodia, Laos, Thailand, Malaysia, and Singapore. Pacific Islanders include much smaller numbers of Indonesians, Filipinos, Hawaiians, Samoans, and Micronesians.

Large Chinese and Japanese ethnic enclaves have long thrived economically in some major cities, like San Francisco, Honolulu, Los Angeles, and New York. More recently, educated, middle-class Vietnamese refugees have established prosperous "little Saigons" in some West Coast cities. Many Cambodians, Laotians,

---

††It will be easier for a Hispanic woman (as well as many women in general) to talk "woman to woman" about health issues related to sexuality. So, if you are male and encounter reluctance in this area, see if a female colleague or nurse can elicit the information.

Hmong tribesmen, and some Vietnamese — formerly farmers or fishermen — were settled by the US Government in rural farming or coastal fishing communities. The incredible variety among and within the Asian American subgroups makes generalizing of only limited use.[54] For example, Filipino culture is strongly influenced by its Spanish and American colonial heritage, as well as Catholicism.[55] This is in contrast to the rest of the Asian Pacific nations, where Buddhism and Confucianism support cultural values. Thus, depending on where a health care provider is practicing, they might encounter highly educated second to fifth generation Asian Americans who are fluent in English, or poor first-generation immigrants with scant to no English language skills.

API Cultural Values

Despite the cultural and linguistic diversity in the API population, the research literature suggests that there are common values that the health care provider needs to know.[56] Perhaps the most significant commonality among this diverse population is their **collectivist orientation**. Personal identity is defined as being a member of the family, group, or society rather than as an individual (as in the West). In collectivist societies, interdependence and reliance on the group are emphasized. Common to many Asian Americans is the concept of **Tao**, which is a set of unspoken norms emphasizing harmony and equilibrium in relations with others. Religious or philosophical beliefs that are derived from Buddhism view life as a series of trials, struggles with desire, and inevitable suffering. Another concept is **Karma**, which states that "performance" in previous lifetimes determines one's fate (and the trials) one needs to bear in this lifetime. Acceptance of Tao and Karma may predispose believers into a fatalistic acceptance of life conditions. Also from childhood on, one is expected to suppress one's inner needs or personal emotions, except indirectly, and then only to a trusted person inside the family group.

These concepts have several ramifications for the health care providers. For example, a com-

mon belief is that stresses in the family, or physical or emotional illness, such as psychiatric problems, substance abuse, or domestic violence, must be endured privately. Acceptance of the concept of Karma disposes people to believe that disease or mental health problems are the result of — some say punishment for — past actions in this lifetime or a previous one, or poor guidance from the family.[57] The emphasis on family loyalty, maintaining "face", and the fear of being stigmatized may turn such problems into "family secrets" to be kept from outsiders.[58] Many also believe it is "bad luck" to talk about illness and death even within the family. For instance, it would be improper for a son or daughter to verbally discuss death and dying issues with their elderly parents. Instead both sides might express their concern through nonverbal **silent communication**.

In general, these cultural characteristics will predispose API persons to underutilization of Western health care.[59] Other reasons for the under utilization of Western medicine by first generation immigrant Asians and Pacific Islanders may be 1) unfamiliarity with Western institutions and their rules and regulations, which may be part of the culture shock experienced by foreign born Asians, especially Southeast Asian refugees;[‡‡][60] 2) possible mistrust caused by discrimination — assumed or real — by the White dominated society; and, 3) the shortage of culturally sensitive and bilingual health care personnel. API persons, especially foreign-born ones, are often discouraged by this lack of understanding of their cultural values and styles of interaction. For all these reasons, they tend to turn first for health and mental health problems to practitioners within their respective cultural community who can communicate with them in their own language and who will use familiar methods, such as herbal medicine or acupuncture.[61]

Health care providers, who have API families as their patients, have recognized that they need

---

‡‡This may include unacknowledged post-traumatic stress disorder among refugees from Vietnam, Cambodia and Laos.

to modify their approach to patient accountability. For example, informed consent by the patient is a legal requirement and responsibility of the individual patient, as long as they are competent to make such decisions. However, the collectivist orientation will make independent health care decisions difficult for an API patient. Thus, an API patient may resist giving informed consent or sign advance directives. When this cultural dilemma goes unnoticed by health care providers, it can create misunderstanding or conflict, and the patient may be labeled "non-compliant" or "difficult." Instead the health care provider needs to recognize that the whole family needs to be involved in the decision making on health care. Often the family will designate the eldest son of a patient to communicate with health care personnel after consultation with the family. He will relay decisions back to the health care team.[62] Advance directives can also become a point of conflict between the legal requirements of health care facilities to approach all patients to obtain signed instructions and the cultural resistance to discuss death. Since Karma determines the length of one's life, API patients may see advance directives as interfering with fate, and may actively resist accepting or completing the forms.

Techniques for Effective Communications and Interactions

How do these beliefs and behaviors about physical and mental health care issues affect a health care provider's interaction with Asian Americans? If a patient population tends to use Western medicine only as a last resort, the provider is likely to encounter higher percentages of patients with advanced or life-threatening medical conditions or serious mental health problems than in the rest of the population.[63] For example, Vietnamese women living in the United States are five times more likely to suffer cervical cancer, and Asian Americans are three times as likely to develop liver cancer and to have higher rates of breast cancer.[64] The fear of stigma of some physical illnesses for both the patient and the family is so strong that such problems are denied until they can no longer be

ignored. Personal problems that are not to be discussed are instead expressed via silent communication through meaningful glances into the distance or tilting the head forward and looking at the floor, which in their culture would convey that something is indeed wrong, but that it is a taboo subject. A Western born health care provider not sensitive to such subtle signals may feel frustrated in their effort to obtain a clinical and psychosocial history. One effective way to open a dialogue is to "normalize" the cultural reluctance to discuss such problems with a comment like, "I understand how hard (or embarrassing) it must be for you to talk about something like this. A lot of people find it difficult. I am glad that you are here so I can help you."

The emphasis on family loyalty can be used to your advantage in establishing rapport and gaining cooperation. You can empathize with the patient by asking how the patient's illness is affecting the family. You can convey that you want to help the patient resume a useful role within the family as quickly as possible. Depending on the response, you can then tell the patient that information is needed from the patient, so that proper care can be given. You should assure patients that any information is only for medical purposes and is completely confidential. Box 2-1 lists additional points for establishing rapport. Although members of cultures with a high reliance on their own group or community may delay use of Western medicine, once inside the health care system they "may abdicate decision making to the physician, who is seen as a wise and benevolent authority figure."[65]

Health care providers practicing in an area with a large population of Asian Americans should study Asian American culture and develop a list of interpreters to contact in emergency situations. (In some cities with large multicultural populations, such as Seattle, professional medical interpreters may be called on.)[66] Such interpreters may also teach you to read the silent communication of their particular API subgroup. This will enhance your ability to detect the subtle signals that a patient or family might have a taboo medical problem. To address

---

Box 2-1 Considerations for a First Visit

Upon meeting with a patient from a different culture, the health care provider might use the following sequence for establishing rapport. When asking questions convey genuine interest, and listen attentively. One way to assure your patient that they are being listened to would be to nod and say Uh-huh more frequently than most Americans tend to.*

1. Introduce yourself, speaking slowly and distinctly. Then ask the name of the patient, and where they are from.

2. Then talk about totally neutral matters for a few moments.

3. Then shift to questions of a different nature. When did the family come to the United States (if you are talking to immigrants)? Where is or was home for the patient (if American subculture)? Where did they grow up? How many members are in the current family? What and who did they leave behind? What had their lives been like in their home country (or birth place)? Why did they leave? If refugees, how did they survive or overcome the difficulties?

4. Find out about their present living situation. How many in the dwelling? Who is working at outside jobs? How many children in school, and how are they doing?

5. If from the above information you find character traits, like persistence, courage, hard work, faith, or accomplishments by the children, then compliment the patient at this point.

6. Slowly bring around the conversation to health related questions. You would ask what, if any, traditional healing methods the patient might have used prior to coming to you. After respectfully taking note, you could assure the patient that you do not intend to countermand or compete with traditional healing practices. However, make it clear that you need to know what they are doing or taking to make sure that one effort does not interfere with or cancel out the other.

7. Recognize that the first visit is designed to establish rapport and trust. Building rapport may take more than one visit. But if the patient felt you treated them with respect and sensitivity, it is likely that the next time they will be more open with you.

---

*In many other cultures, nodding and vocalizing, as often as once every 20 seconds, are used to convey to the speaker that you are listening or attending to what he /she is saying. For example, in Japanese culture, the listener will not only nod almost constantly, but will also repeatedly say, "Yes, yes", "Is that so?" or "Yes, that's so." These aizuchi do not convey agreement with what the speaker is saying, but are merely affirming that the listener is paying close attention.

---

the reluctance of this population to use Western medicine, using a team approach, including social service agencies, can help establish preventive health outreach programs for health screening. This approach has been shown to be effective in some locations.[67]

RURAL VS. URBAN AMERICANS

The State of Rural Health Care

Millions of health care consumers live in rural parts of America. One of the main characteristics of this population is their poor health status including being at high risk for some conditions, relative to the rest of the population. They face particularly multiple barriers to health care peculiar to their rural status. These barriers adversely affect the health status of rural women and children. Statistics show that rural areas have higher infant mortality rates, higher than expected maternal deaths, rapidly increasing incidence of HIV infections in women and children, excessive rates of death from violence, high frequency of adolescent pregnancy, high incidence of tuberculosis, and deaths from injuries.[68,69] Patient Profile 2-3 shows how one might need to be alert to conditions, like Lyme disease, that one would rarely encounter in an urban setting.

PATIENT PROFILE 2-3

I'm So Tired

SETTING: *Larry is a 36-year-old unmarried male who works in a paint manufacturing plant in a rural county in Tennessee. The chart reads: "continued fatigue, feels worried." He has come in to see Mark, his physician assistant, who has been treating Larry for several years and has seen him change in the last 4 months. Mark notices that Larry has gone from almost perfect attendance at work to coming in once every couple of weeks complaining of feeling "poorly" with low energy and joint pains. Larry usually requests an excuse for a few days of medical leave due to fatigue. Mark notes that Larry is a relatively quiet and somewhat fatalistic person. However, over the years he has moved up in the company to a line supervisor. He has never had a serious relationship and seldom dates. He pretty much keeps to himself. He has a rather impressive collection of Civil War relics and spends his free time attending battle reenactments around the East Coast. Mark reviews the lab results, which had been completed to evaluate his unexplained chronic fatigue: CBC with differential, ESR, basic metabolic chemistries, BUN, ALT, thyroid function tests and urinalysis. All results were reported normal.*

Larry: Hi, you must be sick and tired of seeing me every couple of weeks.

Mark: Well, Larry I'm not sick of you, but I am very concerned that I haven't found out why you feel so tired. All the testing has come back with normal results. *(I wonder if he is having a problem that he is reluctant to mention because he is embarrassed. Larry is a very proud and somewhat private person and may not tell me what is really bothering him.)* Is there anything else you need to tell me? Is there something else bothering you?

Larry grins shyly.

Larry: I am dating an old friend from high school and yes, I am feeling a little "bothered".

They both laugh together.

Larry: Well, I was reading an article about Lyme Disease and wondered if I had it?

Mark: That's a good thought. Have you been in the woods at any time when you remember seeing ticks on your clothing or skin?"

Larry: No, but you know I sometimes help my Mother with her dogs. Everyone knows that dogs carry ticks! That's why that article got me scared about Lyme Disease.

Mark: Do you remember having a recent round red mark or rash on your skin that got bigger and perhaps looked like a rifle target?

Larry: No, nothing.

Mark: You did the right thing to come in and share your concerns. I think it's best to investigate this possible diagnosis. It does require another blood test. *(Why didn't I think of Lyme Disease? Could it really be Lyme? Certainly he does not report any of the symptoms of the acute infectious stages. But when did he first tell me he felt so tired? That was only a few months ago. Fatigue, tiredness, malaise ... these symptoms can be common to so many diagnoses. And then there is his joint pain. I must go with the possibility of Lyme Disease now. Larry's concern could prove to be right.)*

The lab report confirms the diagnosis of Lyme Disease. During a follow-up visit, Larry and Mark talk about the course of the disease, the prognosis and treatments available. Larry is discouraged. Mark asks him to try and remember when he started feeling so tired. Larry says about two years ago. Mark asks Larry why he didn't tell him about feeling so tired when his symptoms first developed and became persistent. Larry says he held back from saying anything because he feared the stigma of being labeled lazy.

Larry: I just got up and dragged myself through each day. It's been a real struggle. I also didn't want to make you angry or try to tell you how to do your job.

Mark: *(His identity has been in terms of being a hard working person and he probably feared that I thought he was seeking disability as has been common in so many families. Also his fatalistic attitude prompted him to just endure his fatigue and not talk with me about it. Did I do anything or say anything that might have added* *to his fear that I'd get mad at him if he told me his ideas about what might be wrong with him? No, I don't think so because I have talked easily with Larry over the years about many of his concerns and personal interests.)* There are some consequences that may occur with this disease. You need to be aware of some of them now...Perhaps the article you read described how the body is affected by the disease.

Larry: Yes, it did mention fatigue and the chances of lots of infections. It also said stress can affect how you feel. I wonder if I will be able to do my job. Some people with chronic Lyme disease need retraining.

Mark: Today I am starting you on the recommended medication and will see you back in the office in two weeks. At that time we will discuss any of your new concerns or questions about the disease.

POINTS TO CONSIDER:

- When Mark gives Larry the negative test results, he also shares his genuine concern for Larry's symptoms of fatigue. Mark remembers that Larry is a quiet and private person and may need some gentle persuasion to share his true concerns.

- They both have joked about Larry being the single man in town so Larry's comment about dating an old high school friend and their laughter helps relieve some tensions.

- Mark takes Larry's statement about Lyme Disease seriously and orders the appropriate diagnostic laboratory tests.

- Mark reviews the nature of their relationship and the personal values and characteristics of Larry.

• •

One of the continuing barriers to rural health care is poverty. The average family income in most rural areas is below the federal poverty line.[70] Job opportunities in general, and well paying positions in particular, are scarce in rural areas.[71] For decades, young people have left their rural communities for better jobs in the cities. This exodus

has left behind an increasingly aging population, many of whom are living in poverty because they are dependent on Social Security payments, which often are inadequate, due to life-long low earnings. Lack of insurance or inadequate insurance is a major barrier to regular or preventive health care.[72] If they meet the very low income guidelines, the poor can obtain health coverage through Medicaid. Medicare usually covers the elderly for 80% of medical care costs, but many cannot afford secondary insurance to supplement Medicare. Another barrier to medical care in rural areas is accessibility. This is a function not only of fewer providers and medical facilities, but also of distance coupled with lack of transportation in sparsely populated areas.[73] The time and effort (a function of distance and availability of transportation) involved getting to the nearest doctor or clinic also prevents many rural people from having routine medical check-ups. When they do need help, their lack of familiarity with doctors and hospitals and poor socialization skills can make them appear fearful, shy, and awkward. In response to this "crisis" of health care in rural America and criticism from advocacy groups,[74] federal and state governments have worked together to launch various initiatives to address some of the problems of the disparities in access and coverage for rural populations. These include forgiving student loans to encourage more health care providers to practice in rural areas. The Children's Health Initiative (CHIP) has provided more extensive insurance coverage for poor children. The successful use of telemedicine has improved access to specialists that would not normally be available in rural areas. Other programs based in rural health clinics are available via TV through health education provided on the Internet.[75]

Rural Values

The dominant White centered world view was previously defined. That world view is centered mostly on the values and behaviors of urban Americans. However, from rural New England, through Appalachia, to Midwestern farming states, the rural South and the far Northwest, health care providers will encounter values, health care attitudes, and behaviors that are similar to each other, but are quite different from those in cities. Depending on which side of the rural-urban divide you were raised, problems communicating with patients from the opposite background may arise. Patient Profile 2-3 illustrates one such example.

RURAL VALUES

Many values associated with a rural population are due to the isolation, as well the small size of the communities.[76] As such, many of these values transcend regionalism or culture or national or ethnic origin.[77] For example, in many rural areas, work usually still centers around farming, lumbering, or mining. Children may be socialized to value manual work over academic learning. As a consequence, many rural residents are likely to have limited education. They will also have a tendency towards **traditionalism**, i.e., holding onto the beliefs and practices handed down from one generation to the next. Among these beliefs are strong ties and identification with the land and the people, and the experiences associated with the **home place**. Another belief is in traditional gender-based family roles, where women are expected to do the childrearing and domestic chores while the men do the "heavy" work, but are less likely to do any "housework". **Familism** is the strong reliance on the kinship ties of the extended family, a necessity coming out of poverty and isolation. In many instances, several generations of the family will live within a short radius, with children being given a plot to build a house, or place a mobile home on the same property. **Neighborliness**, or the tradition of hospitality and helpfulness, comes out of the experience of interdependence, living in isolation, and the need to help each other building houses, raising barns, or getting the truck pulled out of a ditch. **Friendships** are highly valued and often are forever (feuds and enmities can also extend over generations). Friends often become part of the kinship network. An invisible network of word-of-mouth communication is swift and effective in passing on new information through-

out the community.[§§] The other side of this friendliness is **xenophobia**, or fear and distrust of strangers. Until you have been placed in "context" by having some connection with extended family or mutual friends, you are likely to be distrusted as an outsider. In many rural areas, you will find an outward expression of **rugged individualism**, especially by men. This may be likened to machismo, i.e., appearing tough, self reliant, and seemingly unaffected by anxiety or fears. But this posture may be counterbalanced by an inward attitude of **fatalism**, a passive and apathetic acceptance of life and poverty, as well as an avoidance of confrontation or disagreement. In some areas, like Appalachia, which has a history of domination by the coal and timber industries, you also may encounter a sullen but unquestioning response to authority (e.g., doctors, welfare bureaucrats).[||||] Religion traditionally has played a major role in the lives of rural people, and still does so today.[78] In many rural communities, the church is a social institution that draws persons often separated by considerable distance from each other into communal activities.[79] The "little white church" so characteristic of rural America is a strong social support and a solace in crisis.[80] For example, in the farm crisis of the 1980s, churches provided leadership in countering the far reaching negative consequences of the economic depression on farm families.[81] In general, religion as a socializing influence in rural America has tended to reinforce the traditional values listed above.[82]

Techniques for Effective Communications and Interactions

Some of these values strongly influence health attitudes of rural Americans. From the

---

[§§]Persons coming from cities sometimes find it hard to get used to the lack of privacy because of the "goldfish bowl" effect of living in a small rural community where everyone seems to know what everyone else is doing.

[||||]A history of economic exploitation has created a similar sense of fatalism among many Hispanic migrant workers in the rural Southwest.

emphasis on individualism comes a reluctance to ask for help or to admit to any health problems. So, when an urgent health problem forces a rural resident to ask for help, an inner sense of ambivalence may result in the patient giving desultory, evasive, or ambiguous answers during a clinical interview. Along similar lines, the stigma about mental illness, substance abuse, developmental disabilities, or retardation makes it difficult for many rural persons to be open about these problems. Instead, patients may talk about a case of *bad nerves* — which could encompass anxiety disorder, panic attack, or even schizophrenic behavior. Similarly any family member with developmental problems or retardation may be called a "slow learner" or "backward." Health care providers may notice that patients have inadequate understanding of physiological body functions and anatomy. Body shyness, poor self-observation and awareness skills, and the cultural reluctance of rural patients to self-disclose information to a stranger, can inhibit patients from explaining their health problems. All the above factors can be very frustrating to health care providers who are trying to gather clinical information. Sometimes it may appear that such a patient wants the provider to read their mind, so they won't have to go through the discomfort of revealing personal or family secrets. Open-ended questions can lead you to more specific inquiry, which can yield more useful information.

Conclusion

One common theme running through the above descriptions of subcultures is that these groups tend to underutilize standard Western health care for prevention or maintenance. Thus, they tend to present with more advanced or acute illnesses and to have higher mortality rates than urban Whites.[83] One reason is that each subcultural group has different values, behaviors, beliefs, and attitudes about health and health care, which leads to distrust of the health care system (as with African-Americans) or even

avoidance of the health care system (as with Native Americans). Poverty combined with the lack of insurance is a second reason for underutilization of the health care system. A third reason is that members of various subcultures believe they will encounter prejudice or discrimination, or lack of understanding from health care providers and the American health care system. Federal and state initiatives,[84] as well as cooperative partnerships with a large spectrum of professional associations[85,86] and foundations to create outreach programs for underserved minorities are trying to address the first two. But only you, the health care provider, can change patients' perceptions of the health care community. This chapter's brief sketches of some subcultures hopefully will increase your tolerance, understanding, and empathy for patients who are attempting to communicate sometimes painful information to a stranger from another culture.[87]

The next chapter discusses in detail how health care providers can establish effective communications and listening skills when taking medical and psychosocial histories as well as how to discuss treatment options with patients.

REFERENCES

1. Hechter M (1987). *Principles of Group Solidarity.* Berkeley: University of California Press.
2. Stark R (1998). *Sociology, 7th Ed.* Belmont, CA: Wadsworth. 275.
3. Swigonski ME (1999). *Challenging Privilege through Afro-Centric Social Work, in Multicultural Issue in Social Work: Practice and Research.* Washington, DC NASW Press. 51.
4. Sowell T (1994). *Race and Culture: A World View.* New York: Basic Books.
5. US Census Bureau (2000). The Foreign-Born Population in the United States: March 2000 (P20-534). Available on the Internet at http://www.census.gov/population/www/socdemo/foreign.html
6. US Census Bureau (2001). Chapter 16, Race and Ethnicity. In America at the Close of the 20th Century. Available at http://www.census.gov/population/pop-profile/1999/chap16.pdf
7. Lee CC. (1997) 2nd ed. Cultural Dynamics: The

Importance in Culturally Responsive Counseling in C.C. Lee (Editor) *Multicultural Issues in Counseling: New Approaches to Diversity 2nd ed.* Alexandria, VA: American Counseling Association Press.

8. Taylor SE, Peplau LE, Sears DO (2000). *Social Psychology, 10th Ed.* Upper Saddle, NJ Prentice Hall.

9. Achterberg J (1985). *Imagery in Healing: Shamanism and Modern Medicine.* Boston: New Science Library.

10. Dossey L (1997). *Healing Words: The Power of Prayer and the Practice of Medicine.* New York: Mass Market Paperbacks.

11. Vontress CE, Naiker K S (1995). Counseling in South Africa Yesterday, Today and Tomorrow. *J Multicultural Counseling,* 23, 149-157. Alexandria, VA: American Counseling Association.

12. US. Department of Health and Human Services (1985). *Report of the Secretary's Task Force on Black and Minority Health: Vol I.* (Heckler Report). Washington, DC: Dept. of Health and Human Services.

13. Hawkins DR, Rosenbaum S (1993). *Lives in the Balance: The Health Status of America's Medically Underserved Populations.* Washington DC.: National Association of Community Health Centers.

14. Weiss LD (1997). *Private Medicine and Public Health: Profit, Politics, and Prejudice in the American Health Care Enterprise.* Boulder, CO: Westview Press.

15. Adams D (1995). *Health Issues for Women of Color: A Cultural Diversity Perspective.* Thousand Oaks, CA: Sage Publications.

16. Center for Health Economics Research (1993). *Access to Health Care: Key Indicators for Policy.* Princeton NJ: Robert Wood Johnson Foundation.

17. Ewalt PL, et al (1999). *Multicultural Issues in Social Work: Practice and Research.* Washinton, DC: NASW Press.

18. LaFromboise T, Coleman HLK, Gerton J (1993). Psychological impact of biculturalism: Evidence and theory. *Psych Bulletin,* 114:395-412.

19. Swigonski ME (1999). Challenging Privilege through Afro-Centric Social Work, in *Multicultural Issue in Social Work: Practice and Research.* Washington, DC: NASW Press.

20. Sanders JL (1999). Advocacy: A voice for our clients and Communities: Advocacy of behalf of African American clients. *Counseling Today* Jan. 1999. p. 28.

21. Patterson O (1982). *Slavery and Social Death: A Comparative Study.* Cambridge, MA: Harvard University Press.

22. Myrdal G (1944). *An American Dilemma: The Negro Problem and Modern Democracy.* New York: Harper & Row.

23. Weitz S (1972). Attitude, voice and behavior: A repressed affect model of interracial interaction. New York: Oxford Press.

24. Tuch SA, Martin (1997). *Racial Attitudes in the 1990s: Continuity and Change.* Westport, CT: Praeger.

25. CDC (2000). Table 53. AIDS cases according to age at diagnosis, sex, detailed race and Hispanic origin: Unites States, selected years 1985-1999. In *Health, United States, 2000.* National Center for Health Statistics. US Dept. of Health and Human Services. 223.

26. Tapper ML (2001). Increasing High-Risk Behavior: It's Not Just Gay Men. A report on the 8th Conference on Retroviruses and Opportunistic Infections (February 6, 2001). Retrieved on July 23, 2001 from Medscape at http://psychiatry.medscape.com/Medscape/CNO/2001/RETRO/Story.cfm?story_id=2032&CME_story='false'

27. CDC (2001). 20 Years of AIDS: 450,000 Americans dead, over 1 million have been infected. Press Release June 1, 2001. Retrieved on May 22 at http://www.cdc.gov/od/oc/media/pressrel/r010601.htm

28. CDC (2000). Table 54. AIDS cases according to race, Hispanic origin, sex and transmission category: selected years 1985-1999. *Health United States, 2000.* National Center for Health Statistics. US Dept. of Health and Human Services. 224.

29. CDC (2000). Tables 47, 63, 68. in Health, United States, 2000. *Health United States, 2000.* National Center for Health Statistics. US Dept. of Health and Human Services.

30. Anderson MF (1994). *Black English Vernacular.* Rainbow Books

31. Dossey L (1997). *Healing Words: The Power of Prayer and the Practice of Medicine.* New York: Mass Market Paperbacks.

32. Kamo Y (2000). Racial and ethnic differences in extended family households. *Sociological Perspectives,* 43,2:211.

33. Rodney HE, Tachia HR, Rodney LW (1999). The Home Environment and Delinquency: A Study of African American Adolescents. Families in Society: *J Contemp Human Services,* 80, 6:551.

34. Wilkinson CF (1987). *American Indians, Time and the Law.* New Haven CT: Yale University Press.

35. Adrian F (1990). *The Protestant Work Ethic.* New York: Routledge.

36. Locust C (1988). Wounding the Spirit: Discrimination and Traditional American Indian Belief Systems. *Harvard Educational Review.*

37. Gover K (2000). Remarks of Kevin Gover, Assistant Secretary-Indian Affairs, Department of the Interior, at the Ceremony Acknowledging the 175th Anniversary of the Establishment of the Bureau of Indian Affairs, September 8, 2000. Retrieved on July 2, 2001 from http://www.doi.gov/bia/as-ia/175gover.htm

38. Morisette PJ (1994). The holocaust of first nation people: Residual effects on parenting and treatment implications. *Contemp Fam Therapy,* 21 352-360.

39. Jaimes MA (Ed) (1992). *The State of Native America: Genocide, Colonization, and Resistance.* Boston: South End Press.

40. Weaver HN (1999). Indigenous People in a Multicultural Society: Unique issues for Human Services, in *Multicultural Issues in Social Work: Practice and Research.* Wash DC: NASW Press. 88.

41. Herring RD (1994). Native American Indian Identity: A People of many Peoples. In Salett EP & Koslaw DR (Eds.). *Race, Ethnicity, and Self: Identity in Multicultural Perspective* 170-197 Washington, DC.: National Multicultural Institute.

42. Garrett MT, Wilbur MP (1999). Does the Worm Live in the Ground? Reflections on Native American Spirituality," Spiritual and Religious Issues in Counseling Racial and Ethnic Minority Populations. *Journal of Multicultural Counseling and Development:(Special Issue)* 27,4:193-206.

43. Williams EE, Ellison F (1999). Culturally Informed Social Work Practice with American Indian Clients: Guidelines for Non-Indian Social Workers. In *Multicultural Issues in Social Work: Practice and Research.* Washington, DC: NASW Press. 78-84.

44. Harwood A (1981). *Ethnicity and Medical Care.* Cambridge, MA: Harvard University Press

45. Williams EE, Ellison F. (1999). op cit. p 82.

46. US Census (2001). Table 4. Difference in Population by race and Hispanic or Latino Origin, for the United States: 1990-2000. Census 2000 PHC-T-1. Retrieved on July 2, 2001 at http://blue.census.gov/population/cen2000/phc-t1/tab04.pdf

47. Delgado M, Barton K (1999). Murals in Latino Communities: Social Indicators of Community Strengths, in *Multicultural Issues in Social Work Practice and Research.* Washington DC.: National Association of Social Work Press. 229-244.

48. Estrada SL, Trevine FM, Ray LA (1990). Health Care Utilization Barriers among Mexican Americans: Evidence for HHANES 1982-1984. *American Journal of Public Health,* 18:17-33.

49. CDC (2001). Tables 53, 54 in *Health United States, 2000.* National Center for Health Statistics. US Dept. of Health and Human Services.

50. Lozano-Applewhite S (1995). Curanderismo: Demystifying the Health Beliefs of Practices of Elderly Mexican Americans. *Health and Social Work,* 20:247-253.

51. Rodriguez R (1995). Searching for Roots in a Changing Society. In Henslin JM (Ed) *Down To Earth Sociology: Introductory Readings, 8th Ed.* New York: Free Press.

52. Bureau of Primary Health Care (1996). *Models that Work: Compendium of Innovative Primary Health Care Programs for Underserved and Vulnerable Populations.* Bethesda, MD: United States Department of Health and Human Services Health, Resources and Services Administration.

53. US Census Bureau (2001). Retrieved on July 2, 2001 from www.census.gov/population/www/socdemo/race/api.html.

54. Zane NWS, Takeuchi DT, Young NJ (1994). *Confronting Critical Issues of Asian and Pacific Islander Americans.* Thousand Oaks CA: Sage Publications.

55. Baysa E, et al (1980). The Filipinos. In Palafox N, Warren (eds). *Cross-cultural caring: A Handbook for Health Care Professionals in Hawaii.* 197-231. Honolulu: Transcultural Health Care Forum.

56. McLaughlin LA, Braun KL (1998). Asian and Pacific islander cultural values: considerations for health care decision making. (Special Issue on Cultural and Ethnic Diversity) *Health and Social Work,* 23:2–116

57. Shon SP, Ja DA (1982). Asian families. In McGoldrick M, Pearce IK, Giordano J (Eds), *Ethnicity and Family Therapy.* New York: Guilford (208-228).

58. Fugita S, Ito KL, Abe J, Takeuchi DT (Eds) (1991). Japanese Americans in North Mokuau in *Handbook of Social Services for Asians and Pacific Islanders,* New York: Greenwood Press, 61-78.

59. Yamashiro, G, Matsuoka JK (1999). Help Seeking among Asian and Pacific Americans: A Multiperspective Analysis. In *Multicultural Issues in Social Work: Practice and Research* Washington, DC.: National Association of Social Work Press 458-472.

60. Nicholson BL (1999). The Influence of Pre-immi-

gration and Post immigration Stressors on Mental Health: A Study of Southeast Asian Refugees. In *Multicultural Issues in Social Work Practice and Research* Washington DC.: National Association of Social Work Press. 635-653.

61. Yamashiro G, Matsuoka JK (1999). Help Seeking among Asian and Pacific Americans: A Multiperspective Analysis in *Multicultural Issues in Social Work: Practice and Research* Washington, DC.: National Association of Social Work Press. 458-472.

62. McLaughlin LA, Braun KL (1998). Asian and Pacific islander cultural values: considerations for health care decision making. (Special Issue on Cultural and Ethnic Diversity) *Health and Social Work*, 23,2:116

63. Zane WWS, Takeuchi DT, Young CNJ (Eds) (1994). *Confronting Critical Health Issues of Asian and Pacific Islander Americans*. Thousand Oaks, CA: Sage Publications.

64. Satcher D (1999). Shaping the world together: The Surgeon General demands equity in health care access. *Harvard Alumni Med Bull*, 73,2:16-19.

65. McLaughlin LA, Braun KL (1998). Asian and Pacific islander cultural values: considerations for health care decision making. (Special Issue on Cultural and Ethnic Diversity) *Health and Social Work*, 23,2:116.

66. Cross Cultural Health Care Program (n.d.) CCHP Interpreter Services. Retrieved July 23, 2001 from http://www.xculture.org/interpreter/index.html

67. Sent L, Ballem P, Paluck E, Yelland L, et al (1998). The Asian Women's Health clinic: addressing cultural barriers to preventive health care. *Can Med Assoc J*, 159,4:350-54.

68. Center for Health Economics Research (1993). *Access to Health Care: Key indicators for Policy*. Princeton, NJ: Robert Wood Johnson Foundation.

69. Weiss LD (1997). *Private Medicine and Public Health: Profit, Politics, and Prejudice in the American Health Care Enterprise*. Boulder, CO: Westview Press.

70. Haque A, Telfair J (2000). Socioeconomic distress and health status: the urban-rural dichotomy of services utilization for people with sickle cell disorder in North Carolina. *J Rural Health*, 16(1):43-55.

71. Glenn LL; Burkett GL (1999). Equal dependence of the high prevalence of health problems on age and family income in rural southern areas. *South Med J*, 92(10):981-8.

72. Schoen C (1997). Insurance matters for low-income adults: Results from the Kaiser Commonwealth Foundation Five-State Low Income Survey. *Health Affairs*, 16:163-171.

73. Ricketts TC (2000). The changing nature of rural health care. *Ann Rev Public Health*, 21:639-57.

74. Davis KE, Aguilar AA, Jackson VH (1998). Save low-income women and their children first. (Editorial) (Special Issue on Cultural Diversity). *Health and Social Work*, 23 n2 p83(3).

75. Bureau of Primary Health Care (1996). *Models that Work: Compendium of Innovative Primary Health Care Programs for Underserved and Vulnerable Populations*. Bethesda, MD: United States Department of Health and Human Services Health, Resources and Services Administration.

76. Maurer BB (Ed) (1984). *Mountain Heritage*, 4th Edition. Parsons, WV: McClain Printing Co.

77. Weller J E (1965). *Yesterday's People: Life in Contemporary Appalachia*. Louisville, KY: University of Kentucky Press.

78. Winter M (1991). The Sociology of Religion and Rural Sociology: A Review Article. *Sociologia Ruralis*, 31, no. 2-3: 205-6.

79. Moberg DO (1962). *The Church as a Social Institution: The Sociology of American Religion*. Englewood Cliffs, NJ: Prentice-Hall.

80. Swierenga RP (1997). The little white church: religion in rural America. *Agricultural History*, 71: 415(27).

81. Danbom DB (1995). *Born in the Country: A History of Rural America*. Baltimore: Johns Hopkins Press, 265.

82. Bultena L (1944). Rural Churches and Community Integration. *Rural Sociology*, 9: 257-64.

83. CDC (2000). Table 71, Health care visits to doctor's offices, emergency departments, and home visits within the past 12 months, according to selected characteristics: United States 1997-1998. In *Health United States, 2000*. National Center for Health Statistics. US Dept. of Health and Human Services. p. 259.

84. US Dept of Health and Human Services (1998) President Clinton Announces New Racial and Ethnic Health Disparities Intiative. White House Press Sheet (February 21, 1998). Retrieved July 23, 2001 from http://www.omhrc.gov/rah/sidebars/sbinitPres.htm

85. American Medical Association (2000). AMA teams up with U.S. Surgeon General Satcher to eliminate disparities of care and improve country's

health. Press Release of December 5, 2000. Retrieved July 23, 2001 from http://www.ama-assn.org/ama/pub/article/1616-3546.html

86. American Public Health Assocication (2000). Influential and Diverse Leaders Join Steering Committee of APHA/HHS Campaign to Eliminate Racial and Ethnic Health Disparities: In a Pledge to the Campaign and to Their Nation, Leaders Sign Historic Document. Press Release from APHA (October 6, 2000). Retrieved on July 23, 2001 from http://www.apha.org/news/press/2000/elim_dispar.htm

87. Three Rivers A (1990). *Cultural Etiquette: A Guide for the Well Intentioned*. Indian Valley, VA: Market Wimmin.

CHAPTER 3

Life Span and Human Development

The study of human development examines the different stages of life from infancy past the "golden years." Expanding on the information presented in Chapter 1, we use the psychosocial perspective as a focusing lens on the life course and the developmental tasks of each stage. Of special relevance to the health care provider is how organic and psychosocial factors can either enhance or interfere with stage appropriate tasks. We also look at how expected events and unexpected shocks and traumas can create dysfunctional behavior patterns and set up susceptibility to certain physical disease conditions or psychopathologies.

Theories of Human Development

Theories of human development have tended to organize and prioritize large amounts of information usually with a specific focus on one of five major components of development: 1) physical, 2) cognitive, 3) emotional, 4) social, and 5) moral. More recent textbooks have shortened the list to 1) physical development and health, 2) cognitive development, and 3) psychosocial development.[1] In the area of physical development, changes in body, the brain, sensory capacities, and motors skills are based on empirical observation, and thus, there is relatively little disagreement on them. A combination of milestones are generally used to divide the physical development from infancy to late adulthood.

Different theorists, each highlighting different elements, have examined measurement of emotional, cognitive, social, and moral development. However, common to the concept of stage theories is that there are sequential **develop-mental tasks** at each stage that are building blocks for the subsequent stage. We briefly outline the essentials of four major stage theorists, Sigmund Freud, Erik Erikson, Jean Piaget, and Lawrence Kohlberg (Table 3-1). Most readers may recall these names from their basic Psychology class, and so we will only summarize each theorist's developmental model. Each theorist addresses a different perspective of human development. Each makes a crucial contribution to the understanding of specific aspects of human development. None is comprehensive. This is why most college courses in Child and Human Development use a chronological approach in which each stage is analyzed through the lens of these theoretical models. Until relatively recently, the study of Human Development tended to focus primarily on the period from infancy through adolescence. As theorists began to look more holistically at life span development, marriage, the middle years,[2] and older adulthood[3] were added. Box 3-1 lists age graded periods into which human development is studied over the life span.[4] To the usual list we have added the college years, because millions of young persons spend anywhere from four to seven years between adolescence, adulthood and career in what we call "extended adolescence."

FREUDIAN MODEL OF PERSONALITY DEVELOPMENT

Sigmund Freud developed a **psychodynamic** model of personality development of considerable complexity.[5] Many of his terms, such as the **id, ego,** and **superego** have become part of our language. Freud conceptualized human develop-

TABLE 3-1	Stage Theories of Human Development			
The Life Cycle	Freud's Psychosexual Stages	Piaget's Cognitive Structural Stages	Erikson's Psychosocial Stages	Kohlberg's Moral Development Stages
Infancy	Oral Anal	Sensorimotor	Trust vs. Distrust Autonomy vs. Shame	
Early childhood	Phallic	Preoperational	Initiative vs. Guilt	Level I: *Preconventional Morality* Stage 1. Avoid punishment Stage 2. Obtain rewards
Middle and late childhood	Latency	Concrete Operational	Industry vs. Inferiority	Level II: *Conventional Morality* Stage 3. Social Approval Stage 4. Rules oriented
Adolescence	Genital	Formal Operational	Identity vs. Role Confusion	Level III: (if reached) *Postconventional Morality*
Early adulthood Middle adulthood	I I	I I	Intimacy vs. Isolation Generativity vs Stagnation	Stage 5. Morality of Individual Ethics. Tolerance. Stage 6. Morality of universal ethical principles
Late adulthood	↓	↓	Ego Integrity vs. Despair	

ment as being driven by the **libido**, or biologically based sex drives. His stages of **psychosexual development** refer to the movement of the libido from one eroticized body zone to another during the first five years of life, in order to meet biological needs for satisfaction. Thus, in the first year of life during the **oral stage**, the infant is dominated by sexual needs and desires centered in the mouth. These are satisfied by taking in nourishment, eating, sucking, or by mouthing toys or other objects. During the second year, as toilet training is introduced, the child becomes preoccupied with the libidinal pleasures of the anus. Two to three year olds may become fascinated with the "products" of their body, and enjoy expelling and playing with their feces. Freud also postulated an **aggressive drive**. Thus, when a child is angry in the oral stage, it might bite (the nipple). The anal stage is also marked by ambivalence: the pressure of social conditioning during the anal stage can lead the

child to either want to conform or to resist toilet training. The label "terrible twos" reflects the child's open rebellion, and the terms **anal retentive** and **passive-aggressive** apply to the child's quiet resistance at this stage. The **phallic stage** has probably aroused the most controversy and fierce criticism from feminists.[6] According to Freud, this is when the libidinal drives, interests and pleasures shift from the anus to the genitalia. These needs are satisfied by self-stimulation, masturbation, as well as fantasies about adult sexuality and reproduction. Fiercely debated is Freud's assertion that in their sexual fantasies about the opposite sex parent at this stage, the child wants to take the place of the same sex parent. Named for figures from ancient Greek tragedies, the boy's sexual fantasies and longing for his mother are called the **Oedipus complex**, and the girl's longing to be loved by her father as the **Electra complex**. When the child has resolved or repressed these conflictual urges,

Box 3-1 Developmental Periods in the Life Span

Age Period *	Name of Stage
Conception to Birth	Prenatal Stage (impact on couple)
Birth to Age 3	Infancy and Toddler
3 to 6 years	Early Childhood
6 to 12 years	Middle Childhood
12 to 20 years	Adolescence
18 to 22-27	College or "Extended Adolescence"
20 to 40 years	Young Adulthood (includes career)
40 to 65 years	Middle Age (includes menopause, "midlife crisis")
65 years and older	Late Adulthood

* Because we view development from the perspective of the family, these periods are different from those used by the American Academy of Pediatrics, which focuses on the changes within the individual.

they enter the **latency** period. This period just prior to puberty is when the sexual urges lie more or less dormant. They are reawakened by the hormonal urges of adolescence in, what Freud calls, the **genital stage**. An important part of Freud's theory is that psychological conflicts and trauma, which are not resolved at each stage, become the determinants of the motivations and behaviors throughout the life span.[7]

ERIK ERIKSON'S MODEL OF EGO STRENGTHS OR VIRTUES

Erik Erikson also uses a stage model to track the development of the **autonomous ego**, or what he calls the **healthy personality**.[8] While Freud believed that our emotional and ego development is basically completed by the time we reach adolescence, Erikson assumed that growth and development continues throughout our life.[9] Each of his seven stages has its specific psychosocial task or dilemma. To achieve — and in adult life maintain a positive sense of self — each

human being must successfully resolve sequential **developmental challenges** to reach a position of **virtue** or **ego strength**. Thus, in infancy how well or how poorly our needs are met determines where along the **Trust vs. Mistrust** dichotomy we will be. How our drive for individuation is handled and how we are disciplined in the toddler stage can produce either **Autonomy** or **Shame** or **Doubt**. How the curiosity, creativity and imagination of our middle childhood is treated by the adults around us, determines how we will fare on the **Initiative vs. Guilt** dichotomy. Learning in school, getting along in our family, and the creation of peer friendships, up to puberty is called the **Industry vs. Inferiority** challenge. Our struggle in adolescence to find out who we are is the **Identity vs. Role Confusion** stage. As we move toward forming intimate adult relationships, creating a family and moving into the work world, we face the **Generativity vs. Stagnation** dilemma. Finally as we age, we become concerned about leaving a legacy, confronting the challenge of **Ego Integrity vs. Despair**.

JEAN PIAGET'S MODEL OF COGNITIVE DEVELOPMENT

Jean Piaget, based his sequential stages of cognitive development in children on over 50 years of observational research. In Piaget's view, the ability to process information (which he calls intelligence) is adaptive, arising out of the interaction with the psychosocial environment.[10] He sees four stages of increasing complexity moving from sensorimotor, preoperational, concrete operations, to formal operations. In other words, the more we interact with the environment, the more cognitive complexity our brain can handle. In the **sensorimotor** stage the infant is engaged with the world through the senses, primarily touch, sight, and sound. A key aspect of this stage is that for the infant, reality and objects exist only through the child's sensory experience. According to Piaget, this principle of sensory reality is illustrated when a toy or ball is removed from sight, and the infant loses interest, indicating that for the infant the object no longer exists. During the **preoperational** stage, the child develops the ability to represent things in the mind, through language and fantasy play. Thinking comes from within rather than only from sensory perceptions. At the **concrete operational** stage, the child can sort and classify objects. The limitation here is that the child tends to think mostly in terms of concrete reality, rather than "what ifs." Only when we reach the **formal operations** stage are we able to think conceptually and abstractly, and use formal logic. We can discuss assumptions, work with higher level symbols, such as scientific formulae, and mathematical equations. According to Piaget, only those who have sufficient physical, social and intellectual stimulation and nurturance at each stage will develop the complex cognitive structure required to reach the final stage. More sophisticated research has shown that Piaget's notion of age graded stages is not as rigid as he had thought. However, the main concept that our cognitive abilities move from relative simplicity at birth to ever greater complexity, forms the foundations of much of Western educational theory. For example, his emphasis on adequate early stimulation is the rationale behind childhood enrichment programs, like Headstart.

LAWRENCE KOHLBERG'S MODEL OF MORAL DEVELOPMENT

Lawrence Kohlberg, influenced by Jean Piaget, developed a sequential model of **moral reasoning**.[11] The model suggests that we evolve in our capacity to discern ethical issues and to make moral judgments. Kohlberg says we move from preconventional through conventional, and then possibly but not necessarily to postconventional morality in six stages. In Stage One of **preconventional morality**, the young child acts in obedience to the superior force of parents (or adults generally). The primary motivation is to avoid punishment. A slightly older child obeys parents (adults) to obtain rewards (Stage Two of this level). At the level of **conventional morality** (usually attained between ages of 10-13), the

child is motivated to be "good" in order to please parents and to gain social approval (called Stage Three). As they become adolescents, some begin to conform to "the rules" for the sake of upholding authority and the order of social institutions, including the norms of their peer group or gang (Stage Four). While some people may never move beyond this stage, others develop **post conventional moral** reasoning. We conform out of respect for others, even when we disagree with some of their values. At this fifth stage, we can tolerate and respect conflicts of interest and moral dilemmas in decision making. In Stage Six we make decisions on the basis of self chosen ethical principles, rather than blindly following conventional societal principles. Psychosocial conditions and opportunities largely determine whether we advance past the "either - or", "all or nothing" thinking of the preconventional level, to being motivated to follow the rules to uphold the conventional order, or to making decisions based on moral reasoning derived from internal evaluation and reflection.

Summary

We have presented four theories of human development to acquaint you with the notion of tasks and stages. Persons who have not mastered or completed certain tasks or stages often present special problems for health care providers. For example, patients caught in a struggle between dependence and independence may develop serious transference problems with their health care provider. They may become overly dependent on their health care provider. Some may find it difficult to make decisions and will want to put that responsibility on their health care provider. They may blur boundaries by seeking advice or friendship in inappropriate ways. They may exaggerate symptoms in order to get attention. They may schedule frequent appointments to gain the attention and nurturance from their health care provider, which they did not receive as an infant. In some cases, the search for love and acceptance can turn into improper sexual advances. On the other hand, persons with avoidant attachment patterns may have difficulties establishing rapport with their health care provider. They may feel that they are not getting their needs met, and may end up "doctor shopping". Still others may become argumentative, belligerent, or critical. Chapter 13 discusses ways of treating patients with such deep seated developmental issues.

The Life Course Model

Even though the focus of this book is on psychosocial and behavioral factors, we have included the major theorists and stages of human development so that health care providers will be familiar with the terminology used by pediatricians and child psychologists. We will now depart from this traditional approach and instead use the **life course** model. As in the stage theories outlined above, the life course model has specific phases or stages which are defined by events or the psychosocial circumstances. Similar to stage theory, they are characterized by certain tasks or challenges, in relation to which we move through the various stages of the life course. Some of these life events are **normative** while others are **non-normative**. Normative events are those that are either biologically based, or that happen as a matter of course in most lives. For example, physical growth and development of secondary sex characteristics are normative. Experiencing declining capacities in old age fits into the same category. Going out into the workforce as an adult similarly is a normative development. Non-normative events are those that occur unexpectedly. They can range from adolescent pregnancy, divorce, loss of job to accidental death of a family member. Both normative as well as non-normative events tend to force us to adapt as an individual, and to adjust to an altered psychosocial environment. We will again emphasize how our early experience of nurturance and socialization within the family context influences how we approach and resolve these tasks and challenges. Such knowledge leads to better understanding of patient behavior at various stages of development, which in turn helps to plan more effective care strategies for patients at any phase. We suggest that dysfunctional behavior patterns in each stage can affect the person's attitude towards health care, towards the provider, and towards treatment compliance. The reader should keep in mind the cautions issued in other chapters — namely that all persons are individuals whose unique perceptions shape their reactions to the changes, challenges, and crises of the different stages in their own life course.

FAMILY AS THE CONTEXT

We will use the **family as the context** to proceed through the life course model. In Chapter 1 we elaborated on the importance of the family. We listed various family constellations and described the difference between functional and dysfunctional families. We noted that there is no specific family constellation or living arrangement that is inherently functional or dysfunctional for the personal growth and development of the constituent members (See Box 1-3 in Chapter 1). What matters is how or whether the members master the transitions and tasks at each stage. Functional families tend to proceed through each stage by adjusting and adapting to changes in a healthy way. Dysfunctional families tend to have problems mastering the tasks at each stage and accommodating to the changes in roles. Both normative as well as non-normative events can upset the progress from phase to phase in either type of family. Whereas most functional families tend to return to an adaptive equilibrium after such events, dysfunctional families may be driven further into chaotic or mutually harmful patterns. Because the family is the context, we begin our examination of the life course at the point where the family forms — which is usually when two people begin to live together as a couple.

FORMATION OF A COUPLE: TASKS AND CHALLENGES

A major challenge for a new couple, whether married or not, heterosexual or homosexual, is to balance individual patterns and traditions with an emerging sense of themselves as a couple. A newly formed couple needs to blend two separate sets of family values and traditions. They also need to reach agreement on how to divide household chores (the number one friction point),[12] manage money, establish a mutually satisfying sexual relationship, and find a balance between being together and the privacy and independence needs of each partner. They need to cope with the inevitable disillusions, differences, annoying habits, and imperfections that usually become apparent only after living together.[13] If each partner comes from a different religious background, the couple needs to decide which faith to follow and if they decide to have children in which faith their children will be raised. One essential task at this stage is to find ways to achieve agreement or compromise and resolve conflict on these issues.[14,15]

Research has shown that socioeconomic factors affect this adjustment process.[16] Upper and middle class values tend to emphasize love, intimacy and companionship. By contrast, couples coming from backgrounds marked by poverty and lack of education tend to be characterized by greater emotional distance and limited communication skills. In general, lower class couples have a stricter division of labor based on gender stereotypes, with the authority for decision making — at least nominally — vested in the male. There is little joint planning. Many working class couples tend to see the partner as unpredictable, difficult to understand, and inconsistent. Often their lives are sharply segregated, with women seeking to stay connected to their mother, sisters, or women friends. They may seek intimacy through motherhood and then fulfill their emotional needs through their children.[17] As Melvin Kohn's research has shown, lower class parents in their child rearing practices tend to place greater emphasis on obedience, and to discipline children with corporal punishment as opposed to middle class families where withholding affection or time outs tend to be used more frequently.[18]

How the new couple will relate to their families of origin and the community is another task for the first few years of marriage or between committed couples. Whose family gets visited on weekends or over holidays needs to be resolved. Normally, a shift in loyalties away from their families of origin and towards the new partnership evolves gradually, as the couple deepens their commitment to each other.[19] There is also a shift in the role required of the families of origin, who need to surrender their control as parents, and let the couple establish themselves as a separate and independent unit. This can be difficult if the couple continues to live in same household with one set of parents, or lives in close proximity to the parents. In recognition of the primacy of the couple relationship, each member will need to modify the amount of energy devoted to pre-existing relationships, whether they be same gender friends, or romantic friends.

● ●

PATIENT PROFILE 3.1

THE SMALLEST THINGS

SETTING: Henrietta is a 20-year-old, recently married woman with Type One Insulin dependent diabetes at 15 years of age. She has been receiving ongoing medical care for the diabetes, mild hypertension, and weight control from Catherine, her physician assistant. She remains 22 pounds overweight. Today, she presents with the chief complaint of "problems in my marriage."

Catherine: Good morning Henrietta. I see here that you are having problems in your marriage. How long have you been married now?

Henrietta: About 9 months. At first it was great but now we fight over the smallest things and I get upset. Then I eat something I shouldn't.

Catherine: Hmm. That doesn't sound good. *(First I need to find out what the fighting is about, rule out any domestic violence and then check her blood glucose level and hemoglobin A1c.)* Can you give me an example of what you fight over?

Henrietta: Well, it seems so silly to be talking about this but it's about Sundays — whose family to visit on Sundays.

Catherine: That's not silly at all, and I can understand why it is upsetting to you. This often happens in young marriages. Whose family to visit on your days off can become a pretty big problem unless you work it out. Is the fighting violent? Does he ever hit you or push you?

Henrietta: Oh, no, we just "have words". We've tried talking about it, but we just end up arguing. He wants to visit his family and I want to see mine. Frankly, I kind of miss them, and I think he misses his family. I feel pulled in two directions, and sometimes I just want to chuck it all.

Catherine: *(It sounds like they are both missing their families of origin and maybe needing some extra "parenting". They did marry kind of young. I wonder if these little fights stem from some unfinished business with their parents.)* Yes, I can see that you'd feel like chucking it all. Let's check your blood glucose level and make sure you're OK in that area, then we'll talk about how you two might make these kinds of decisions in a better way.

POINTS TO CONSIDER:

- Since the presenting problem is "problems in the marriage", Catherine identifies the nature of the problem first and rules out domestic violence right away.

- By getting more information about the problem, Catherine is able to assess the relationship between the marital problems and an increased blood glucose level. Chronic emotional upsets may lead to poor compliance with insulin injections, diet, and exercise.

- Being aware of what developmental tasks need to be completed in early adulthood helps identify the possible causes of marital discord.

- Patient education and counseling for Henrietta and her husband are important not only to resolve the marital conflicts but are an essential part of the management of Henrietta's diabetes and hypertension.

• •

Difficulties in Couple Relationships

Harville Hendrix in his Imago Theory of Relationships states that unresolved childhood issues are a source of major friction in couple relationships.[20] According to Hendrix, we tend to be attracted to an adult partner (the Imago) who in many ways is similar to major attachment figures in our childhood, such as our parents. Once in a relationship, we place expectations on the partner to fulfill needs that were not satisfied in childhood. When the partner does not "deliver" on these idealistic childlike expectations, disillusionment, resentment, and power struggles may develop. For example, research has shown that adult romantic attachment tends to be patterned on the early infant-mother attachment imprint, i.e., either *secure, avoidant* or *anxious ambivalent*.[21] An adult, who as an infant received insufficient or inconsistent nurturance, may tend to be either avoidant or overly needy of affection and dependent upon the other person. Such unfulfilled needs may put a strain on the new relationship, making it difficult to develop a sense of equality.[22] Instead the relationship may be marked by an undercurrent of inappropriate parent-child dynamics.[23] Both partners, though usually not conscious of the dynamics, may be dissatisfied. Efforts to change the other to conform to the internal expectations will often produce chronic resentments.[24] Such resentments may spill over into the relationship with a health care provider, and show itself as surliness, or passive non-cooperation.

Poor communication, rigidity, or unrealistic beliefs about the marriage relationship[25] can produce power struggles[26] that often prevent agreement on the tasks for the newly formed couple listed above. Such struggles can consume a young couple. As a provider you may hear from one member of the partnership: "We fight over the silliest things" (See Patient Profile 3-1). This type of statement can be a "red flag" for the health care provider that some unresolved childhood development issues are haunting the relationship. Couple's therapy may be indicated.

PARENTING

Some couples may consider becoming parents at some point in their relationship. Others may choose to postpone becoming parents or choose not to have children at all. For the latter, the focus of the first years of the couple relationship may be exploration of career and job options, and other interests. Some couples who want children may be unable to conceive. Those with sufficient financial resources, can avail themselves of various new reproductive technologies or turn to adoption. A successful pregnancy or adoption automatically affects the relationship of the couple, both positively and negatively.

Tasks and Challenges

The birth of children into a partnership requires reorganizing the family division of labor to include care giving for the infant. For example, because the care needs of an infant are paramount, both parents generally have to adjust the amount of intimacy time they have with each other.[27] Care demands on parents are often exhausting in part because of the lack of sleep from attending a newborn infant's needs around the clock. Health and temperament of a newborn also affect the couple. If there are serious health or developmental problems (e.g., developmentally or speech-delayed, chronically ill, or disabled children), the challenge for parents is to find the energy and love to support each other to fulfill the care demands of such a child. The extended family may be able to lend support at this crucial time. Boundaries established in the formation of the couple now need to be renegotiated with extended families.

Difficulties

Difficulties arise when the couple has not reached mutually satisfactory agreements on roles, division of tasks, and relations with others prior to having children. In such couples, the pregnancy itself may exacerbate conflicts over these issues.[28] The partner may regard the pregnancy as a threat to his primacy in the relationship. It is no accident that domestic violence often begins or becomes more severe during pregnancy. (See Chapter 10.) Socioeconomic factors also play a major role in the ability of the couple to negotiate the transition to parenthood. In general, statistics tell us that age, amount of education, as well as financial status are key variables in how well couples handle the challenges of parenting.[29] Unfortunately, very young, uneducated, and poor parents with poor coping skills, tend to have higher levels of domestic violence and child abuse.[30]

Young mothers can be overwhelmed with the needs of an infant. This is especially true if the infant is "difficult," e.g., colicky. Sleep deprivation alone can lead to feeling low and depressed.[31] You also need to be on the alert for signs of postpartum depression.[32] The parent whose own needs for nurturance are not being sufficiently met, in the medical interview is likely to talk about her own problems more than about how the infant is doing. If the parents' educational level is low and social support is weak, they may not have adequate knowledge of the health care and nutritional needs of their child. Ignorance about normal developmental markers of their infant or baby might predispose them to have unreasonable fears about small changes in their baby's behavior, such as when "teething" may cause discomfort and crying. New parents in general need frequent reassurance, and support. Through careful questioning, you can determine the extent of the parents' knowledge and parenting skills, and if necessary, focus on educating the parents on these topics, either personally or by referring the parents to one of a number of family support programs now offered through social service agencies.

PRESCHOOL TO MIDDLE SCHOOL AGE CHILDREN: TASKS AND CHALLENGES

The tasks confronting parents at this stage focus mainly around the ongoing development of their children. Young children begin to reach out and have relationships with other family members. After the infant stage, children seem to move quickly from one developmental milestone to the next: creeping, crawling, scooting, standing, walking, speaking, toilet training, feeding self, accepting limits, to name a few. The child's "job" at the preschool stage is to develop a sense of self, and to discover and explore the world, the people in it, and how to relate to them. Through imitation, play, and games they learn to individuate and to take the role of the other and see themselves through those eyes. Gender role identification and gender appropriate behavior is generally learned at this stage through socialization from parents, older siblings, and especially peers.[33] The role of parents is to guide this growing independence while setting appropriate discipline limits. Early childhood is also the time for socializing the child into the family core beliefs and values. The moral and ethical standards of behavior modeled by parents, peers, and teachers are absorbed or picked up by imitation by the child. Ideally in a functional family, the couple will have the maturity to adjust to evolving demands of a growing child, and the concomitant changes in parental roles from total care giving during infancy to providing guidance and support as the growing child develops a sense of independent selfhood and separates from the parents.[34]

Difficulties

Difficulties emerge when parents lack knowledge about the changing phases of child development or have their own unresolved issues with dependency. They may resist the child's natural process of individuation and may try to keep the child dependent upon them. Sometimes disagreements and conflicts between the parents over childrearing practices and division of labor may lead to inconsistent parenting, and poor limit setting. Parental fears and anxieties about who and what influences their children may lead to rigid efforts to control the child's peer contacts. As a health care provider, you may then see the effects of such parenting. They can manifest in the child as depression, problems with anger control, disinterest in learning, or discipline problems in school.

As the child moves into middle childhood (9-11), peer groups become dominant, children tend to congregate in same sex groups. They are particularly vulnerable to peer rejection.[35] Inclusion or exclusion from groups can cause the child to experience alternately success and acceptance or self doubt and fears of rejection or failure. Health care providers need to be alert for signs of depression, anger, substance abuse, or thoughts of suicide. You may need to educate the parents that the child's reaching out for new friends is normal, and remind them that it is their task to monitor the child's social activities. To help parents counteract their fear of losing control over what their children are doing, you can suggest that they contact the parents of their children's friends, and coordinate rules and set limits with them.

The school environment may present parents with a maze of new information that sometimes conflicts with their educational background. Parents from cultural and language backgrounds other than White American may find themselves in unfamiliar territory when it comes to school expectations of them and of their children. Everything from bus drivers' rules, the learning process of the child, homework, as well as the course subject matter, and grading policies may be alien to them. Often they need interpreters to relate to teachers, aides, principals, school social workers and nurses. Also, parent-child friction can develop when children begin to behave and express values that differ from the cultural norms practiced at home.

Problems and Difficulties for Children

Children with learning disabilities are at risk and need special support.[36] Being labeled "hyper" or "slow" can be a confusing and stressful situation for both the child and parents. Early recognition, treatment or assignment to special classes are essential processes to prevent long range damage to self esteem, and possible development of behavioral problems, like **Oppositional Defiant Disorder** (ODD).[37] If you are treating such a child, you may be able to facilitate getting the child assessed promptly, and connecting the parents with organizations or support groups that focus on helping parents to obtain the services their child needs.

Pre-school and middle children are also vulnerable to the stress of non-normative events. Disruptions in the family context, such as divorce or custody battles, chronic illness or death of a close family member, or loss of job by income providers can cause financial difficulty. The family may have to move to less expensive housing, and do without comforts previously enjoyed. Families, poor in communications skills and/or social support, may not cope well with such disturbances in the family equilibrium. They may lapse into dysfunctional adaptations, such as substance abuse or domestic violence.[38] In some cases where parents never successfully completed their own early developmental tasks, one or the other parent may inappropriately use their child to fulfill their own dependency needs, i.e., using the child as a confidante. This places an undue burden on children at a time when their developmental task is to become independent and move out into the world. In response to such conflicting messages, some children develop psychosomatic "illnesses" such as stomach or headaches. As a health care provider, you must be alert to such family dynamics when you encounter symptoms of illnesses without organic cause. Of special concern are situations of physical or sexual abuse for which we provide guidance in Chapter 11.

PUBERTY AND ADOLESCENCE

The term adolescence did not even exist until the turn of the 20th century. Up to the Industrial Revolution, even childhood, as we know it, hardly existed. As Ed Shorter describes in his classical study *The Making of the Modern Family,*[39] children were seen as a legitimate supply for the labor market as domestics or farm workers from age four or five on. By age 13-15 most children had either been sent to work and live outside the home, or had left. With the advent of machine technology, the demand for child labor decreased sharply. Later, child labor laws prohibited placing children in factories and in the labor market. As the wealth of the parents increased, fewer young children had to leave home to work

and thus, there was no longer the abrupt transition from childhood to adulthood. Stanley G. Hall is generally credited with inventing the term adolescence and applying it to those children from 11 to 18 years old, who no longer had to work.[40] Mandatory education laws were in place in all States by 1918.[41] Today children from all economic levels are expected to complete 10-12 years of primary and secondary education.

Tasks and Challenges

Adolescence ushers in a major transition for the family and the children.[42] Prior to this period, the child had relied mainly on the parents and family as the main source of nurturance and sense of connection. Developmental tasks of adolescence are shown in Box 3-2. They fall into three major categories: 1) personal tasks, 2) relational tasks, and 3) socioinstitutional tasks.[43] Their search for autonomy and personal identity is often marked by experimentation with new roles and behaviors. Their search for a social identity includes testing themselves in partner and group relationships. They may pair up with a boyfriend or girlfriend. They form beliefs about intimacy, commitment and couple relationships.[44] They meet their needs for independence (primarily from parents), as well as their affiliative needs by being part of cliques, clubs, teams, or gangs. They also are developing skills associated with learning and succeeding in the school environment. Peer influence at this point can easily overshadow parental influence on such issues as sexual behavior, substance abuse, and other risk taking behaviors.[45] This is also a time to try out new reasoning powers, and to develop their moral compass. Indeed, they may "practice" their new found cognitive powers on their parents by challenging and arguing about the reasons for parental rules. Often adolescents give parents hostile verbal messages that they want to be left alone to set their own limits, while at the same time not admitting that they crave the guidance and love of their parents.[46]

The challenge for the parents is to stay engaged with their adolescent, to continue to provide guidance, and to set limits and bound-

---

Box 3-2 Tasks of Adolescence

Personal Tasks:

- Acquiring autonomy: relating to family rules, deciding on curfew, what clothes to wear, defending own rights
- Coping successfully with everyday life situations: going to disco or cafe alone or with friends, handling own money, spending vacation without parents or other adults, going alone to a doctor, staying home alone when parents are away for a weekend
- Dealing with pubertal development: accepting one's physical changes
- Developing self-awareness: being aware of own strengths and weaknesses, taking account of another's judgment regarding oneself
- Finding reference values: having an opinion or a preference regarding political parties, choosing own life philosophy or religion, having an opinion regarding social issues such as abortion, death penalty

Relational Tasks:

- Establishing a stable relationship with friends: having a steady group of friends, having a best friend
- Establishing an intimate relationship: having a boy friend/girl friend, how far sexual intimacy should go in a relationship

Socio-institutional Tasks:

- Successfully completing one's school career: bearing responsibility for successfully completing school
- Preparing oneself for integration into a work setting: choosing a profession, having a job
- Achieving economic independence: being financially independent
- Preparing oneself for the responsibility of having one's own family: living on your own, having own family and taking care of them

---

aries.[47] For example, working through unpleasant confrontations between parent and adolescent can teach the adolescent valuable lessons in conflict resolution. Parents can model and support their adolescents in problem-solving and decision-making, helping them achieve autonomy in healthy ways. Parents need to recognize that the rapid physical growth, sexual maturing, and cognitive changes of this period are likely to produce quick fluctuations in mood and behavior. By maintaining good communication skills, they can instill positive guidance on civility and social graces, sexual behavior, and spirituality and help their adolescents resist negative influences from peers, the media, and advertising. They also need to send positive messages about learning to their children, and take an active interest in their academic progress.[48]

Difficulties

Difficulties can arise from several sources. Where communication is poor, parent-adolescent relations may become frayed to the break-ing point. Sometimes extended family members or parents of friends can act as neutral mediators to exercise a moderating influence.[49] In some instances, you, as the health care provider, may find yourself listening to the complaints of either the adolescent or the parents. By being a good listener, you may be able to influence adolescents in ways that they might not accept from their parents. For example, you can play a key educational role that can moderate sexual risk taking.

Some parents, who want to minimize dissension, abdicate their parental role and give in to demands by the adolescent to be left alone. A hands-off attitude may leave the adolescent without a counterweight to peer and media pressures. Without guidance, there is greater risk of "falling into bad company," and temptations for deviant behavior are harder to resist. Such dangers may be exacerbated, if there is gang violence, drug trafficking, and street violence in the neighborhood. In the medical setting, you may see adolescents for drug overdoses, injuries from violence, gang rape, STIs including HIV, as well as severe stress caused by witnessing violence.

Another barrier to successful transition for adolescents during this period is when parents have not resolved issues from their own youth. For example, parents who did not successfully resolve struggles for independence during their own adolescence, may have difficulties in setting proper limits for their adolescent children. Rigid *or* inconsistent parental efforts to control or set limits, can lead to protracted power struggles, and alienation from the family unit and/or the community. The emotional volatility and impulsivity of adolescence pitted against inflexibility of rigid parents can lead to verbal or physical fighting in the family. "They treat me like a child and I AM NOT" is a common frustration voiced by adolescents about their parents. Such conflict can escalate into serious behavioral and academic problems possibly leading to school drop out.[50] Such problems may impede or prevent the mastery of crucial tasks of adolescence, including goal setting and decisions related to entering into adult life such as job/career choices and making commitments. Other problems can arise when adolescents resenting interference from parents take subterfuge by leading a dual life. They pretend to their parents that they are following the "rules," while secretly engaging in rebellious or deviant behavior. In some instances, the adolescent can turn to other sympathetic adults and go through this period without developing major behavioral problems.[51]

Often both adolescents and parents may prefer to stay in denial rather than to confront the adolescent's deviant behaviors. Health care providers need to be alert to overt and hidden conflicts because they can lead to covert but unhealthy ways for adolescents to rebel against parental authority.

In treating adolescents, the health care provider also needs to understand the role of regression as a response to stress. For example, some adolescents entering puberty, may have had little or no advance preparation for the changes in their bodies. Some may be frightened or embarrassed by these changes. Others may be

overwhelmed by the prospect of adulthood, and its attendant responsibilities. In response to such anxieties, they may regress into behaviors from a time in childhood when they received more nurturance from the family unit. Signs of regression in younger adolescents may include holding on to their "blankies", puzzles, and toys. Or they might engage in games with younger children of the same sex (e.g., playing with dolls, video game collections, rock star adoration). They seem to be resisting growing up, wanting instead the dependency and simplicity of childhood. For some parents who want their adolescents to move on into life, to take more responsibility, and to express more independence, such regression can be frustrating. Other parents, who have their own unresolved independence needs, may actually encourage such regression in order to keep the child close by them. Family traumas that impact normal development, like death, divorce, or illness can also trigger regression in adolescents (as well as in children of any age). In general, health care providers treating adolescent patients or their parents need to be alert to signs of dysfunction such as alienation, conflict, or regression. If, in taking the social history of the patient, you come across evidence of serious problems between parent and adolescent, it is appropriate to speak to both of them about the issues. In complicated cases, a referral for family counseling is indicated.

Regardless of what else is going on, you should question any adolescent from age 11 onwards on the issues of substance abuse, sexual behaviors, relationship issues and identity formation including gender orientation. Although drug use appears to be fairly widespread among adolescents from all social strata, adolescents living in inner cities, are more likely to also be exposed to the trauma of daily violence.[52] The more threatening the neighborhood, the more common the symptoms of depression, anxiety, oppositional defiant disorder, and conduct disorder.[53] Adolescents and their parents can be challenging patients for the health care provider. Adolescents in their distrust of adults or authority figures may be surly and non communicative when you question them about health problems. Indications by either adolescent or parents of tension or alienation should lead you to be more assertive in assessing and interviewing parents and adolescents.

COLLEGE AND "EXTENDED ADOLESCENCE"

The upper age level of adolescence has never been clearly defined, and in our society there are no recognized rituals to demarcate the transition from adolescence into adulthood.[54,55] Coming out of adolescence, young adults face many challenges and divergent ways of accomplishing them. One major decision involving the desire for independence is whether to get a job or postpone independence by continuing education. This choice is influenced by family values, economic circumstances, and personal preferences, strengths, and limitations. Middle class values and economic status tend to steer a large proportion of high school students towards college as preparation for career entry.[56] While many from lower socioeconomic status realize that education is essential for upward mobility, for many others, the need for education is not self evident.[57] For some young people, primary and secondary education may have been an unpleasant experience marked by failure due to psychosocial factors, such as lack of family support for studying, family discord and instability, or poverty and the need to work. Also, endogenous factors, such as low intelligence, learning disabilities, inability to concentrate due to **Attention Deficit Disorder,** behavioral problems due to hyperactivity or childhood trauma may have made learning difficult or frustrating. For those who have developed an aversion to academic learning, the end of mandatory school attendance often comes as a relief. For whatever reason, the end of secondary education marks the beginning of the adult or work phase of life for many. In general, those less educated also tend to marry earlier, have children sooner than those who seek more education.[58]

Those from more affluent homes tend to continue their education past high school at much higher rates than those from poor homes. They do so because in large part they came from more favorable psychosocial environments, i.e., they were encouraged to learn and study by their families, and thus their learning experience may have been more rewarding and successful. They generally accept that education is the key to preparing themselves for a career.[59] By going to college or technical school, millions of young persons postpone adult tasks like forming a family or embarking on a career. This last historical evolution has created another level of development between adolescence and adulthood.

How can one classify this large population of college students? Judging by the publicity given to some extra-curricular activities of college students, such as partying, binge drinking and high interest in sexual activity, as well as financial dependence, we could argue that this period is an extension of adolescence. If, on the other hand, one uses biological or cognitive developmental markers, one would conclude that these college students are adults. The truth lies somewhere in between.

Tasks and Challenges

Some of the developmental tasks faced by college students may be quite similar to those in the formation of a couple, albeit in different form. For those going away to college, it is the first time they are separated from their family of origin. They have to test their ability to live and get along with roommates in dormitories or apartments. This includes division of chores and adopting mutually acceptable behaviors, from sharing bathrooms, noise levels of TV or CD players, allotting study time, to when to go to sleep at night. College students who form romantic attachments have to make choices between maintaining separate residences (but sleeping over at his or her place), cohabitation, or marriage. These types of relationships test the ability of the participants to arrive at mutually satisfying levels of commitment, emotional nurturance, and sexual activity. Indeed many participants in such relationships view them as proving grounds for eventual marriage or committed partnerships.

During the college years many also question beliefs, values and behaviors derived from their families of origin. It is also a time when their own identity undergoes change.[60] Pressure to change comes from various sources. The more diversity existing on campus, the more exposure to ideas, values and behaviors that may challenge their childhood beliefs. Within the student subculture, there are norms and behaviors that are different from those of society at large. For some this means binge drinking, using drugs and partying. But for the vast majority of students, it is learning to fit into a competitive environment to achieve academic success. The challenge of the college curriculum may lead to new insights and different ways of reasoning and perceiving the world. Faculty members, who take a personal interest in students, may provide powerful new role models that influence the emerging identity of the students. Some students reach a new maturity level of cognitive reasoning called *post-formal thought*, in which logic is illuminated by intuition.[61] Schaie asserts that young adult students acquire knowledge at this stage not only for its own sake, but to become competent and independent.[62] In general, for most students, college is a positive and healthy formative experience. It gives them a chance to explore different career goals. The academic and social challenges of this period also produce major intellectual and moral growth as they progress through their college "career." In addition to acquiring technical know-how relevant to their career field, they are polishing communication, decision making, and social skills for life in the career world.

For those who pursue post-graduate or professional degrees, there is another delay. However, being in graduate school no longer seems to postpone forming families and establishing separate households. This is usually made possible by assistance from parents, student loans or scholarships. In many cases one spouse may work to put the other through school, or both may be working part time while one or both get their professional or postgraduate training. However, some adult tasks may still be on hold for those students. For example, true autonomy and financial independence, as well as separation from family of origin often have to wait until entry into the career path.

Difficulties

Those who chose to end their education after high school may find themselves stuck in low paying jobs. Some may drift into unhealthy life styles: poor nutrition, unsafe sexual behavior and/or substance abuse. Single parenthood may relegate many young women and their children into lifelong poverty. Lacking job skills, stuck in low paying jobs without health insurance coverage, such women may not be able to obtain regular health care. Thus, their health problems, when they do present in health care settings, may be more acute or complex.

Some of those who choose to continue their education may also experience difficulties. Freed from family influences through distance in many cases, and allied with like-minded peers, some college students engage in alcohol or drug abuse and other unhealthy behaviors. For others, separation from the family of origin, combined with shyness or poor social skills, can produce feelings of isolation and alienation from the college social scene. Research seems to show that competitive pressures in college and fears of doing poorly in their classes and major fields have produced levels of anxiety among college students that are higher today than a generation ago.[63] Suicidal ideation or attempts are not uncommon.[64] When you are the health care provider for college students, it is important to routinely ask questions related to their behaviors, academic progress, and emotional well being.

• •

PATIENT PROFILE 3.2

MY HEART IS GOING TO BURST

SETTING: *Louisa, a 37-year-old married woman is being seen for chest pain, fatigue, and numbness in both arms. James, her physician assistant, has* been treating her since he came to the suburban clinic several years ago.

James: *(Entering the examining room, I see Louisa sitting with her head down. She does not look up at me. This is odd because she usually greets me with a cheery although formal "Good morning Doctor.")* Louisa, what's going on today?

Louisa: It's my heart. Sometimes it feels like its going to burst.

James: What does it feel like? *(I am concerned about the word "burst". She has difficulty finding the words to describe "burst." I inquire about the onset, duration, frequency and characteristics of the chest pain. She offers limited information. I ask specific questions about the numbness in both arms and the severe muscle fatigue. I perform a thorough cardiovascular examination as well as a thoracic, musculoskeletal and neurological examination. No significant findings. Even with no pertinent physical findings, I must first rule out cardiovascular disease. Order a STAT EKG and then obtain chest x-ray, and routine blood chemistries with lipid levels. Also must consider cervical or thoracic spine disease, degenerative disease and esophageal disorder. No comorbid history. I suspect there is more. Something, perhaps my gut instinct, tells me there is something else going on here. As I prepare her for the EKG, she looks at me directly for the first time. The sadness in her eyes and weariness in her facial expression hit me hard. I remember that Louisa is a proud and private person and may need some encouragement to speak what is on her mind.)* Louisa, you look sad. How are you feeling? *(She sighs and shakes her head from side to side but remains silent. I gently try again.)* Louisa, do you want to share some of it with me?

Louisa: *(She nods, then haltingly tells me what is going on.)* My 20-year-old daughter is a sophomore in college. Her first year as a freshman was the first time she was away from home. She didn't get good grades and this year she isn't doing very well either. She is going with a 22 year old known "druggie". Under his influence, the two of them have stolen my sister's coin collection, sold it, and probably spent the money on drugs. I was mortified when my sister told me. I felt so hurt and ashamed. I just wanted to die. I tried talking with my daughter about it, but she wouldn't listen to me. I felt I'd lost any influence or control over her. I wake up at night in a panic, sweating and my heart pounding. I worry about her future. Will my daughter ever have children? Will I ever have grandchildren? Or even worse maybe my daughter might die from a drug overdose.

James: Have you talked with anyone about this situation?

Louisa: No, I couldn't talk with any other family members or friends. I'd be too embarrassed. They might think I failed as a mother. My husband is drinking again. I feel all alone with this problem. And I am so afraid!

James: Louisa, I can understand that you are worried about this situation and your physical symptoms. Most likely you are having a stress reaction so I am going to limit testing today to an EKG, a chest x-ray and some blood work. But I'd like you to see our wellness counselor and talk with her a few times. Maybe you can get a better perspective on this problem. *(As Louisa is talking, my instinct is reinforced. It becomes clearer to me that the pressures of Louisa's life and lack of support from her husband are causing her symptoms. Psychosomatic stress is more likely the cause of her symptoms than the other non-cardiac disorders. And I learned to trust my intuition and follow up on it. My intuition led me to ask more questions and stopped me from getting side-tracked into diagnostic assessments that may not be completely relevant. After I broadened my interview to include questions about her family life, and her concerns about them, the course of treatment became clearer.)*

Louisa: Well, if you think it will help.

POINTS TO CONSIDER:

• Being alert to nonverbal communication of one's patients provides vital information for assessment.

- James sets up appropriate diagnostic testing.
- James not only looks at his patient, but he really sees her and is tuned into the expression in her eyes.
- After James learns more about the situation with Louisa's daughter, he tells her that he will limit the diagnostic testing to the routine studies.
- A referral for brief counseling in this case can help Louisa gain a better perspective on her daughter's actions and in turn this can help reduce her uncomfortable physical symptoms.

• •

ADULTHOOD: TASK AND CHALLENGES

Adult development occurs in multiple dimensions over a long period of time. Many developmental tasks and challenges can be divided into five broad spheres of activity throughout adult life: family, work/career, social relationships, health, and spirituality. While for purposes of examination we can identify specific tasks and challenges in each sphere (see Box 3-3), we need to remember that the level of competency in one sphere is likely to affect task fulfillment in the other areas. Because of the extended period of time (ages 20-60 plus), as well as the possibility of non-normative events, the sequence of development is neither age graded nor uniform.

How each person manages adult tasks and challenges is affected by several factors. First, individual genetic predispositions, such as intelligence, temperament, and physical health characteristics, consciously or unconsciously affect whether and how a person approaches certain tasks. For example, early academic success or failure due to endogenous factors will expand or limit the choice of work or career. Second, core beliefs and values from the family of origin, and possibly a separate subculture, are key factors in how we look at and relate to the world. Thus, childhood socialization (discussed in the first two chapters) is another key determinant of adult development. Third, our **cohort**, i.e., the generation or group with which we grew up,

influences us. Different names for certain cohort groups, like the *beat generation*, *hippies*, the *baby boomers*, or the *gen-Xers*, indicate the people born around the same time. The historical and cultural events and pressures of their formative years shaped their values and attitudes. Fourth, we are also affected by the events, cultural fashions, or patterns of our current times. For example, family structure has undergone profound changes in the last forty years. Practices that were once frowned on and were rare have now become commonplace according to the latest census figures.[65] Among these are cohabitation without marriage, births to single mothers, family formation by same sex couples and divorce. A fifth influence on the sequence of adult development is the normative and non-normative events that require adaptation or change. Typical normative events of adulthood are getting married and entering the work force. Examples of non-normative events are the bride or groom that gets left at the altar, or the middle aged employee who loses his job through "downsizing." Similarly a sudden life threatening illness such as a heart attack or breast cancer, or the death or disability of a child or significant other can also disrupt normal development. How we respond to such shocks determines whether or how we will approach developmental tasks of mid-adulthood.

Poverty As a Challenge to Normal Task Fulfillment

All of the above factors are directly affected by a sixth factor: socioeconomic status. Moving through the normative tasks of adulthood may be easier for those with adequate economic resources than for those whose financial situation makes life a struggle for survival. Lack of access to health insurance is a significant stressor, as is lack of education or marketable job skills. With housing costs in many large cities high, setting up a separate household is difficult even with relatively good wages. For many the choices are: living with the family of origin, living in a low rent area far from the job, and/or sharing housing costs with several others. Many

Box 3-3 Adult Developmental Tasks

Family Tasks:

- Making choices about whether to stay single or get married
- Deciding whether and when to start a family
- Deciding whether one parent stays at home for full-time parenting or works while children are in child care
- Deciding how to divide parenting responsibilities
- Reaching agreements on child rearing practices including how to discipline for misbehaviors
- Adapting to and encouraging the growing independence of their children and supporting their educational efforts
- Keeping open communication patterns within the family while maintaining intimacy within the couple relationship
- Providing financial support as children make choices to establish their own households, or pursue vocational training or higher education
- Deciding about the level of involvement with their adult children as the children form their own families
- Balancing family responsibilities with the demands of work or career goals
- Relating as adult children to their own parents and extended family
- Cooperating with other adult siblings about providing care for aged parents in declining health
- Assuming the role of elders in the family as parents die
- Facing their own aging, decline in health and death.

Work/Career Tasks:

- Deciding what type of work or career is desired
- Getting and maintaining skills to perform the job
- Doing the job well
- Maintaining good relations with coworkers and supervisors
- Deciding an amount of time, effort and ambition to devote to advancement

- Coping with changes in status: transfers, promotions, demotions, layoffs
- Balancing work demands and loyalties with family responsibilities

Social Relations Tasks:

- Choosing friends
- Deciding on time and effort to devote to activities or involvement with friends
- Balancing activities with friends with demands of family
- Deciding on level of involvement in volunteer community activities, such as coaching, being classroom parents, or PTA

Health and Well Being Tasks:

- Prioritizing health, i.e. whether to actively protect and promote health or to ignore and neglect self care
- Deciding about potentially harmful habits such as smoking, substance abuse, poor diet, insufficient exercise, unsafe sex
- Making choices about preventive health care: getting regular medical check ups
- Adopting health promoting habits: good diet, regular exercise and sufficient rest

Spirituality Needs and Tasks:

- Finding personal answers to questions like: "Why am I here? What is my purpose? What comes after this?"
- Adopting a personal set of beliefs about God or the supernatural, and your relationship to those beliefs
- Deciding on the level of involvement in formal religious activities: church, synagogue, temple, mosque
- Deciding on whether and how to integrate spiritual practices into everyday life
- Involving family in spiritual practices: prayers at meals, bed time, attendance at religious services
- Possibly choosing religious education for children

may have no choice but to live in low rent but unsafe neighborhoods in crowded or unsanitary living conditions. Thriving or achieving autonomy under such circumstances of economic hardship can become an elusive task. The emotional and physical stress may be hard even on healthy persons. However, for persons who are physically, mentally or psychologically challenged, the task of autonomy or economic self sufficiency may be extremely challenging if not impossible. Those without family support systems may find the struggle overwhelming and end up on disability or welfare, or homeless. If they are on anti-psychotic medication, compliance with dosage and frequency regimen is generally poor and they may drift in and out of community mental health centers and homeless shelters.

A key task for adults with low levels skills and low income is to solidify their job positions. The barriers faced by those entering the job market in the post industrial information age, without adequate training or education, are formidable. With the disappearance of manufacturing jobs due to globalization, the prospects for those with only a high school diploma or less, of climbing the ladder of success in today's technology oriented economy are poor. Job changes often consist of a lateral change in job positions rather than upward mobility. Job stagnation and the feeling of being trapped in a dead end job may lead some people into depression and/or substance abuse. Others who recognize that advancement is not possible without additional technical training or college, may opt for further education. The presence of community and technical colleges, as well as the availability of government assistance or student loans, make the phenomenon of the returning older student a common one. Going to college — either part time or full time — for these students often brings additional stress, as they juggle the demands of family, work, and study.

If you practice in a low income area, you will find that the patient's stress of coping with poverty will manifest in presenting problems that may be in an advanced state of progression

due to the inability to afford regular health check ups. You are likely to encounter high rates of serious emotional problems ranging from depression, anxiety, to post traumatic stress disorder either from the exposure to violence in the neighborhood, or due to the higher incidence of child abuse and domestic violence. In such situations, you need to treat the immediate symptoms, but must also take action to resolve the underlying psychosocial stressors. This may mean referral to a mental health clinic, or reporting the abuse to the appropriate state social service agency. However, you can also insure that struggling low income families who are often faced with choices between food, rent, health care, or medication are connected with social service agencies. There are a number of safety net programs ranging from housing assistance, child care subsidies, job training, to health insurance programs for children (CHIPS).

CAREER PHASE: TASKS AND CHALLENGES

Let us return to those who after years of professional training or education are entering their career path. One initial task will be to find a balance between career and time for family, leisure, emotional, social and spiritual growth. As an emerging health care provider, you may be in this stage of development. The pattern established early in your career path will likely affect your long range physical and emotional health. The desire for advancement and financial success often leads to setting priorities in which career comes first. Too much of an emphasis on work is likely to lead to a neglect of personal health, trouble in relationships with significant others, and emotional distance from the children. (We will discuss how such patterns can affect you in Chapter 6 "Stress Management and Self Care for the Healer".) Stressful career patterns may also lead to a weakening of ties to both sides of the extended family.

The so-called midlife crisis may be precipitated by a number of factors. It may be a crisis of values, when after going along on an automatic career oriented path, persons experience a disillusionment or dissatisfaction with the pattern or direction of their lives.[66] Having placed a high priority on career, many find that their significant and family relationship have suffered. Alienated and feeling resentful about the lack of love and attention from the other, either partner may look elsewhere for emotional comfort. Whether this midlife reevaluation leads to closer family relationships or to further estrangement or divorce, depends on such factors as internal models from childhood, as well as the levels of maturity, commitment, and communications skills. The midlife crisis may look different to a woman.[67] If she is also working outside the home, it is likely that she will also be working the "double shift," i.e., managing the household after coming home from work. She may feel disenchanted by the stress load, and the estrangement from her significant partner and family. For stay-at-home mothers, lack of appreciation for her role, and or emotional neglect from a husband preoccupied with career may lead to an intense focus on children. In such cases when the last child leaves home, women may face a crisis of identity, referred to as the "empty nest syndrome." The task for them becomes to establish a new and separate identity at that point. They may resolve this by leaving the home for work or by plunging into volunteer work, going to college, or getting divorced.

In many instances, midlife reevaluations actually produce stronger marriages, and the couple starts enjoying a life unencumbered by children in the house.[68] They may focus on intergenerational solidarity within the extended family. Visiting to and from their adult children, enjoying and helping with grandchildren, as well as visiting or helping their own aging parents can become part of a satisfying routine. Other tasks at this stage may include solidifying economic security, perhaps paying off the home mortgage, and planning for retirement years by making long range investments.

Difficulties and Effects on Health

The adult couple's plans for the enjoyment of their middle and later years may be disrupted by unexpected events. For example, an out of wedlock birth or the divorce of an adult child may force the couple to take in the daughter and her offspring for a period of time. The adult couple may be called upon to provide additional help with the grandchildren, or even to become surrogate parents, while the adult child works or seeks additional training for the job market. If the family has only moderate income, the extra financial burden as well as the pressures of the additional people all living under one roof can cause significant emotional stress. Another unexpected event might be the illness or sudden death of one member of the adult couple. If death took away the major income earner of the household, the loss of income may cause abrupt changes in life style, such as having to move into less expensive housing. The same is often true after a divorce. In the aftermath of divorce, poverty usually marks the household headed up by the divorced mother of children. Another shock to the stability of the middle years may be the crisis of a disabling illness of an older parent. The difficult care decisions faced by the adult children of an aging parent and end-of-life issues will be presented in Chapter 8.

Job disruptions may also cause immense personal and family stress. Over the past few years, we have seen massive job layoffs not only for blue collar workers, but also for highly skilled professionals due to mergers, consolidation and restructuring of industries. Often such layoffs come with little advance warning. With high debt loads, and little or no income, some families may see cars or even family homes repossessed. Often they will experience downward mobility. Periods of unemployment are especially stressful and depressing for the chief income producer. If prolonged, unemployment can lead to intra-family tension, conflict, and health problems. The impact on the health of the various midlife stressors in large part depends on how individuals perceive them and how they react to them. As we will discuss in the chapter on stress management, persons with good coping skills and good support systems can minimize the damaging effects. Given the wide range of possible shocks and crises in midlife, it is essential that you do routine psychosocial assessments to get the information on the stressors underlying physical or emotional problems. There is no common denominator for the wide variety of physical problems that can occur during this extended period. For example, although in general menopause has no serious direct health impact on women, it may cause a period of physical discomfort and emotional lability for some women.[69] The concern about osteoporosis and vaginal thinning in post menopausal women can cause a decisional crisis on whether or not she should go on hormone replacement therapy. Common among many women going through menopause is the feeling that health care providers do not understand them, are not willing to listen to their concerns, or to give them adequate information for them to make a decision.[70]

The most common emotional problems seen in adults of both genders by the health care provider are depression and anxiety. In most instances, the emotional and behavioral reactions to stressful events are transitory. The DSM-IV calls such short lived responses to "an identifiable psychosocial stressor or stressors" an "Adjustment Disorder."[71] However, the health care provider must learn to regard evidence of depression and/or anxiety as clues to the psychosocial stressors that need to be explored, rather than to treat the symptoms only pharmacologically. In many instances, adjustment disorders are successfully resolved with short term counseling. A referral to a professional for such counseling may be appropriate.

• •

PATIENT PROFILE 3.3

AROUND AND AROUND

SETTING: *Martin, a 63-year-old married man, has come to the urban doctor's clinic to see Romney, his physician assistant, who has been treating Martin for high blood pressure and arthritis for the last several years. Martin's presenting problem is "difficulty getting to sleep at night".*

Romney: Good morning Martin. How can I help you today? *(He looks exhausted!)*

Martin: Hi Romney, how about doing some babysitting for us?

Romney: Oh, ho — those two grandchildren getting to you?

Martin and Romney banter back and forth briefly about the "joys" of grandparenting. Romney can see that Martin is relaxing and he asks him:

Romney: What is the problem with your sleep?

Martin: Our daughter Bonnie left her husband and is getting divorced. She had to come home but that's another story. She decided to go back to school. She's an LPN and wants to get her RN. We're caring for her children while she works and goes to school. They're great kids but ages 7 and 8. Well. They're pretty active and by the end of the day Marie is exhausted.

Romney: Hmmm. Before you leave today, let's make an appointment for Marie too.

Martin: That's a good idea. She's been meaning to call for an appointment, but, well, she gets busy too.

Silence falls and Romney notices that a worried look flashes across Martin's face. *(Romney thinks: I do need to check on Marie but for now, I'll focus on Martin.)*

Romney: Let's return to your sleeping problem. How long has this been going on?

Martin: Two months — when Bonnie returned home. You see after working all day, I come home and give Marie a break. I occupy the children while she fixes dinner, then we walk a little and put the children to bed and fall into bed ourselves — exhausted. That's when my mind starts ticking away.

Romney: What else are you worried about?

Martin: Marie's parents are ailing and she runs over to help them while the kids are in school. I'm worried that her fibromyalgia is worsening.

Romney: It may be. She probably isn't getting enough rest. What else?

Martin: There's this new guy at work who is a management consultant. I don't agree with his recommendations. They may take the company into a questionable direction. I'd hoped to be heading for retirement by now but we just cannot afford it. After the last rain, we discovered our gutters are damaged and that they need replacing and our car is 11 years old and needs a new transmission. So I worry. All these problems just swirl around and around in my head and I just don't see an end to them.

Romney: That's quite a lot of worries. Is there anything else?

Martin: NO! That's enough!

Romney: It sure is. No wonder you have a hard time falling asleep. *(I need to rule out any additional sleep problems.)* Let me ask you a few questions which will help me understand what is going on.

Martin: OK.

Romney: Do you wake up in the middle of the night?

Martin: No.

Romney: Wake up earlier in the morning than you need to?

Martin: No, although some mornings I'd sure like to sleep in.

Romney: Do you feel rested when you do get up?

Martin: Sort of. It depends on what time we went to bed.

Romney: How is your appetite?

Martin: Fine.

Romney: Do you enjoy eating?

Martin: Yes, you know Marie is a great cook.

Romney: Are you and Marie enjoying your sex life?

Martin: Our desire is reduced somewhat by exhaustion, but when Bonnie takes the kids to my parents for a day, we usually have relations.

Romney: You two still enjoy walking?

Martin: Oh yes, and the kids are a real treat to walk with.

Romney: *(He doesn't sound depressed. I wonder about anxiety.)* Do you worry a lot during the day?

Martin: No, I'm too busy.

Romney: Do you have shortness of breath?

Martin: No.

Romney: Panicky feelings?

Martin: No.

Romney: Tightness in your chest or in your stomach?

Martin: No, just the worrying.

Romney: Do you drink caffeine or alcohol in the evenings?

Martin: No, I only drink one cup of coffee in the mornings. We used to have a glass of wine with dinner but we stopped that several years ago.

Romney: Martin, I've ruled out depression and anxiety. Your difficulty getting to sleep stems from the stresses in your life that we call situational, which is a temporary condition.

Martin: What do you mean "temporary"?

Romney: I know the problems your family has may seem endless but they will change some day. Sometimes it helps to talk this over with a psychotherapist in order to learn to cope better with the stress of worrying. Would you be willing to do that?

Martin: OK.

POINTS TO CONSIDER:

- Noting Martin's exhausted appearance, Romney jokes with him about grandparenting.

- Inquiring about the worries yields useful information about Martin's burdens.

- Romney identifies the situational nature of Martin's difficulties in getting to sleep and makes appropriate recommendations.

● ●

Conclusion

We reviewed the most widely used stage theories in order to acquaint you with the terminology used by pediatricians or child psychologists in their discussion of specific patients. However, as mentioned at the onset of this chapter, this survey of the life course has purposely departed from the traditional approach to the study of Human Development. Hence, the many references to contextual influences like the family or peers, to past and present events, to physical and emotional development, socioeconomic conditions, and how such factors can and do influence the patient's potential for illness, their attitudes toward health, and their response to treatment. In order to sensitize you to these psychosocial issues, we have made some broad brush generalizations. We caution the reader to look at each patient's individual response pattern to the tasks and their concomitant stresses in the life course. We do want to emphasize that because most illnesses occur within or are caused by the psychosocial environment, you need to go beyond treating symptoms. You need to take into account the stage of life and find out what kinds of stressors the patient is experiencing that may be causing physical or emotional health problems, i.e., enuresis in a child, identity related anxiety or depression in adolescents, or stress-related illnesses in adults. The patient's lack of awareness, or lack of coping skills may produce depression or anxiety related to mastering a stage specific task or the feelings triggered by normative or non normative events.[72] Following your assessment of the psychosocial issues, you may be able to educate and reassure the patient (or parent of a child) about the "normalcy" of such stage specific difficulties and how to resolve them. As will be explained in the Chapter on Communications, patient understanding of what is going on and why they feel the way they do is one of the crucial components of successful treatment interaction.

In this chapter we have not included the care giving stage and end-of-life issues that come in the older adult years. These issues are so complex that we have addressed them separately in Chapter 8.

REFERENCES

1. Papalia DE, Olds SW, Feldman R (2001). *A Child's World: Infancy Through Adolescence.* (10th Ed) New York: McGraw-Hill.
2. Erikson EH (1985). *The Life Cycle Completed.* New York: Norton.
3. Neugarten B (1977). Personality and Aging. In Birren J, Schaie KW (Eds) *Handbook of the Psychology of Aging.* New York: Nostrand, 626-649.
4. Papalia DE, Olds SW (1992). *Human Development* (5th Ed) New York: McGraw-Hill.
5. Freud S (1953). *A General Introduction to Psychoanalysis.* New York: Perma-books.
6. Masson JM (1984). Freud and the Seduction Theory: A Challenge to the Foundations of Psychoanalysis. *Atlantic Monthly,* 253, 2:33-60.
7. Freud A (1946). *The Ego and Mechanisms of Defense.* New York: International Universities Press.
8. Erikson, EH (1959). Growth and Crises in the Healthy Personality . In EH Erikson, *Identity and the Life Cycle, Selected Papers,* 50-100. Psychological Monograph No. 1. New York: International University Press.
9. Erikson EH (1964). A Schedule of Virtues. In Erikson, *Insight and Responsibility,* 111-157. New York: WW. Norton.
10. Piaget J (1952). *The Origins of Intelligence in Children.* New York: International Universities Press.
11. Kohlberg L (1969). Continuities and Discontinuities in Child and Adult Moral Development. *Human Development,* 12:93-120.
12. Kluwer ES, Heesink JAM, Van de Vliert E (1997). The marital dynamics of conflict over the division of labor. *J Marriage Fam* 59:635-53.
13. Beach SRH, Tesser A, Fincham FD, Jones DJ, Johnson D, Whitaker DJ (1998). Pleasure and pain in doing well, together: an investigation of performance-related affect in close relationships. *J Pers Soc Psychol* 74:923-38.
14. Fincham FD, Beach SRH (1999). Conflict in Marriage: Implications for Working with Couples. *Ann Rev Psychol,* 1-47.
15. Burleson BR, Denton WH (1997). The relationship between communication skill and marital satisfaction: some moderating effects. *J Marriage Fam,* 59:884-902.
16. Kohn ML (1963). Social Class and Parent-Child Relationships — An Interpretation. *Am J Sociol,* 68:471-480.
17. Perry-Jenkins M, Folk (1994). Class, Couples, and Conflict: effects of the division of labor on assessments of marriage. *J Marriage Family;* 56:165-181.
18. Kohn ML, Schooler C (1983). *Work and Personality: An Inquiry into the Impact of Social Stratification.* New York: Ablex Press.
19. Germain CB (1991). *Human Behavior in the Social Environment: An Ecological View.* New York: Columbia University Press, 167.
20. Hendrix H (1988). *Getting the Love You Want: A Guide For Couples.* New York: Henry Holt & Co.
21. Hazen C, Shaver PR (1987). Romantic love con-

ceptualized as an attachment process. *J Personality Soc Psych*, 52:511-524.

22. Senchak M, Leonard KE (1992). Attachment style and marital adjustment among newlywed couples. *J Soc Pers Relat*, 9:51-64.

23. Feeney JA (1994). Attachment style, communication patterns and satisfaction across the life cycle of marriage. *Pers Relat*, 1:333-48.

24. Mikulincer M (1998). Adult attachment style and individual differences in functional versus dysfunctional experiences of anger. *J Pers Soc Psychol*, 74:513-24.

25. Bradbury TN, Fincham FD (1993). Assessing dysfunctional cognition in marriage: a reconsideration of the Relationship Belief Inventory. *Psychol Assess*, 5:92-101.

26. Beach SRH, Tesser A (1993). Decision making, power and marital satisfaction: a self evaluation maintenance perspective. *J Soc Clin Psychol*, 12:471-94.

27. Fincham FD (1998). Child development and marital relations. *Child Dev*, 69:543-74.

28. O'Leary KD, Malone J, Tyree A (1994). Physical aggression in early marriage: prerelationship and relationship effects. *J Consult Clin Psychol*, 62:594-602.

29. Cummings EM, Davies P (1994). *Children and Marital Conflict*. New York: Guilford Press.

30. Feder L, (Ed.) (2000). *Women and Domestic Violence: An Interdisciplinary Approach*. Binghamton, New York: Haworth Press.

31. Kendall-Tackett KA (2001). *The Hidden Feelings of Motherhood: Coping with Stress, Depression and Burnout*. Oakland, CA: New Harbinger.

32. Kennedy R, Suttenfiled K (2001). Postpartum Depression. *Medscape Mental Health*, 6(4), 2001.

33. Adler PA (1994). *Peer Power: Preadolescent Culture and Identity*. New Brunswick, NJ: Rutgers Univ Press.

34. Giannetti CC, Sagarese M (1997). *The Roller Coaster Years: Raising Your Child Through the Maddening Yet Magical Middle School Years*. Derry, NH: Broadway Books.

35. Harris JR (1998). *The Nurture Assumption: Why Children Turn Out the Way They Do*. New York: Free Press.

36. Wenz-Gross M, Siperstein GN (1997). Importance of social support in the adjustment of children with learning problems. *Exceptional Children*, 63, 2:183 (11).

37. Taylor HG, Anselmo M, Foreman AL, et al (2000). Utility of Kindergarten Teacher Judgments in Identifying Early Learning Problems. *J Learning Disabilities*, 33 2:200.

38. Lasch KE et al (2001). The relation of family violence, employment status, welfare benefits, and alcohol drinking in the United States. *Western J Medicine*,174, 5: 317-324.

39. Shorter E (1975). *The Making of the Modern Family*. New York: Basic Books.

40. Hall GS (1904). *Adolescence: Its Psychology, and its Relations to Anthropology, Sociology, Sex, Crime Religion and Education*. New York: Appleton.

41. Hellinger D, Judd DR (1991). *The Democratic Facade*. Pacific Grove, CA: Brooks-Cole.

42. Montemayor R, Adams G, Gullotta T, (Eds.) (1994). *Personal Relationships During Adolescence: Advances in Adolescent Development*, (Vol. 6). Newbury Park, CA: Sage.

43. Dekovic M, Noom MJ, Meeus W (1997). Expectations regarding development during adolescence: parental and adolescent perceptions. *J Youth Adolescence*, 26, 3:253-273.

44. Dowdy BB, Kliewer W (1998). Dating, parent-adolescent conflict, and behavioral autonomy. *J Youth Adolescence*, 27, 4:473-493.

45. Santelli JS, Lindberg LD, et al (2000). Adolescent Sexual Behavior: Estimates and Trends From Four Nationally Representative Surveys. *Fam Plan Perspect*, 32, 4:156-165, 194.

46. Epstein JH (1998). Nurturing teenagers to a better future: massive study confirms importance of parental care. *The Futurist*, 32,2:14-16.

47. Bluestein J (2001). *Parents, Teens and Boundaries*; Albuquerque, NM: ISS Publications.

48. McGrath EP, Repetti RL (2000). Mothers' and Fathers' Attitudes Toward Their Children's Academic Performance and Children's Perceptions of Their Academic Competence. *J Youth Adolescence*, 29, 6:713.

49. Richardson B (2000). *Working with Challenging Youth, Lessons Learned Along the Way*. Philadelphia: Brunner-Routledge.

50. Janosz M, LeBlanc M, Boulericem B, Tremblay RE (1997). Disentangling the weight of school dropout predictors: a test on two longitudinal samples. *J Youth Adolescence*, 26, 6:733-763.

51. Greenberger E, Chen C, Beam MR (1998). The role of "very important" nonparental adults in adolescent development. *J Youth Adolescence*, 27, 3:321-344.

52. Reynolds LK, O'Koon JH, Papademetriou E, et al (2001). Stress and Somatic Complaints in Low-

Income Urban Adolescents, *J Youth Adolescence,* 30, 4:499.

53. Aneshensel CS, Sucoff CA (1996). The Neighborhood Context of Adolescent Mental Health. *J Health and Social Sciences,* 37:293-310.

54. Kett JP (1977). *Rites of Passage: Adolescence in America, 1790 to the Present.* New York: Basic Books.

55. Mahdi LC, Christopher NG, Meade M, (Eds.) (1996). *Crossroads: The Quest for Contemporary Rites of Passage.* Peru, IL: Open Court Publishing Co.

56. Biblarz TJ, Raftery AE (1999). Family Structure, Educational Attainment, and Socioeconomic Success: Rethinking the "Pathology of Matriarchy"(1). *Am J Sociol,* 105, 2:321.

57. Manski CF (1992-1993). Income and Higher Education. *Focus,* 14, 3:14-19.

58. Gilbert DL (1997). *The American Class Structure in an Age of Growing Inequality.* Belmont, CA: Wadsworth.

59. Eskilson A, Wiley G (1999). Solving for the X: aspirations and expectations of college students. *J Youth Adolescence,* 28, 1:51.

60. Samuolis J, Layburn K, Schiaffino KM (2001). Identity Development and Attachment to Parents in College Students. *J Youth Adolescence,* 30, 3:373.

61. Labouie-Vief G, Hakim-Larson J (1989). Developmental Shifts in Adult Thought. In Hunter S, Sondel M (Eds) *Midlife Myths.* Newberry Park, CA: Sage.

62. Schaie KW (1978). Toward a stage theory of adult cognitive development. *J Aging Hum Dev,* 8, 2:129-138.

63. Twenge JM (2000). The Age of Anxiety? Birth Cohort Change in Anxiety and Neuroticism, 1952-1993. *J Personality Social Psychology,* 79, 6:1007-1021.

64. Alfeld-Liro C, Sigelman CK (1998). Sex differences in self-concept and symptoms of depression during the transition to college. *J Youth Adolescence,* 27, 2:219-245.

65. US Census Bureau (2001). Households by Type. Table DP-1 Profile of General Demographic Characteristics for the United States, 2000. Census 2000. Located at www.census.gov/prod

66. Hermans HJM, Oles PK (1999). Midlife Crisis in Men: Affective Organization of Personal Meanings, *Human Relations* 52, 11:1403.

67. McQuaide S (1998). Women at midlife: success in midlife transformation. *Social Work,* 43,1: 21-32.

68. Lang SS (2001). Midlife crisis less common than many believe. *Human Ecology,* 29,2:23.

69. Avis NE, Stellato R, Crawford S, et al (2000). Is there an association between menopause status and sexual functioning? *Menopause: The Journal of The North American Menopause Society,* 7, 5:297-309.

70. National Institute on Aging (1992). Ongoing Research. In *Menopause* (A Consumer Publication) Bethesda, MD: NIH.

71. American Psychiatric Association (1994). *Diagnostic and Statistical Manual of Mental Disorders* (4th Ed) DSM-IV, Washington DC: APA.

72. See special issue on Depression in *Journal of Family Practice,* June 2001, v 50 i 6.

CHAPTER 4

Basic Counseling and Communication Skills

The purpose of this chapter is to sensitize the reader to the various aspects of communication and how they affect the interaction between health care providers and patients. This chapter examines the key role of nonverbal communication in the total message. The Bayer Model of Complete Clinical Care[1] is used to clarify medical interview-assessment tasks. In this model, the communication tasks, *Engage, Empathize, Educate,* and *Enlist* are used to address the biomedical tasks of Find it, and Fix it. The last section of this chapter addresses issues of dual relationships with patients, professional boundaries, transference, counter transference, and termination of a patient relationship.

Overview

Communication is the key to understanding the exchanges between you and your patient. That seems self evident. Yet patient surveys indicate that misunderstandings about what to expect, treatment options, and treatment instructions are often blamed on the health care provider.[2] Patients who sue their providers often report feeling rushed, receiving no explanations, feeling ignored, or that insufficient time was spent on their care.[3] But as we know, communication is a two way street. Communication is complex because it occurs on different levels. For example, our body image is the basis for how we present ourselves nonverbally to others. Body image forms the basis for self image. We live in our bodies and they communicate how we feel about ourselves to others. The fact that disease rests in the body, and we live in our bodies creates special configurations of information, perceptions, attitudes, emotions and thoughts. When disease occurs, body shame can be a powerful problem in the communications process. As Patient Profile 4-2 illustrates, the health care provider needs to be alert that there are conditions or diseases where body image and self image interact powerfully: skin diseases, facial disfiguration or changes, obesity, cancer related changes (loss of hair or breast, edema), and breast/penis size (as it relates to perceived attractiveness or sexual function/dysfunction).

Factors Affecting Patient Communication

There are many internal reasons why a patient may misunderstand, misinterpret, or simply be unable to hear what you are saying. Previous chapters have discussed how psychosocial issues, cultural beliefs, and language barriers can strongly color the patient's perceptions of you, of the clinical setting, of patients' roles in providing personal information in the medical interview, and of the treatment plan which you expect them to follow. You also also need to be reminded that your own beliefs, values, stress/fatigue levels or inner conflicts may interfere with your ability to listen, or to ask the right questions. In the case in Patient Profile 4-1, the patient had several internal thought processes that interfered with her listening abilities. Also, if you as a provider feel uncomfortable about discussing issues like domestic violence, sexual abuse, or abortion, you may not respond to and follow up on either verbal or nonverbal clues the patient may be giving you about those issues. Notice the word *clues*, because often you have to piece together bits of information that are not always conveyed in words by the patient.

• •

PATIENT PROFILE 4.1

A MIND OF HER OWN

SETTING: Jamar, a physician assistant, has just examined Mrs. Wier, an 80-year-old widow, for gall bladder problems. She has been relatively healthy for the past three years but today there is concern about her gall bladder. Jamar knows her well; she tends to be strong-willed and opinionated. At times they have joked about it.

Mrs. Wier: *(What is he talking about now? My gall bladder? What I should be careful of eating? Who is he to tell me what to eat? I have been deciding what I eat for 80 years now and he thinks he knows everything. Maybe I'd better ask him about my diet.)* Now, young man, tell me again why I should avoid fried foods?

Jamar: *(I am not sure she was listening when I first told her. I know she is headstrong and may not follow my advice but if I explain it to her again, maybe she will.)* Mrs. Wier, eating fried foods is taking in too much fat and cholesterol. It is not healthy and can cause your gall bladder to not function properly. You can help yourself and your gall bladder to stay healthy by making a change in your diet. This change is to not eat fried foods. It can be as easy as just changing the way you cook certain foods, try broiling or baking instead of frying. I know you can do it. Otherwise we might have to consider surgery. With your mind set and strong will, you should not have any difficulty making the change.

Jamar grins and she grins back.

Mrs. Wier: You bet! And I wouldn't have it any other way. And you know I don't want surgery. Tell me again about the changes I have to make in my diet.

Jamar repeats the dietary changes needed.

Jamar: *(Maybe if she has something in writing, she'll study it when she gets home and is more comfortable. She may not want to listen here because of the pressure to get out of here in time for the bus to pick her up.)* I also have a brochure about cholesterol and the gall bladder. You can take it home to read leisurely. Would you like that?

Mrs. Wier: Yes, I read better when I'm more comfortable. *(That was nice of him to understand my creature comforts...)* I'll read the brochure and then decide what to do. You know how I am.

Jamar tells her about the medication.

Mrs. Wier: *(She slumps in her chair. I am so tired. Ooo. What did he just say about that medicine? I'm to take it when? How much? Why? What does it do? Oh, he called it XYZ? Isn't that the pill my sister Sarah took, and it killed her? How much is it going to cost? I can't afford any more medication. How much water am I supposed to drink with this pill? Maybe I just won't take it, and tell him I did. Maybe I should have listened to what he said about diet. I could just eat right and not take the pill. Would he know?)* I'll read the material on the medication.

Jamar: Yes, read it carefully. *(She looks tired. Maybe that is enough for today. I can always talk with her on the phone later after she's read the brochure.)* I'll call you in a few days. I know you like to talk on the phone in the afternoons.

Mrs. Wier: Let's do that.

POINTS TO CONSIDER:

• Jamar knows his patient well. He knows she is strong-willed and has a tendency to not listen. He takes the time to explain the dietary changes a second time.

• He reinforces the importance of making dietary changes, so as to avoid surgery.

• Jamar understands the stress involved in the appointment and gives her a brochure to read at home when she is more comfortable.

• He recognizes she is tiring from the office visit. He offers a telephone visit in a few days to review the patient education brochure and answer any questions.

••••••••••••••••••••••••••••••••

COMMUNICATION CHANNELS

Verbal communication is the content of what a person says. Experts tell us that no more than 30-35 percent of social meaning is carried by words.[4] The rest comes from our perception of nonverbal behavior and our interpretation of the context in which the communication takes place. **Nonverbal communication** comes to us either in a visual, kinesthetic or auditory channel.[5] The visual form consists of expressive behaviors, such as facial expression, gestures, posture, and appearance. Nonverbal behavior also includes eye contact and how much personal distance is maintained. Our auditory channel of perception monitors the **paralanguage** of the communication. This includes pitch of voice, voice tone, volume, rhythm, inflections and hesitations. For example, a mother can distinguish fairly easily whether her baby's cry is from hunger, anger, or frustration. She will tell you *why* she knows her baby is sick. It may be the cry is different, the baby is not feeding as usual, is sleeping more, or is acting differently. In such a situation, you need to listen and believe the mother, who is keyed into her baby, and thus is usually correct in her interpretation.

FACTORS INFLUENCING COMMUNICATION OUTPUT

Communication output in all three channels may be influenced by the immediate situation, as well as by psychosocial issues or cultural factors. For example, stress induced by any of these can make our facial expressions more strained, or erratic — or in the case of fear or trauma — almost frozen. In the paralinguistic channel, a higher pitch in our voice may indicate anxiety, excitement, or lying. Increased volume, or stri-

dency may signal anger, emphasis, excitement — or it may only be a hearing loss. The context in which we see or hear these nonverbal signals, and whether they are congruent with the verbal message, is how we as listeners determine their meaning. Normally this is an unconscious process of evaluation of the total message. Generally when we are dealing with persons with whom we are familiar, we tend to be quite accurate in interpreting the verbal and nonverbal messages. However, since our perceptions are determined by our cultural upbringing, we may be thrown off target when we face a patient from a different culture, or even a different social class. Tone and pitch of voice, pauses or hesitations, personal distance, eye contact, hand gestures, or postural changes all may have different meanings in their culture or class. For example, you might be tempted to conclude that a patient who avoids eye contact, and who hesitates every time before speaking, is evasive. In fact, they may be acting from a cultural obligation to show respect.

In general, nonverbal communication may be more accurate than verbal, because most of the time it is unintentional and uncensored.[6] This is why we need to be alert to **nonverbal leakage**.[7] This is when emotions *leak out*, despite a person's effort to conceal them.[8] One type of leakage is the **respiratory avoidance response.** This is a frequent clearing of the throat, even when no phlegm or mucus is present. A variation of this is the **nose rub.** This is a light rub on the nose with the dorsal surface of the index finger. Each action can signify rejection, disagreement with the verbal statement being made, or ambivalence about the statement being heard. For example, you are asking a teenager "How are things at home (at school)?", and the teenager responds "Fine" while clearing their throat or rubbing their nose. The message may be "No way is it fine" "Why are you asking? or Do you know about Dad's drinking?" In fact, the home life may be chaotic but be covered up by the family secret rule. As we will see in later chapters, there are times when it is essential not only to listen for incongruencies in consistency or plausibility of the verbal information but also to tune in to signals from the various nonverbal channels. Such incongruencies provide clues that a patient may be withholding important but embarrassing information, or may be fabricating.[9]

Communications and Biomedical Tasks

With this short primer on the essentials of the active parts of communication, let's take a closer look at the Model of Clinical Care in Box 4-1. This model, developed by the Bayer Institute for Health Care Education,* shows the communication tasks as well as biomedical tasks health care providers need to accomplish in every encounter with a patient. The four communication tasks: **Engage, Empathize, Educate** and **Enlist** become the tools for allowing you to successfully **Find** and **Fix** the biomedical problems.

ENGAGING THE PATIENT

In engaging the patient, health care providers need to recognize that medical education has given them a way of thinking and expressing themselves, which is quite different from how most of our patients think and communicate. Health care providers have mastered a unique vocabulary of medical terms in their training process. Providers also tend to think deductively using the diagnostic decision tree or the algorithmic approach to arrive at a diagnosis. Many patients, who come to a health care provider's office, are unfamiliar with medical terms for physiological functions, body parts or symptoms. If they come in with a serious medical problem they may also have an impaired ability to listen or

*This first was published as an article by Keller VF, Carroll JG (1994). A new model of physician-patient communication. *Patient Education and Counseling*, 23, 131-140. The Bayer Institute for Health Care Communication in West Haven, Connecticut, has been sponsoring nationwide workshops on Clinician-Patient Communication since 1989.

Box 4-1 Model of Complete Clinical Care

COMMUNICATION TASKS	BIOMEDICAL TASKS
Engage	Find It
Empathize	Fix It
Educate	
Enlist	

Reprinted with permission from Clinician-Patient Communication To Enhance Health Outcomes, Workshop Manual. Bayer Institute for Health Care Communication (1998) p 8.

---

focus. They are likely to be preoccupied with emotions such as grief, discomfort, anxiety, fear, terror, embarrassment, or shame. Patients may have an illness that threatens to bring about changes in lifestyle, altered roles, impaired functioning or even the prospect of death. Flooded by feelings, patients may only comprehend bits and pieces of what the health care provider is trying to communicate. A patient in such a state may not be in a position to give coherent answers or give informed consent.

These feelings at the beginning of an appointment may be complex as illustrated in Patient Profile 4-1. As discussed in Chapters 1 and 2, patient reactions are shaped by their core beliefs about themselves, as well as familial or cultural messages about illness, their bodies, or about seeking help from an "outsider." One way to get in touch with what goes on in our patients is to imagine, or think back to a time, when you as a health care provider were in such a similar situation, and an unfamiliar health care provider asked you "personal" questions about your health habits, looked at your body, and perhaps probed body parts you consider private or about which you may feel shame. Maybe you can remember some of the feelings you had. One point is that the patient's emotional state at the time of the interview can create an ambivalence or barriers to their understanding. Your memories, feelings, or associations about "sensitive" topics may make you reluctant to discuss certain topics with your patients. (This will be discussed in more detail in later chapters.)

A second point is that the heightened emotional arousal may cause patients to alternate between anger/resentment at themselves for being ill, or at you for being dependent on you, or to display passive helplessness. Attending to the various verbal and nonverbal cues allows us to tune in to the feelings of anxiety or ambivalence the patient brings to this first encounter with us. For example, we can alleviate some of these feelings by acknowledging them with a statement like, "Is being here a little stressful for you? It is for most people coming to a clinic (or to meet a new doctor.)" Sharing with the patient that most other persons in a similar situation have the same feelings is called "universalizing." It is a very effective technique because it allows the patient to feel heard, and to know that feelings of distress are "normal," which in itself tends to reduce anxiety.

ENGAGE: BUILDING RAPPORT

A major task of a first appointment with new patients is to welcome them, to develop rapport and to "join" with them. The major goals here are to help them feel more comfortable with their health care provider and the clinical setting, as well as to furnish the provider with holistic and impressionistic information about how the patient thinks, communicates, and functions. The first appointment is an opportunity to get to know the patient as a person rather than as a "medical problem". It also lets the patient observe and get to know their provider as a person rather than as a remote authority figure. This is a special time *before* beginning the medical interview and typically lasts up to five minutes. It is best that this take place before a patient gets undressed and dons an examination gown. Taking this time may seem to be a luxury that is not justifiable with the pressures of a busy practice. Unfortunately, all too often health care providers give in to such time pressures.

Start with an attitude of warm welcome using a pleasant, consistent tone of voice. The health care provider is like a host creating a warm setting. Be certain the patient is comfortably seated. The health care provider needs to sit at eye level with the patient, leaning towards their patient when appropriate, and avoiding any barriers — such as a desk or even a clipboard.

A crucial part of these first few minutes of establishing rapport is to listen attentively and without interruption. Although good eye contact is recommended, it is also vital to sense if "too much" eye contact is making the patient uncomfortable. On the other hand, too little or poor eye contact may signal that the health care provider is not interested in the patient. This can happen during this rapport building phase when the health care provider instead of giving full attention to their patients is taking notes, reading the patient's chart, gazing out the window, or frequently looking at a clock or a watch. Being curious about the patient is as important as attention given to their presenting complaint. With a new patient, the health care provider could say: "Before we talk about your XYZ, tell me something about yourself." Find out *who* they are within the context of *their* family, community or even ethnic heritage. This is not idle chitchat about the weather or sports. The aim of establishing rapport is to find some common linkage in experience, background, identity, or acquaintances that will produce a feeling of comfort and trust with the patient. If the problem is urgent or acute, then other tasks take precedence.

• •

PATIENT PROFILE 4.2

AM I A BAD PERSON NOW?

SETTING: *Alice is a 28-year-old married woman and a new mother. She has returned to the HMO for a follow-up assessment of a skin lesion. She will be seen by a nurse practitioner, Mrs. Wu, who is just meeting Alice for the first time.*

Alice is waiting in the examination room thinking:

(Will it cover my whole body? When I first talked about it with someone here, I mainly got a diagnosis and some information about it. Hadn't I washed enough in those summers

when I worked in the garden and sweated so much? I've always thought of myself as being very clean. A few months later I noticed the patch on my right breast was getting larger. What did that mean for me? For my husband? Had he noticed it?)

Mrs. Wu: Good morning Alice. My name is Mrs. Wu. How can I help you today? *(Mrs. Wu notices that Alice does not make eye contact. Her arms are crossed over her chest and she is seated in a tense posture.)*

Alice: Well, I have a few questions about this tinea versicolor — I'm not sure — *(What will Mrs. Wu think of me?)*

Alice's voice trails off into a whisper.

Mrs. Wu: *(She's not looking at me and she seems tense. There — her voice dropped. I wonder if she's embarrassed about this skin infection. I'll approach her gently.)* Yes, sometimes a person can have questions about skin disorders.

Mrs. Wu leans forward and nods for Alice to go on.

Alice: This is a little embarrassing to talk about — you know — private. *(I want to talk about my sexual relationship with my husband but I hardly know her. Had it "turned him off"? Should I hide it and turn the lights down so he doesn't see it? Am I a damaged person now? Tainted? Will our love making be the same or will it deteriorate? What does it mean for me as a wife?)*

Mrs. Wu: Alice, I know you just met me and sometimes it is hard to talk with a stranger, but rest assured, I am here to listen and help you.

Alice: *(Well — this is the reason I came in today. Here goes...)* I'm worried about how my husband will feel about me. You know, will this skin disorder affect his desire for me? He's always liked my perfect skin and now it is blemished.

Mrs. Wu: Usually in a marriage, one's intimate relationship is part of a larger picture — companionship, and acceptance. Do you feel you and your husband trust each other?

Alice: Yes, we've always really liked each other's company and trusted each other.

Mrs. Wu: It sounds like your relationship is based on more than him liking your skin?

Both of them laugh.

Alice: Well, looking at it that way. Of course! *(How about me as a Mother? Should I stop breast feeding my son? Will he get it from me? This sounds crazy. She's a woman, maybe she'll understand my question.)* I was also wondering if I should stop breast feeding my son. I know this sounds like a silly question, but will he get it from me?

Mrs. Wu: That's not a silly question at all. Other mothers have asked that very same question. You can continue to breast feed your son as long as the area of infection does not come in contact with his mouth or face. For added protection, I recommend that you use a soft cotton patch over the nipple area while he is feeding. This skin infection can be easily treated with a topical medication. However, before we discuss the medication, do you have any other questions today?

Alice: No, and thank you for understanding.

POINTS TO CONSIDER:

• Mrs. Wu recognizes the patient's nonverbal communication, including voice tone and volume and adjusts her communication accordingly.

• When Alice mentions she wants to talk about something private, Mrs. Wu reassures her appropriately.

• Mrs. Wu reminds Alice of some characteristics of a strong marriage.

• When Alice discounts her question as silly, Mrs. Wu mentions that other mothers have asked that question thus normalizing Alice's concerns.

• Mrs. Wu provides patient education and management plans for the skin infection.

● ●

Set Agenda

Setting or eliciting the patient's agenda is another important pre-interview task. Just as one normally does not go to the supermarket to buy one item, most patients come in with more than one complaint. Three or more is typical. As providers with long years of experience have found, the "chief complaint", or reason for coming in frequently is the socially or culturally acceptable "cover" for other — possibly taboo — medical or psychological problems.[10] It is vital to discover *all* of the complaints, otherwise you may find yourself holding the doorknob at the end of the interview, while the patient tries to "quickly tell" you about the other complaints. To make sure that the chief complaint is not the "cover", you could ask: "Is there anything else on your mind?" "What else has been going on with you?" or "Anything else you would like to tell me?" Once all of the complaints are out in the open, you could ask "What are you hoping to accomplish today?" Essential to this task is the necessity to inform the patient how much time there is for today's appointment and then negotiate which complaint(s) are most important to address today. The patient may only need reassurance on some issues, but other lesser complaints can be investigated during another appointment. Setting an agenda together may happen almost immediately, or only after the patient has told their story. But doing it cooperatively — as suggested above — is one way of letting the patient know they are heard and are active participants in the interview process.

ROLE OF EMPATHY

The quality of empathy needs to be brought into this encounter. As Coulehan and Block define it, "being empathic means listening to the total communication — words, feelings and gestures — and letting the patient know that you are really hearing what he or she is saying."[11] They assert that being empathic is scientific "because *understanding* is at the core of objectivity." (Emphasis added.) Empathy is a key skill for health care providers for several reasons. First, it is an active concern and curiosity about the emotions, values, and experiences of the patient that allows them to see and hear their patient. Their empathic response lets their patient know *what* is being heard by them[12] Second, empathy

allows a safe psychological space to be created. This is accomplished by inviting the patient to talk about what they are thinking and feeling, and then acknowledging those feelings without judgment. Third, it gives the patient the assurance that their health care provider is paying attention to them. Several verbal and nonverbal behaviors contribute to an empathic understanding. Some behaviors are obvious and some are more subtle. One suggestion is not to listen and write at the same time. If the health care provider is taking notes while their patient is speaking, it may give the impression that they are not listening. In fact, the provider may miss important verbal and nonverbal information because they cannot fully attend to the patient while writing. The health care provider needs to trust that they are recording with all their senses, as they let the patient tell their story. Such empathic listening will give the provider information about the patient's thoughts and feelings, which can guide them on how and what to ask about while eliciting the medical history. Some readers may feel uncomfortable with this emphasis on empathy. Doubts and concerns about the use of empathy fall into the following four areas:

1. **Am I expected to be able to empathize with everyone? What about someone I just don't like?**

True empathy is not about liking nor is it sympathy or pity. For example, Olson[13] noted that nurses find it difficult to empathize with patients whom they held responsible for their own disease, such as smokers with emphysema. Empathy is the ability to see things as the patient sees them from their perspective. It is the ability to understand the patient's emotions, difficulties even if you have never shared the patient's experience or "walked in their shoes", such as being addicted to nicotine or losing a child. You imagine how it would feel if you were in that position. It is a learned ingredient in communication, and it must be practiced before it becomes a comfortable and indispensable part of every encounter.

2. **What do I do after I share my empathy with the patient?**

It is usually best to remain silent. Wait a few seconds for the patient to absorb empathic reflection, and the feeling of being understood. Resist the urge to fix things, or make the patient feel better. For example, if you have empathically reflected back to a patient how frightening it must be to have just received a diagnosis of cancer, your quiet presence while the patient processes this information, can provide invaluable solace to the patient. Immediately "rattling off" the available tools used to "fight" or "lick" this medical problem probably comes more out of your need to bring yourself back to the safety of factual territory, than reassuring the patient.

3. **Wouldn't my empathic response trigger emotional breakdowns by patients?**

Rarely. More often an appropriate empathic response increases trust. The patient who feels understood, usually does not need to "escalate" to obtain acknowledgment of their emotional distress. It does take time to listen to the patient's story, to reflect back to them your perceptions of what they are saying and feeling, and to allow the necessary pauses for the patient to digest what has just been paraphrased. Patience, often the antithesis of academic training to be efficient, needs to be practiced. The axiom, "Silently count to ten" may well apply in such situations. Over-concern with uncontrollable emotional outpouring — possibly coming out of your own discomfort with emotions — can inhibit an empathic response.

4. **Wouldn't empathizing with a patient's anger just make it worse?**

Usually anger will lessen if you show that you understand the underlying emotions behind it, such as the patient's sense of frustration, fear, disappointment. For many, anger is a difficult emotion. A common response to anger is to ignore it. It can stand in the way of liking or empathizing with a patient. It can also raise fears of being sued by the patient. A misconception is that if anger is acknowledged, the patient will be reinforced in their resentment and desire to seek revenge. However, when you communicate understanding of the patient's reason for being angry, you are not signifying agreement or approval of inconsiderate or angry behavior but are defusing the anger. The following dialog illustrates how the empathic reflection of the feeling of abandonment de-escalated the feeling of anger or hostility:[†]

Patient: I couldn't reach you when I was home and hurting.

PA: I see.

Patient: I don't know if you do see! You had promised that you'd be there if I needed you. I needed you and you weren't there!

PA: So you were home with the pain and it was frightening and you couldn't get me on the phone.

Patient: (*Angry look.*)

PA: And you felt alone and abandoned and angry with me.

Patient: That's about the size of it.

PA: I can imagine how upsetting that was for you.

Patient: I know that phones are busy sometimes, but I really needed you.

PA: And you couldn't find me.

Patient: Exactly! I guess it doesn't do me any good to get angry with you, though. It's the system, not you. I know you are concerned with my welfare.

PA: Thanks for saying that. Maybe we can set up some guidelines for you to get help if you need it in the future and can't reach me.

Patient: OK.

---

†Adapted and reprinted with permission from Bayer Institute for Health Care Communication.

ENGAGE: PATIENT HISTORY AS TOLD BY PATIENT

The patient's story is their experience of an injury, illness or health concern, and their provider needs to listen to it without interruption. As research shows, many practitioners find it difficult not to jump in with questions. Typically, the patient is interrupted for the first time after only 18 seconds of telling their story.[14] Health care providers need to resist the urge to "organize" it with factual *what*, *when*, *where* and *why* questions. They need to hear the story from the patient's perspective and be open to learning more from listening rather than from shaping it too soon into treatment goals. If the health care provider asks such questions too early, the story may become distorted as the patient unconsciously begins to shape their responses to what they perceive the provider wants to hear. Instead, the provider needs to focus on empathically acknowledging the feelings, values and thoughts of the patient. Empathic comments like: "That must have been difficult (frightening, stressful, painful)" convey to the patient that you really understand. Building such an emotional bridge of understanding is effective in moving patients past their fears and helpful in getting them to *join* their provider in a cooperative partnership. The facts of the medical history will make more sense with an empathic understanding of the patient's perspective of their key concerns.

Sometimes a patient will ramble or go off on tangents. Observe thought processes, and use open-ended clarification questions and reflective listening to refocus the story: "Tell me more about... I am curious about." Or you can use reflective listening statements like: "Let me see if I heard you correctly", and then after repeating what you heard, asking: "Is that right?" Similar kinds of questions can be used to reflect concerns or fears that the patient may not express verbally but which you see in their nonverbal language. "You seem nervous (scared, worried) about the possibility of surgery, is that right?" Once the patient says "Yes, I guess so", you know the circle of understanding has been completed, and that trust is being established.

Medical History

Obtaining a detailed medical history is a critical function. It has been estimated just the history alone provides most of the basic information required for a correct diagnosis.[15] As one author writes:

> Careful history taking actually saves time. The history provides the roadmap; without it the journey is merely a shopping around at numerous garages for technological fixes. When detailed historical data are lacking, [a health care provider] may be paralyzed into inaction or resort to improper therapeutic options.[16]

The secret to collecting such data then is this process of engaging the patient and empathic listening. Short circuiting this process may not only produce incomplete or misleading data, but may foster negative judgments about patients. The patient's ambivalence, mistrust, or resentment in a first encounter can affect the health care provider personally. A perception of non-cooperation could then lead the provider to categorize the patient as a "problem patient." Research has shown that providers tend to make judgments fairly early in an encounter whether a patient is manageable, treatable or likable.[17] **Manageability** relates to the perception of the patient's willingness to participate in the goal of getting well, of their motivation to do so, and of their willingness to accept and carry out directions. **Treatability** is an estimate of the likelihood that the patient will benefit from the treatment. Aside from factors inherent in the seriousness of the disease condition, it includes an appraisal of the patient's ability to understand and to carry through on goals and instructions. If the patient displays a *yes .. but* attitude, the provider may question their patient's commitment to healthy outcomes. **Like-ability** deals with the perception of whether the patient is pleasant to treat. (Hispanics use the term *simpatico*.) It is related to manageability and treatability in that failure is an uncomfortable experience in a medical setting. Hence when the provider gets the impression that a patient is not going to cooperate, they may not invest as much effort into a person with a "bad attitude". They need to especially guard against dismissing persons from minority cultures who may not be skilled in communicating with health care providers, and/or whose distrust or suspicion of them and the health care system may produce ambivalence in their first encounter. This also applies when a person is reluctant to tell their story. Remember that it is not acceptable to talk openly about certain health or mental health conditions in many families or cultures. This means that the provider needs to be alert to indirect language, euphemisms, or a story about a "friend" to *hear* what the patient may be too uncomfortable to say openly about a taboo health condition. When such indirectness is encountered, respond indirectly by talking positively about persons who have such a condition or disease. The aim is to *normalize* the condition and thereby disarm any stigma or shame imposed by their belief system. The provider may wish to empathize aloud how difficult it must be to face a situation that is, however, fairly common (or at least not unique). The provider may then add that the condition could or needs to be treated, and give the patient an estimate of the effectiveness of treatment. Once the patient feels that they are not judged and their fear of the cultural stigma lessens, they are more likely to open up and communicate the details needed for a complete assessment and treatment.

Educating the Patient

The third task in effective patient communications and completing the biomedical tasks is to educate the patient. By virtue of academic training and experience, health care providers have an abundance of knowledge. Sometimes that fund of knowledge can lead them to conclude, that only they know how to interpret the patients' symptoms. However, in every encounter with patients, education is a two way street. The patient has information the provider needs. This goes beyond a recitation of symptoms. Whenever a health problem develops, patients like to figure out what

is going on. Some patients may go into denial, hoping that by ignoring it, or "toughing it out" it will go away. In any case, there is at least some internal processing about what is happening cognitively and emotionally. Patients sometimes seek advice from those close to them. They may relate it to something they saw on TV or read about. The point is that by the time they seek out a health care professional for the complaint, they will have ideas and some feelings about what is going on with their body. So, the health care provider can assume that the patient will have formulated a self-diagnosis. The patient's internal belief system will determine how they think about cause and effect, and how it is going to affect their functioning, relations with others, as well as the symbolic or moral meaning. The health care provider's task is to learn what the patient thinks and feels about what they know. A simple question will often bring this out. After hearing their story, a good question to ask is: "What do you think is going on?" or "Do you have any thoughts or ideas about your condition?"

Their response will allow the provider to assess their understanding of what is going on and how they have been responding to their health challenge. This is important because the patient's insight into their own problem may give their provider a key piece to the puzzle of the task of finding the biomedical complaint. Keller and Carroll[18] bring out another reason for finding out the patient's view. The way the patient conveys that understanding, including concerns, fears, or dismissals, provides clues to the patient's attitude towards willingness to change health habits, and to follow a treatment regimen. It also communicates a picture of the patient's internal map of reality. "It is the patient's map that is central, and will impact patient behavior, not the physician's map," Keller and Carroll add. That map may be incomplete, and the patient may have anxiety about those gaps, or unanswered questions in their mind.

Keller and Carroll suggest two ways of dealing with the patient's "unanswered" questions. First, is to encourage the patient at all times to ask questions. The goal of patient education is not simply to impart information, but to create understanding. Keller and Carroll cite studies that show that under most circumstances, patients will walk out the door having forgotten about half of what has been said. However, when the patient is actively involved in the process of eliciting the information, the information their health care provider gives them is more specific to their needs. The patient can digest the information, which creates more understanding. General understanding rather than specific terms tend to be retained in memory better. This understanding is the foundation for enlisting the patient's cooperation and responsibility for treatment adherence. A simple way to encourage the patient to join in this process of what is going on is to ask: "Is there anything else you have been thinking or would like to ask me?"

However, many patients may be reluctant to articulate their questions. Keller and Carroll suggest that health care providers assume that all patients are concerned about their situation and about what the health care providers actions are doing to them. The writers group these concerns into the following eight questions. Part of the task of educating the patient is for you to incorporate answers to these questions into the interview protocol with every patient. This is especially urgent the more serious or complicated the pending diagnosis appears to be. About their situation the patient wants to know:

1. What has happened to me?

2. Why has this happened to me?

3. What is going to happen to me, in the short term, in the long term?

About your actions you can assume they want to know:

1. What are you (they) doing to me (examination, tests)?

2. Why are you (they) doing this — rather than something else (diagnostic or treatment options)?

3. Will it hurt, or harm me, and how much and for how long (diagnostic tests and treatment)?

4. When and how will you know what these tests mean?

When these questions are automatically incorporated into the educational effort, you not only create understanding but also reassurance. Of course, you will not always or immediately have the answers to what is going on with the patient. It helps to share with the patient that "at this stage" you do not have adequate information to draw a conclusion. When you tell the patient what you are about to do and why — whether it is simple touch and palpation, or some more invasive procedure — the patient can be prepared and that assists you in understanding more about what is going on. However, even if you are conscientious in answering the "assumed" questions, you need to keep in mind that the patient may have additional questions. Throughout the examination, you can repeatedly invite the patient to join in finding answers, with "Are there other answers you need?" This may reveal frustration or other emotional reactions that the patient may have. It is better to respond to those early and thereby prevent an internal build up of anxieties, fears or even resentments for being "left in the dark." Also remember, if the goal is understanding, you may need to find out what and how much the patient understands before you proceed to *enlisting* the patient into participating in the treatment process. One way to discover this is to acknowledge your own fallibility: "I sometimes may not make myself clear in what I say. Would you tell me what you understand at this point, so I am sure we are both understanding each other." Such open ended questions are much better than: "Do you understand?" The latter are usually answered with a "Yes", whether the patient understands or not. A "Yes" or "No" gives you little information about the internal processes of how the patient handles the information you have given them.

Enlisting the Patient

The Bayer Health Care Communication model divides enlistment into two parts: *decision making* and *encouraging adherence*. The goal of both parts is to increase the patient's responsibility and competence to care for their health. A large study consisting of 1057 audio taped encounters between primary physicians, surgeons and their patients undertaken in 1993, was published in the Journal of the American Medical Association in December 1999.[19] The authors found that only about 9% of patient decisions conformed to the criteria for informed decision making. More alarmingly, physicians rarely explored whether patients understood the decision (0.9%-6.9%). The study seems to indicate that the old model of "doctor knows best" still ruled these encounters. Today we hear more about informed consent, patient participation, and advanced directives. But to some, these are merely legal terms, rather than basic assumptions on how to partner *with* patients in arriving at diagnoses and treatment decisions.

Health care providers are not the only ones struggling with these changes. Patients too are finding it difficult to adjust to the new paradigm of participatory health care. Many patients still see the health care provider in a position of omniscience, reflected in such statements "I'll do what you think is best." Or "Whatever you say..." Whenever you hear such utterances, you have to resist the urge to say "OK, then let me tell you what you need to do". Instead, you need to actively enlist the patient in the decision making process. Here is another opportunity to get their "self diagnosis" ideas and to solicit suggestions about treatment. For example, some useful phrases are: "I have arrived at one explanation of what the problem is (briefly go through your explanation). How does that fit in with what you have been thinking?" When the patient shares explanations, you need to maintain a curious but neutral stance. Do not ignore, or judge the input of the patient or the treatment suggestions made by others, like the spouse, relatives, friends, TV, or magazines. Hearing themselves recite such suggestions can lead the patient to recall what they or a relative did in a previous similar situation, and how the "solution" worked. New and unsolicited information may change your thoughts and direction of treatment or lead to practical solutions. If the patient feels that you valued the information, it is likely to enhance treatment adherence.

It is suggested that you also inform the patient that you want them to think this through *together* with you and arrive at an agreement about the various issues in treatment. As you listen to the patient's own ideas, your aim is for agreement and increased compliance. Patients often have a preference for treatment. Influences for such a preference may range from not wanting to miss work to fear about certain medical procedures. How they think about treatment may in fact, influence how they think about diagnosis. For example, a patient with cardiac insufficiency may offer a lesser diagnosis in the hope of avoiding hospitalization or surgery. This calls for being alert to how a patient ties his own diagnosis to treatment. The important point to remember here is that agreement or at least understanding about the diagnosis improves the chances that treatment regimens will be followed.

ENLISTING TREATMENT ADHERENCE

The second step is enlisting adherence to the agreed upon regimen. As pointed out in the *JAMA* study above, most patients leave the encounter without sufficient knowledge or understanding of the treatment decisions to which they agreed. Therefore it is not surprising that about 50% of patients do not follow the treatment recommendations. The Bayer model suggests the following six specific actions to raise the level of patient adherence to the treatment regimen agreed upon:

1. **Keep the regimen simple.** The fewer the required behaviors, the more likely that they will be remembered and carried out. If a complicated regimen is required, you need to

break it down into sequential component steps.

2. **Write out the regimen for the patient.** Say it out loud as you write it down. If you use pre-printed forms, go over the regimen with the patient. Using a highlighter or pen, personalize the instructions for the patient. If a specific technique is involved, demonstrate it to the patient.

3. **Motivate the patient and give specifics about the benefits and timetable.** Many patients leave without knowing *why* they are doing what they have been asked to do whenor *what* benefits or improvements they will receive from adhering to the instructions.

4. **Make sure that the patient knows the potential side effects and what to do if they occur.** This is not only a key to informed consent, it also prevents patients from giving up on adherence without exploring other options. Side effects that are anticipated are less likely to lead to abandonment of the treatment. The *JAMA* study showed that one of the most common omissions is for the clinician not to inform the patient about possible or likely side effects of key prescription medications.

5. **Discuss with the patient any obstacles to carrying out the various parts of the treatment.** This is the time to explore the various barriers to treatment that might interfere with following through. These barriers may range from personal doubts, cultural beliefs to psychosocial factors such as lack of money to purchase the prescription drugs or supplies, or transportation to and from therapy.

6. **Get feedback from the patient.** It is essential that you have an assurance that the patient understands the regimen. You can ask the patient to tell you *what* they understand they are to do. As they recite what they remember, you can gently add in things they omitted, or highlight them on the written instructions. It is equally important to ask them during fol-

low up visits to describe the steps in their adherence. Last, you need to discuss with the patient how they feel about following the regimen. If you detect emotional commitment, the outlook is good; if you see ambivalence, or resistance, you need to explore that further until agreement is reached.

This section has identified and explored the communication tasks the health care provider needs to accomplish in any encounter with patients. The model presented here has been proven effective in research and experience. It has been presented under the sponsorship of the Bayer Institute for Health Care Communications to thousands of health care providers in interactive half day workshops over the past few years, with positive feedback. The authors feel confident that health care providers who incorporate this model into their protocol for working with patients, will find it very useful.

Boundary Issues

The focus on the personal involvement in engaging the patient, listening to them empathically, and letting them express their feelings, raises the question of professional boundaries. You might ask, "How can I maintain my professionalism when I am asked to engage my patients on an emotional level? Won't this lead to boundary problems or over-involvement?" These are valid concerns that health care professionals face. It is an American misconception that expressing emotions to one's patients is somehow unprofessional.[20] Yet surveys show that patients view the health care provider who is warm and caring, more favorably on several dimensions of satisfaction than one who is cool and distant.[21,22] For example, when you share your own sincere sorrow and even tears with a patient's family who has just experienced death, you are giving a priceless gift of shared grief and understanding that will provide comfort to the bereaved.[23] Giving this kind of comfort is professional. Allowing patients or their families to see an expression of emotion reassures them that their health care provider has a human or feeling side. Experienced health care providers will tell you that patients, or their families who have seen such an expression of shared grief or concern are much less likely to file a malpractice suit.[24]

The other issue is excessive involvement. In the professional relationship, you need to maintain clear role boundaries. Being friendly and caring does not violate those boundaries. Being a *friend* to one's patients is a boundary violation because it can lead you to do things that as a professional you should not do. It is essential to keep in mind this simple distinction between *being friendly* and *being a friend*.

The greatest threat to professional boundaries arises out of the phenomena of **transference** and **counter transference**. These two terms originate in the fields of psychiatry and psychology. They refer to feelings from our past that are triggered by someone, upon whom we then **project** those feelings. This comes from the natural tendency to identify and categorize new experiences and new persons in relation to what was learned in the past. Transference is a projection from the patient onto the health care provider. Typically, a patient can have some deep-seated feelings or memories about someone in their past. You, as their health care provider, in the present, by virtue of some similarity (or strong contrast), may trigger these feelings or reactions in your patient. The patient will project those feelings onto you, reacting to you, not as you, but *as if* you were the other person out of their past. Not only feelings but certain behavioral responses may be connected to transference issues, rather than to your specific actions. Similarly, counter transference occurs when you project on to a patient some feelings, memories, or behavioral responses related to someone in your past, rather than to the words or actions of the patient in the here and now. Counter transference can seriously interfere with your objectivity, as well as endanger the professional relationship.

One needs to distinguish between negative and positive transference and counter transference. **Positive** transference or counter transference arise out of positive or pleasant memories or associations. For example, a patient may respond to you as if you were a favorite family relative, who always listened to them and treated them kindly. For you, positive counter transference can arise when a patient reminds you of a favorite person in your past. Both cases may automatically lead to a positive perception of the other. Such a positive attitude can be used to facilitate the process of establishing rapport and trust, cooperative treatment planning and adherence to the treatment regimen. **Negative** transference or counter transference comes out of negative or unpleasant memories and associations in one's past. For example, your role as an authority figure can trigger feelings of fear, anger, or rebellion that may be related to a patient's experience with a domineering or critical parent. This can seriously interfere with rapport, trust, and cooperation. Similarly, a patient who reminds you of someone unpleasant in your past is likely to impair your perception of like-ability, manageability, and treatability. In both cases, the negative feelings may lead to unsatisfactory or even hostile communications. This can seriously impair the effort to fully address the health problem.

Having said all that, it is important to remember that transference and counter transference occur frequently. They are inevitable in many relationships with patients. You will often have patients who project thoughts and feelings onto you, either negatively or positively. By the same token, it is likely that with some patients you will counter transfer positively or negatively. The problem is that transference and counter transference tend to happen on an unconscious level. For example, a health care provider may not realize that the strong feeling of warmth and love they have towards a certain patient may come from an unconscious association with a romantic encounter they had in their youth. The danger is that if the motivation for these feelings remain on an unconscious level, they might propel the health care provider into inappropriate intimacy with this patient. Of course, the reverse could also happen. A patient could develop romantic or sexual feelings towards their health care provider, based on unconscious transference issues. This is dangerous territory, and as the records of disciplinary actions taken by professional boards will attest, boundary violations relating to sexual involvement with patients occur with alarming frequency.[25]

How to Manage Transference and Counter Transference

How does one approach the issues inherent in transference and counter transference? First, it is vital to acknowledge that they are a normal and common phenomenon. Pretending that they do not exist, or that one is immune from them is counterproductive. The key to addressing transference and counter transference is to bring them into conscious awareness. Any unusually strong emotional or physical response between the patient and you — that is out of keeping with the interactional context — is the surest sign that some unconscious mechanism brought this on. This requires an alertness to strong feeling reactions both in the patients and yourself.

When such feelings are brought to awareness, several choices emerge on how to address them. For example, when you suspect negative transference from a patient, you might at first examine your own feelings and responses to the patient. Sometimes it is good to bring the issue into the open. You might say, "I notice that you seem angry with me. Did I say or do something to cause you to feel that way?" If the patient cannot account for the feeling or attitude, a follow up question could be: "Sometimes I remind my patients of someone in their past. Can you think of anyone in your past, that I remind you of, that could trigger these feelings of anger (fear or distrust)?" It may be that the patient previously had a bad experience with a health care provider, and is still angry or fearful. But if the patient seems baffled by these questions, you

could ask them to "just think about it" some more. You could also briefly explain how the negative feelings towards you or the health care system could interfere with getting well, and your own efforts in eliciting the relevant information from them and developing a treatment plan together.

When transference or counter transference involve romantic and/or sexual feelings, you need to take immediate action to acknowledge and defuse such feelings. In a situation of romantic transference, a good first step is to inform a trusted colleague of the situation. This automatically brings the problem from the realm of secrets into the open. The act of sharing usually brings with it a sense of relief. Second, the next time a patient makes some romantic comment, the clinician might say, "I sense that you have some warm and loving feelings towards me. This can happen. I do feel flattered. However I am your health care provider, and any other relationship is not possible."[26] After any response from the patient, the provider will want to impress upon the patient that they intend to be a warm and caring health care provider but that they cannot respond to the person's romantic feelings. They can add that their professional code of ethics makes it improper and illegal for them to respond in any other way.

This last point is also important advice for health care providers to give themselves when they find themselves strongly attracted to a patient. While it is inappropriate to burden a patient dependent on their care with an explanation of romantic counter transference, it is advisable to discuss it with someone. This could be either a professional colleague, or perhaps even a spouse. Generally, the act of bringing it out in the open will disarm the impulse to act on such feelings. As an additional precaution, if this happens to you, you may want to arrange that you are never alone with a patient when romantic transference or counter transference feelings are in the air. If it proves difficult to clear the air of such romantic feelings, it would be wise to refer the patient to a colleague, thereby terminating a

---

Box 4-2 Principles for Maintaining Clear Boundaries

1. **Define boundaries for self and patient.** Ask yourself the following questions:
   a. Is this what a health care provider does?
   b. Do I sense how the patient experiences this?
   c. Is what I am doing for the patient, rather than for me?
   d. Is this the healthy side of my patient being supported by my action?

   If the answer to any of these questions is No, it could lead to boundary crossing or ethical violations.

2. **Patient focus.** Part of "engaging" is to find commonalities. The more we have in common, the more we tend to like a patient, increasing the temptation to get into personal topics. A clear signal of trouble is when we start talking about ourselves instead of focusing on the patient.

3. **Personal neediness.** A tendency to work compulsively and delay gratification, may lead a provider to feel undervalued. This makes you vulnerable to personal over involvement from a sympathetic or seductive patient. Be alert to feelings of overwork and under appreciation. (See chapter on Stress Management and Self Care)

4. **Transference.** Your caring is likely to trigger gifts of gratitude, admiration or even romantic love from patients. Personal compliments not related to the care, written notes, phone calls outside office hours, gifts, or invitations are the signals for such transference. Clarify roles and boundaries with the patient. Often a clearly stated explanation will resolve the situation and allow the patient to save face.

5. **Counter transference.** The nature of good health care is akin to loving and caring for someone. You need to be alert to any change from professional caring to romantic caring. Take counsel with someone and bring it out into the open. Similarly, your liking for a patient can tempt you to become a close personal friend. You can be "friendly" but should not be a "friend" to your patients.

6. **Dual Relationships.** Patients may tempt you into a personal, or business relationship with gifts, invitations to social events, or investment opportunities. There may be strings attached - expectations of special favors, such as free care, or drug samples. Dual relationships can easily compromise professional ethics. Clarify with the patient that you will give excellent care without gifts or other favors.

With permission adapted from Principles for Avoiding Seduction. In Platt FW, Gordon GH, (1999). *Field Guide to the Difficult Patient Interview.* Baltimore: Lippincott Williams & Wilkins. p 67.

---

relationship that can no longer be on a purely professional level.[27] Box 4-2 provides guidelines on how to recognize the transference and counter transference dilemmas in boundary issues and how to disarm them.

Termination Issues

Sometimes the professional relationship between a health care provider and a patient comes to an end. This may be due to a change in health insurance coverage, such as when patients change jobs, and are covered by a different HMO. Or patients may get laid off and lose health insurance coverage altogether. They might move out of the geographical area covered by your practice. Or you might move to another practice not covered by their HMO. When the provider-patient relationship has been of long standing, patients tend to have reactions ranging from annoyance, anger, disappointment, to a sense of abandonment. These feelings can be viewed as part of a type of grief and mourning process. Patients may have revealed intimate information that only the provider and they know. Thus, when this long-term relationship is about to end, they may experience a sense of loss. Proper referral procedures should be implemented at this time to assure continuity of cov-

---

TERMINATION — when an established professional relationship between patient and a health care provider comes to an end due to departure of the patient or the provider or a change of insurance coverage.

---

erage. They may include referral for "free" clinics, or clinics that have eligibility for reduced fee payments.)

Termination issues are often overlooked in our highly mobile society. Yet, properly addressing these issues is an essential aspect of relating to patients, as well as good professional practice. For example, if you are going to be absent temporarily, you need to arrange backup with colleagues. If you plan to leave permanently, you need to prepare your patients far in advance of your departure. Leaving without notifying your patients or referring them to another provider is not only unethical, but may put the patients at risk. Often only you know their medical history, as well as such intangibles about how to enlist a particular patient's cooperation and treatment adherence. Ideally, there would be a period of overlap, during which you could personally introduce your successor, allowing your patients to meet and briefly interact with them. You might briefly review the patient's history in your colleague's presence, inviting the patient to add anything. The successor could ask a few questions, thus giving them a chance to interact with the patient.

When a health care practice closes, it is essential that all patients be notified. Current patients who have ongoing health problems need immediate referrals to other health care providers. Patients who have not been seen in some time, need to be notified at their last known address by letter, which should include a choice of referral health care providers. One last point is that health care providers also need to make provision for an orderly and secure transfer of medical records to the practice location of the new health care providers, either during one's temporary absence, or after termination.

PATIENT PROFILE 4.3

ONE COMPLICATED LADY

SETTING: *Irene is a 39-year-old married woman with one adopted daughter. For the past 20 years Irene has been under the care of Dr. Monty, a general practitioner in a busy clinic affiliated with a metropolitan hospital. Irene has a complex medical history. Several specialists are involved in the continuity of her health care.*

Dr. Monty in reviewing her medical history is confronted with difficulty reaching a clear diagnosis. Eight years ago, she came in with recurring UTIs. She had been born with one good kidney and the other one functioning at 40%. She was on BP medication for hypertension. Six years ago she was diagnosed with adult onset diabetes. Medication and proper diet stabilized her glucose level. She reported at that time that she felt depressed and anxious sometimes about her medical problems. Her scores on the BDI-II and BAI (Beck Depression and Anxiety Inventories) indicated moderate depression and mild anxiety. Dr. Monty prescribed Paxil. Her depression and anxiety lessened. Every couple of months she came in with another cluster of symptoms (e.g. headaches, nausea, muscle pains, general fatigue) — none of which had responded well to any treatment regimen. In her psychosocial assessment she reported that her marriage was fulfilling and she loved her husband, Reggie. During one visit, we discussed psychosomatization and how feelings sometimes get "played out" in our bodies. I told her there might be some issues there she needed to work on which she might be translating into her body. Here's the referral to the psychotherapist. Then five years ago she came in complaining of migraine like headaches, numbness in her arms and feet, shooting pains in her chest, and that she'd had "blackouts". Further questioning revealed that she meant she felt "out of it" for a while. Questioning her husband, Reggie, provided no further information. After getting more details on her stress levels and her headaches, I concluded they were tension headaches and referred her back to her psychotherapist for stress management. The headaches were less frequent when she was handling her stress levels better. The referral to the neurologist revealed no definitive diagnosis. Four years ago fainting was recorded as the chief complaint. Dr. Monty remembered one appointment with her where when he entered the examination room, Irene was sort of "propped up" against her husband wearing clothes more suited to a 12 year old. Dr. Monty recalls what was said at that appointment:

Reggie: She has a terrible headache.

Dr. Monty: Irene, what is going on?

(Irene responds in a child like very high voice tone using halting phrases, with that odd, highly constricted voice indicating she was in a great deal of pain from the headaches.)

Irene: I've had - another spell. I don't feel - good. They - keep getting - worse.

Dr. Monty: *(Spells?" That's new. Were these the blackouts? What was going on? Were the headaches related to these spells? I need some answers here! Other causes like renal failure, heart problems and metabolic problems, or her diabetes had been ruled out. She again confirmed that she did not drink alcohol nor took any drugs.)* Reggie, can you tell me what she is like during a spell?

Reggie: She doesn't know herself. Won't eat, drink liquids, and sometimes curls up and won't talk. Sometimes she talks and sometimes not. She kept bowel and bladder control. Sometimes she acts like a teenager and wants to go to bars. She's never violent. We usually try and get her distracted onto something else and keep her at home.

Dr. Monty: I need to talk with her psychotherapist for a minute.

Dr. Monty then remembered stepping out of the examination room and calling her psychotherapist describing her symptoms. Possible alternative diagnoses could be conversion disorder, dissociative identity disorder, or at a minimum some form of amnestic syndrome. We were both puzzled and admitted that neither of us had a clear understanding of what was going on with Irene. My instinct is to refer her back to the neurologist, even though he had previously ruled out a slow growing tumor.

Dr. Monty remembered receiving a frantic call from Reggie four months ago reporting that she had become aggressive and combative. He said she was struggling with him and their daughter, screaming and not making much sense. Dr. Monty told him to bring her in immediately and when they arrived, she was quiet, but vomiting and seemed very ill. Because she appeared so ill, Dr. Monty admitted her to the hospital. She had quietly tolerated various diagnostic tests. That evening, Reggie called to say that she "went wild," had attacked four nurses and the security guard, wrecked her room and terrified her roommate. She was screaming and fearful that they were going to hurt her. She was immediately admitted to a psychiatric hospital. When she "came to herself", and learned what she had done, she was very upset. After a few days, she stabilized and was discharged home with a diagnosis of Acute Stress Reaction. After her discharge, she reports to Dr. Monty that these episodes always "feel like a seizure". She had no specific memories of the episodes afterwards. Just that they "felt like a seizure". However, all neurological examinations did not clinically support the diagnosis of epilepsy.

Today in his office, Dr. Monty keeps hearing her say "seizure" and says to Irene:

Dr. Monty: Sometimes people can have seizures without any findings on the EEG. Since you had some violence and aggressive behaviors in your last episode, you may have temporal lobe epilepsy — partial type.

Irene: I knew it. It felt like a seizure. Can you give me anything to help me?

Dr. Monty: Yes I can prescribe a trial of Tegretol 200 mg. twice a day to see if the episodes resolve.

Irene: Great. Maybe we are getting somewhere.

Two months later during a follow up appointment, Dr. Monty learns that the seizures did resolve.

POINTS TO CONSIDER:

- Dr. Monty continued to be curious about Irene's condition, taking time to review her chart.

- When a patient has a complex medical history, it is essential to consult with other medical and mental health professionals.
- Dr. Monty seeks complete answers to his ongoing concerns.
- He listened to his patient's word of "spells" and sought consultation.
- He listened to his patient's word of "spells" and "seizures" and pursued the possibility of a diagnosis of epilepsy.

● ●

REFERENCES

1. Bayer Institute for Health Care Communication (1999). Model of Complete Clinical Care. In *Clinician-Patient Communication to Enhance Health Outcomes*. (Workshop Manual). p 6. West Haven, CT: Bayer Institute.
2. Entman SS, Glass CA et al (1994). The relationship between malpractice claims history and subsequent obstetric care. *JAMA*, 272, 20:1588-1591.
3. Levinson W, Roter DL, et al (1997). Physician-patient communication: The relationship with malpractice claims among primary care physicians and surgeons. *JAMA*, 277, 7:553-559.
4. Birdwhistell RI (1970). *Kinetic and Context: Essays on Body Motion Communications*. Philadelphia: University of Pennsylvania Press.
5. Fatt JPT (1999). It's not what you say, it's how you say it: nonverbal communication. *Communication World*, 16, 6:37(4)
6. Ekman P, Friesen WV (1974). Detecting deception from the body or face. *J Personality Soc Psych*, 54:414-420.
7. Kraut RE (1980). Humans as lie detectors: Some second thoughts. *J Communication*, 30, 209-216.
8. Vrij A, Semin GR, Bull R (1996). Insight into behavior displayed during deception. *Human Communication Research*, 22, 544-562.
9. Feeley TH, Young MJ (1998). Humans as Lie Detectors: Some More Second Thoughts. *Communication Quarterly*, 46,2:109-118.
10. Lown B (1996). *The Lost Art of Healing*. Boston: Houghton-Mifflin. 16.
11. Platt FW, Platt CM (1998). *Empathy: Miracle or Nothing at All*. JCOM, 5,2:32.
12. Spiro H, Curnen M, Peschel E, St James E, eds. (1993). *Empathy and the Practice of Medicine*. New Haven, CT: Yale University Press.
13. Olson DP (1997). Development of an instrument to measure the cognitive structure used to understand personhood in patients. *Nursing Res*, 46:78-84. Cited in Platt, op. cit. 32.
14. Beckman H, Frankel R (1984). The effect of physician behavior on the collection of data. *Ann Intern Med*, 101: 692-696. Cited in Platt, op. cit. 135.
15. Ramsey PG, Curtis JR, Paauw DSY, et al. (1998) History-taking and preventitive medicine skills among primary care physiand: an assessment using standardized patients. *Am. J. Med*. 104: 152-158.
16. Lown B (1996). *The Lost Art of Healing*. New York: Houghton Mifflin Co. 17.
17. Roter DL, Hall JA, et al (1995). Improving physicians' interviewing skills and reducing patient's emotional distress. *Arch Internal Med*, 155, 1877-1884.
18. Keller & Carroll, op. cit., 135.
19. Braddock III, CH, et al (1999). Informed Decision Making in Outpatient Practice: Time to Get Back to Basics *JAMA*, 282:24:2313-2320.
20. Peterson MR (1992). *At Personal Risk: Boundary Violations in Professional-Client Relationships*. New York: WW Norton.
21. Cardello LL, et al. (1995). The Relationship of Perceived Physician Communicator Style to Patient Satisfaction. *Communication Reports*, 8,1: 27-37.
22. Conlee CJ, et al (1993). The Relationships among Physician Nonverbal Immediacy and Measures of Patient Satisfaction with Physician. *Communication Reports*, 6,1:25-33.
23. Quill TE (1996). *A Midwife Through the Dying Process: Stories of Healing and Hard Choices at the End of Life*. Baltimore: Johns Hopkins Univ Press.
24. Lown op cit.
25. Council on Ethical and Judicial Affairs, American Medical Association. (1991) Sexual misconduct in the practice of medicine. *JAMA*, 266: 2741.
26. Bayer Training Manual.
27. Farber NJ, Novack DH, O'Brien MK (1997). Love, boundaries and the physician-patient relationship. *Arch Internal Med*, 157:2291-2294.

CHAPTER 5

Sensitization to Prejudice and Discrimination

This chapter addresses how prejudices can affect professional objectivity. Subtle forms of discrimination may deny patients the professional care they deserve. We explore the ramifications of prejudice and discrimination based on stereotypes about 1 — race and ethnicity, 2 — sexual orientation, and 3 — age, disability and weight. Specific guidelines on how health care providers can identify and reduce prejudice and discrimination within their profession as well as in the workplace are provided.

Processing Social Information

The last chapter explored how behaviors arising out of a patient's own anxiety, fear, anger, or discomfort at being sick, or being in a clinic, or about meeting a new health care provider could lead the provider to an adverse evaluation of the patient's like-ability, treatability, and manageability. Another powerful barrier that can cloud professional judgment are stereotypes related to prejudices. Without realizing it, most people routinely make snap judgments based on gender, race, ethnicity, religion, age, socioeconomic status, gender orientation, physical and mental disabilities and even physical fitness or appearance. This nearly automatic process of forming impressions is probably best explained by the discipline of Social Psychology. It teaches that human beings form impressions of others fairly quickly after meeting another person for the first time. The process of person perception generally follows the six principles shown in Box 5-1. One reason the process is so rapid is that people seek

certainty about *how* to relate to the other person. We want answers to questions such as: "Is this person good or bad?", and "Do I like or dislike the person?" On the most fundamental level of instinctual survival, we want to know whether the person we have just met is safe to be with.[1]

CATEGORIZING AND STEREOTYPING: AN AUTOMATIC PROCESS

Because humans are social beings, they also display the tendency to group themselves and others as belonging either to an **ingroup** or to an **outgroup**.[2] To understand this tendency, we invite the reader to think back to a time when this process of categorization and the formation of prejudices and discrimination may have played a role in your life. Some will recall the different cliques that dominated the scene in junior high or high school. Each clique, whether at the top or the bottom of the hierarchy of desirability, considered itself an ingroup. Ingroup membership was characterized by a strong sense of solidarity, and also by members referring to themselves as "we." Non members were automatically were referred to as "they" and were considered to be in the outgroup. Most cliques had **prejudices** — or negative beliefs and attitudes about the other groups. For example, those who wore the latest designer label clothes — one clique common in most schools — the "preppies" were likely to look down on the kids without fashionable clothes, often calling them negative names.

When name calling, judgments, or prejudices are translated into actions denying members of specific outgroups the rights and privi-

---

Box 5-1 Person Perception: Forming Impressions of Others[40]

In thinking about how people form impressions of others, it is useful to keep in mind six quite simple and general principles:

1. People form impressions of others quickly on the basis of minimal information and go on to impute general traits to them.

2. Perceivers pay special attention to the most salient features of a person, rather than paying attention to everything. They notice the qualities that make a person distinctive or unusual. This may include racial, ethnic characteristics, or age.

3. Processing information about people involves perceiving some coherent meaning in their behavior. To a degree, the perceiver uses the context of a person's behavior to infer its meaning, rather than interpreting the behavior in isolation.

4. The perceiver organizes the perceptual field by categorizing or grouping stimuli. Rather than seeing each person as a separate individual, the perceiver tends to see people as members of groups — a man wearing a dark blue uniform as a police officer, even though that person may have features that make them quite different from other officers.

5. Inner cognitive structures are used to make sense of people's behavior. Upon identifying a woman as a police officer, the perceiver uses previously stored information about police officers more generally to infer the meaning of their behavior.

6. A perceiver's own needs and personal goals influence how they perceive others. For example, the impression you form of someone you will meet only once is different from the impression you form about a future colleague.

---

leges of the ingroup, it is called **discrimination**. In some extreme instances, the dominant ingroup in a society may categorize target minority groups as less than human, leading to assumptions that they do not deserve to be accorded full human or civil rights. The 20th century had several examples of extreme depri-

vations of civil rights from the Holocaust and tribal genocide in Africa and the Middle East, to ethnic cleansing in Bosnia and Kosovo.

DISCRIMINATION IN HEALTH CARE

Health care providers follow the Hippocratic oath to provide care and to do no harm. It is assumed that care is provided without reservations regarding gender, race, ethnicity, religion, disability, or gender orientation. Thus, health care providers have a special responsibility to be aware of their human tendency to categorize others into stereotypes based on group membership. Health care providers may tell themselves that they are not prejudiced because they believe that good persons should not have prejudices. However, as a matter of human nature, it is almost impossible to be completely free of stereotypes and prejudice. In the socialization process, human beings learn and internalize generalizations about certain groups of people. Many people pick up stereotypical impressions from comments made by their parents, from their peers in childhood and adolescence, from depictions in the media, and from personal experience with members of a specific group or category of persons. Many such generalizations are stored away in the recesses of the mind. Such stereotypes are primed or activated when they meet a person from such a group. The risk for health care providers is that they might — without consciously realizing it — react to a patient *as if* that person were going to automatically exhibit certain character traits or behaviors "typical" of the group.

•••••••••••••••••••••••••••••••

PATIENT PROFILE 5.1

JUST MAKE HIM NICE

SETTING: *Jimmy, a 24-year-old mildly developmentally delayed man, presents to the clinic with his mother, Rose who is also mildly developmentally delayed. Rose reports that Jimmy has been angry and verbally abusive to her lately, especially since he graduated from high school. She* *has heard that there is a pill for angry people that will make them "nice". Nancy, their nurse practitioner, has been providing their health care for 8 years now.*

As Nancy walks into the examination room, she asks Jimmy how he is. Rose immediately answers for him in an angry and pressured manner:

Rose: He's not right in the head. He's never been right in the head. He used to be so nice and all, but now he is so mean to me. I just don't know what to do. I hear there's a pill that will make him nice again.

Nancy: *(There she goes again answering for Jimmy. No wonder he is angry. She doesn't give him a chance to speak. A "nice" pill. That's a new one on me.)* Hello Rose, I haven't heard about a "nice" pill but let's talk and see if we can understand why Jimmy is so angry now. I can understand that you are feeling upset and maybe even confused because Jimmy used to mind you and you both got along so well. *(Maybe I'd better hear what this "nice" pill is that she is talking about, but first I need to make some connection with Jimmy. He is sitting there so quiet and tense.)* Rose, I need to talk just with Jimmy now. Is that OK?

Rose nods.

Nancy: Jimmy, how are you doing with those two puppies you told me about at our last appointment?

His eyes light up. He smiles and says:

Jimmy: They are close to 4 months now and you know how puppies are — just jumpin' and carryin' on.

Nancy: *(Jimmy has such a nice smile. His whole face changes when he smiles. I had better find out about his behavior and his feelings. Mom is getting restless.)* I bet they are. Do you think the puppies have caused your mother to be upset with you?

Jimmy: No. She likes the way I take care of them.

Nancy: Good. So, let's talk about your new behavior that is upsetting your mother. OK?

Jimmy hangs his head and Rose blurts out:

Rose: I just can't do anything with him. He's changed on me. He won't do his chores. He sits and daydreams on the porch. He wanders off and doesn't let me know where he is going. When I ask him where he's been, he snaps back at me.

Nancy: *(I really need to talk with Jimmy more but Rose keeps answering for him. I'll ask her to step out for a minute so I can talk with Jimmy. I can ask her about this magic pill later.)* Rose, I would like to talk with Jimmy alone.

Rose: Oh sure. I'll go back to the room where the magazines are. Some of them have nice pictures.

Rose leaves. Nancy turns to Jimmy who is about ready to explode, obviously wanting to unload his feelings.

Jimmy: I don't want to hang around with my Mother the rest of my life. I want a life. I want friends. I want a job. I want a girlfriend. I love my Mother and she's good to me, but she gets on my nerves and then I get on her nerves and oh, it's just a mess. I was talking with some guys downtown about a training center. Maybe I could learn something that would help me get a job. I like computers.

Nancy: *(Jimmy is ready to move on with his life and his Mother hasn't noticed that. And for that matter, neither did I. Jimmy's been out of school a year and a half now. He deserves a life. I guess I'd just thought he'd live at home with his Mother and that was it. My own thoughts about his mental deficiencies may have hindered me from being aware that he is maturing socially and does want a life of his own. I think he's angry and acting out because he is realizing he can do more with his life. I wonder too if he is developing hormonally now and whether that is a factor with his anger.)* Sure, Jimmy. You are right on the target. Let's bring your mother back in and talk with her about your wants and needs.

Jimmy: Great! *(Oh she understands me and she isn't mad at me. She's nice.)*

POINTS TO CONSIDER:

- Nancy paraphrases and redirects Rose's frustration so that a productive discussion can follow.

- After supporting Rose and settling her down, she realizes she needs to talk with Jimmy alone. The chances of him opening up about what is going on are better in a one-to-one interview especially since Rose tends to answer for him.

- Nancy's own preconceived ideas about Jimmy's abilities had limited her thinking which made it easier to stereotype Jimmy. Having learned of Jimmy's own expectations and goals, she is now eager to support his efforts to have his own life.

• •

In the complex situation of health care, one way health care providers tend to apply stereotypes is when they size up patients for like-ability, treatability and manageability. If a health care provider forms the impression that they are not likely to be successful with patients from certain minority groups, the health care provider may not make as vigorous an effort to engage, empathize, educate, and enlist them. Indeed since certain ethnic minorities, like African Americans and Hispanics are heavily under represented in health care professions, it is likely that patients from those groups will be treated by a provider who does not share their cultural beliefs. Thus, in many instances of cross cultural contact, there is the possibility of miscommunication, fear, mistrust and poor decision making by both health care provider and patient.[3] The completion of the Student Exercise on this page may assist you in identifying your prejudices.

Specific Target Groups

RACIAL AND ETHNIC PREJUDICE

In looking at racial and ethnic prejudice and discrimination in health care, we will take African Americans as a sample minority population. As mentioned in Chapter 2, other racial and ethnic

---

What Are My Prejudices?

Take paper and pencil. On the left hand side of the sheet of paper list each of the target groups listed in the chapter. Leave some room between each. Then, as you focus on one group at a time, record any associations, memories, positive or negative beliefs that appear in your mind. You may come up with blanks on some groups about which <u>you</u> know little, or may not have had any contact. Even in those cases, you may have formed some impressions from the media. After you have written down the stereotype, search your mind for at least one person from each target group, whom you have met, or know by reputation, who contradicts the stereotypes.

Use the image of the person you identified to disarm your personal stereotype by illustrating the fallacy of applying blanket judgments to all members of the group.

---

minority patients from Hispanics, Native Americans, Asian Americans and Pacific Islanders also tend to receive lesser care than members of the dominant ingroup, i.e., White Americans.[4] For example, several ethnic minorities tend to avail themselves of mammography at much lower rates.[5,6] A general finding was that certain expensive high technology health care procedures with preventive features were not offered to minority patients with the same frequency as to Caucasian patients.[7,8] Some of the factors have to do with poverty and access to health care, but even research which controlled for socioeconomic and health status differences found that the health care received by African Americans tended to be worse than that received by Caucasians.[9] Box 5-2 provides a disturbing glimpse of how stereotypes might interfere with communication between health care provider and African American patients.

In care situations, like the lung cancer study, the problem leading to misunderstanding is likely to be on both sides of the ethnic or racial divide.

Box 5-2 Racial Disparity in Rates of Surgery for Early Stage Lung Cancer[41]

The 1999 report of a study of 11,000 lung cancer patients over 65, found that African-American patients were less likely than White patients to get surgery for early stages of lung cancer, and as a result were more likely to die from a potentially curable disease. Since the study found no significant differences in socioeconomic status, insurance coverage, complicating illnesses, or access to care, this differential in care and mortality raises two disquieting possibilities. Either doctors were not recommending surgery to African-Americans as often as to Whites, or African-Americans for some reason were more likely to say "No" to lifesaving surgery.

One explanation offered by the authors of the study is that silent stereotypes may be at work here on both sides. They suggest that White doctors and African-American patients may have trouble communicating with each other, partly because of an undercurrent of tension between the races, and partly because of differences in social class,

education and culturally determined beliefs. Telling someone that they have cancer and must have all or part of a lung cut out, is a wrenching and arduous task in any circumstance. If the health care provider does not understand the African-American patient's cultural beliefs and suspicions about White medicine, they may not present the information in a way that the patient can understand or will trust. Thus, African-American patients may distrust the advice or the urgency of a physician not of their own race. The infamous Tuskegee study of untreated syphilis has made many African-Americans leery of participating in any clinical trials or even large screening programs for sickle cell anemia.[41] Such distrust may predispose them to reject treatment advice, or they might agonize so long, that the cancer might become inoperable by the time they decide. The unfortunate consequences of such distrust and miscommunication are unnecessary suffering and higher mortality rates.

For example, a specialist may assume that a minority group patient is not likely to listen or take their advice for an invasive procedure like an operation for early stage lung cancer. Thus, they may not try to communicate past the expected resistance. In fact, one interpretation of the study cited in Box 5-2 is that doctors in such situations may have found it easier to tell themselves that they tried, and thus, let the minority group patient walk away without communicating sufficient urgency regarding life saving surgery. In addressing this issue, Dr. Talmadge King, Chief of Medical Services at San Francisco General Hospital, editorialized that "this is not good enough." He stated, "We have tended to blame the patient, but I think the problem is on the side of the doctors. It's up to us to understand where the patient is, and learn how to communicate so they can understand what we're saying."[10] Dr. King's point that the health care system needs to take steps to bridge the cultural gaps is well taken.

Innovative outreach projects have demonstrated that when health care information is presented in a culturally congruent manner and set-

ting, in the same language as the patients', underuse of life saving procedures (like mammography, pap smears, or prostate cancer screening) by minority groups can be reduced.[11] Such efforts need to be made especially for non-English speaking patients. Since foreign language abilities are not emphasized in the American educational system, problems arise almost automatically when non-English speaking patients enter the health care system. Inability to speak a common language is a strong barrier to fulfilling the communication tasks described in Chapter Four (engage, empathize, educate, and enlist). It requires effort and patience to either make do with pidgin English and sign language, or to find an interpreter. Rushed health care providers may opt for the former, convincing themselves that they did their best "under the circumstances." As in the lung cancer study cited above, health care providers may simply not make the extra effort to explain fully additional life saving treatment options to non-English speaking patients. Unfortunately the potential for misunderstandings, and recriminations are high in such situations.

HOMOPHOBIA AND HETEROSEXISM

Homophobia is the antipathy or disdain for gay men and lesbians, which is a widespread response to this previously hidden segment of society. Although approximately 10% of the general population is **gay, lesbian, bisexual or transgendered** (GLBT) (with much higher concentrations in some locations), the unique health needs of these patients are often ignored.[12,13] Moreover, the portrayal of lesbians, gays, bisexuals and transgendered persons in health textbooks has often been biased, while discussion of the health care needs of these patients has been either missing or has been influenced by subtle homophobia until recently.[14,15] Inappropriate and inaccurate stereotypes included: viewing gay men as effeminate and creative, lesbians as masculine and sexually frustrated, and bisexuals and transgendered persons as confused.[16] Worse, daytime talk shows "using the low-risk strategy of voyeurism" to sensationalize examples of kinky and outrageous relationships and sexual practices, have blurred any "neat binary division between heterosexual and homosexual."[17] The message from family, peers and religious leaders for a long time was that any orientation other than heterosexual is abnormal, sick, perverted, sinful, and that it contributes to the breakdown of the family. Hate crimes against homosexuals are a still a reality in American society. With so much open hostility, it is not surprising that the vast majority of homosexuals stay hidden.[18]

• •

PATIENT PROFILE 5.2

THIS IS HARD FOR ME

SETTING: *Nora, a 34-year-old woman and security guard at a large detention center for young offenders, comes to an outpatient clinic attached to a large urban hospital. Lars, a physician assistant, has been providing health care for Nora for 2 years now. She has returned to hear the results of laboratory tests confirming that she has a candida infection.*

Lars: Hello, Nora. The results of the laboratory test confirm that you have a candida infection.

Nora grimaces and then says:

Nora: Does that mean I should tell the person I had sex with what I have?

Lars: Yes, and perhaps he needs to see his doctor for treatment.

Nora: *("He?" "His?" Well maybe it's time to tell him I am a lesbian. I have talked with him about some gay and les friends I have. He doesn't seem to overreact or say anything negative. I'm pretty sure it's OK to tell him. He's straight. If he puts on that "holier than thou attitude", I can always go somewhere else for medical care. I hope he accepts me. He does keep asking me if I have a boyfriend. I get so tired of that. My parents used to ask me that until I outed to them. Oh, I get so tired of having to do this. Why can't this society just accept us for how we are?)* Well, there's something I've been wanting to tell you but I — this is hard for me.

Lars: *("Hard" ? — I'd better reassure her.)* Nora, you've known me for 2 years now. You know that you can talk with me about anything. We took care of a couple of episodes of the flu, and that time you broke your clavicle in a tussle with one of the incarcerated youths, as well as the hepatitis scare you had when an active carrier bit you.

Lars sits quietly, leaning forward with a pleasant, mildly expectant look on his face.

Nora: *(Here goes –)* I am a lesbian. There, I've said it.

Lars: *(I had wondered if she was homosexual. She never said anything about dating, or having a boyfriend. I'd better approach this delicately. She said this was really hard for her.)* I am glad you told me. I know that coming out can be very difficult. I appreciate that you trust me enough to tell me about your orientation. I'm sorry that I kept asking about you having a boyfriend. I should have asked you if you had a significant other or a partner. Using a more neutral term might have had us talking about this sooner than now. Well, again, thank you for telling me. Can I ask a few questions? The information may help me provide better and more relevant medical care to you in the future.

Nora: *(Whew! I'm glad that's over and he's being sensible about this.)* Sure, Lars. I'm really relieved that you understand.

POINTS TO CONSIDER:

- Lars picks up on the phrase "hard for me". Although he does not know what it is, he decides to generally remind her of their history together and to give her reassurance.

- By communicating in a pleasant and non-threatening manner to Nora, he continues to encourage her to tell him what she needs to tell him.

- Lars is aware that he needs to respond with sensitivity and professionalism.

- Every time a homosexual tells someone about their gender orientation and the experience is positive, it strengthens their ability to continue to tell others in their life, thus minimizing the pressure their orientation has on them intrapsychically and socially.

• •

Coming out for GLBT persons is usually a gradual and difficult internal process occurring in six stages,[19] requiring enormous courage, and energy. (See Chapter 7.) Persons coming out must constantly evaluate whom they can trust with their sexual identity.[20] Gay youth are particularly vulnerable to internal and external pressures, resulting in higher rates of depression, suicide, substance abuse, and homelessness (due to running away).[21] Suicide is the leading cause of death among gay, lesbian, and bisexual adolescents, accounting for up to 40% of all adolescent suicide attempts[22] and possibly as much as 30% of completed suicides.[23] Lesbians have higher rates of breast and cervical cancer, possibly because they do not get regular checkups. The fear of stigmatization often prevents them from coming out to their health care providers.[24] Indeed the biggest threat to the health of this sexual minority population is that they avoid health care because of the fear of discrimination.

Their fears may be well founded. Studies have shown that health care professionals and staff persons tend to be less tolerant of GLBT patients.[25]

Working for Inclusivity

What can health care providers do to change this situation? One, is to educate themselves on the etiology of gender orientation and to develop an understanding of the unique health and mental health challenges faced by this minority population. (Chapter 7 will deal with the biological etiology of homosexuality in more detail.) Two, is to learn to use *non-heterosexist* language in health care delivery. The health care provider may also need to revise the patient intake form. Most standard intake forms only list *married, single, divorced, widowed.* The simple addition of category "partnered" would show inclusivity. One such example would be in the way the health care provider elicits a medical history. If they automatically assume heterosexuality in a female patient, an answer of "yes" to the question "Are you sexually active?" would automatically lead the health care provider to concerns about contraception, and pregnancy. Such concerns might not only be irrelevant, but might make a lesbian patient uncomfortable, because of the heterosexist assumptions. Simply adding the question "Are your partners men, women, or both?" at the history-taking stage increases the likelihood that the patient will share her identity as lesbian or bisexual. Other neutral questions like: "Are you married, partnered, or single?" and " Is there a significant person in your life?"[26] also demonstrate sensitivity. Literature, signs, or posters placed on bulletin boards can indicate acceptance and inclusivity and can show that an office or clinic is a safe place to discuss GLBT health concerns.*

Policies at many hospitals or residential facilities still exclude persons other than the immediate biological family from visiting patients. This often prevents seriously ill GLBT patients

---

*Discreet literature is available from Wildflowers Inc. at www.bloomington.in.us/~iwish/wildflower/

from getting crucial social support from their partners or friends. Working actively towards changing these policies to allow identified partners to visit is another way to reduce prejudice and discrimination in the health care setting.[27]

Other suggestions for improving health care for this population rest on the general admonition to treat each person as an individual rather than as a stereotype. Using the communication model from Chapter 4, be ready to be informed by the patient's story, rather than having pathology oriented assumptions about homosexuality. Explore the unique aspects of each person's experiences with a non-judgmental attitude. Finally, if you feel discomfort or fear, you need to identify and work through your own attitudes regarding homophobia, homosexuality, bisexuality and transgender issues. A first step to help you with your own feelings of prejudice is to get to know someone who has a brother, sister, son or daughter who is GLBT. Another way to counter your biases is to make the effort to become acquainted with a person of differing sexual orientation. Hopefully you will realize that their sexual orientation is irrelevant to how they perform their professional duties. Finally, if you feel that non-judgmental, respectful, professional care of a patient is difficult for you because of his or her gender orientation, you should refer that person to another provider.

PREJUDICE BASED ON AGE, MENTAL ILLNESS AND OTHER FACTORS

Age

Another target group are persons who do not fit society's norms of "normal." Society often puts the aged, the physically disabled and those with mental disorders into this category. It is said that America lives in a youth-oriented, throw-away culture. The popular media has an obsessive fascination with beauty, and the sex lives of the young, rich and famous. The cosmetics and pharmaceutical industries thrive on selling products to enhance beauty, youth, and sexual drive. By the same token, American society appears

almost phobic about aging. **Ageism** is the term coined for the many negative stereotypes about aging and the subtle discrimination against older people.[28] An example would be adult children assuming that their parents are no longer capable of certain physical activities (including having sex) because they are "too old." Or they start making decisions for them on the assumption that they can no longer do so for themselves.

Health care providers may deny that they hold any prejudice against the elderly. However, some of the unflattering labels by health care staff and professionals applied to older patients reveal a bias coming from underlying unspoken attitudes. Demeaning terms such as: decrepit, rigid, senile, little old lady, dirty old man, old biddy, gummer, frail and useless, grouchy or grumpy old man, or a GOMER (get out of my emergency room) tend to **infantilize** older persons, making them appear incompetent to make decisions. You need to remember that some character or behavioral descriptors apply to a tiny minority of persons in any age group. In point of fact, persons are now living much longer and healthier lives due in part to better nutrition, more awareness of self care requirements, new breakthroughs in pharmacology, and advanced technology in body part replacement. Indeed the large majority of persons entering old age is much healthier than ever before. The graying of America will accelerate dramatically when the large cohort of **baby boomers** enters retirement age in the second decade of this century.[29] These "young old" people are not likely to see themselves as old. They no longer take for granted that they will have degenerative conditions at ages when that used to be the norm. Indeed older patients will resent any hint of negative stereotyping by their health care providers. Health care providers need to be aware not only of the demographic shift in the population, but also of the internal attitude shift of self concept in the population approaching their sixties, seventies or eighties. Health care providers must not assume that older patients are a homogeneous group with similar attributes. Thus, it is essential to complete careful assessments, unbiased by expectations that a pathology condition is automatically age related, and therefore "normal." Health care providers need to engage, educate, and enlist these patients with the same respect, patience, and expectation that they are as fully functioning and competent as any other patient. At the same time, it is self evident that in many respects geriatric medicine is different. Chapter 8 will take a closer look at these differences.

Mental Illness

In American society there is a stigma associated with mental disorders.[30] The American cultural norms of being independent, being in control, of being OK, are seen as violated by someone whose mental and emotional functioning is deemed not "normal." In fact, there is evidence that primary health care providers are reluctant to identify and refer patients even with relatively minor mental health symptoms, like mild depression, anxiety, or adjustment disorders.[31] The negative cultural stereotypes may predispose a health care provider to suspect that such "complaints" may be **factitious**, i.e., made up, to get attention or to malinger. Such an attitude may make health care providers less sympathetic to the plight of patients who may have a dual diagnosis of other physical problems in addition to a mental disorder For example, authors of one study hypothesize that "medical providers' discomfort in treating patients with mental disorders might make them reluctant to offer these patients aggressive treatment (for physical pathologies) even when medically appropriate."[32]

Somatization of untreated psychiatric problems tends to be associated with increased medical services.[33,34] Frequently, psychological problems, like depression or anxiety, arise out of stresses and traumas in the psychosocial situation of the patient. Thus, a health care provider, who is unwilling or uncomfortable about acknowledging psychiatric problems or even belittle such problems may increase their patients' distress. As presented in Chapters 10 and 11, this is especially true in situations of domestic violence or sexual abuse. Chapter 12 provides greater detail in how to identify and work with patients with mental disorders.

Smoking

There are several other categories of patients who sometimes meet with less than sympathetic reception by their health care providers. Some are persons with behaviors that cause their illness or pathology. Thus, health care providers tend to blame heavy smokers who develop emphysema, COPD, or lung cancer. In fact their attitude may harden, if the patient is "unwilling" to immediately follow their recommendation to stop smoking. What health care professionals need to remember here is that nicotine is one of the most addictive substances.[35] Thus, it may be more helpful to acknowledge the dependence and to focus on providing support for patients in their efforts to wean themselves off smoking or to stop smoking, than to go into the mode of "disapproval" or write them off because they are "not compliant."

Obesity

Similarly, some health care providers may find it difficult to provide unbiased care for obese patients. The cultural emphasis on being thin has conditioned many of us to put unflattering labels on overweight persons. Health care providers may blame the patient for health conditions related to obesity. To put obesity into perspective, health care providers need to remind themselves, that unless there is solid evidence for organic or metabolic problems, they need to examine patterns of obesity as the probable result of psychosocial pressures or trauma. Obesity can be a somatic response to childhood sexual abuse, rape, or an unhappy marriage. In women it is often associated with low self-esteem, depression, and suicidality.[36] These factors should be seen as a red flag that may signal a subconscious self sabotage. Thus, health care providers need to be sensitive to assessing for depression and the possible need for counseling. Addressing the underlying psychosocial causes is likely to eliminate unconscious barriers to treatment adherence.

Counteracting Prejudice and Discrimination

It is essential for a personal sense of justice as well as professional self image, that health care providers take proactive steps to disarm their own biases and prejudices. The question "Am I prejudiced?" does not encompass the dimensions of automatic judgments that health care providers routinely make. Most people tend to be unaware of hidden prejudices. As pointed out at the beginning of the chapter, our rapid and automatic information processing of incoming perceptions leads to categorizations based on stereotypes. Some may not directly affect our professional work, while others could interfere with our ability to communicate with members of specific groups, and thus affect the general level of care. Hence, we need to ask ourselves *How prejudiced am I?* This requires a willingness to complete a self examination of our personal beliefs about specific target groups. (See Patient Profile 5.3.)

● ●

PATIENT PROFILE 5.3

WE MIGHT AS WELL BE HONEST WITH EACH OTHER

SETTING: Carleton, a 55-year-old African-American male with lung cancer, has completed one series of chemotherapy and radiation at a large urban oncology clinic. The chemotherapy and radiation treatments were not very successful. Carleton quit a 20-year, two-pack-a-day smoking habit the day he was diagnosed with lung cancer. Mark, a Caucasian male, one year out of his oncology residency, has reviewed Carleton's medical record and is meeting with Carleton today to discuss the results of his treatments and future treatment options.

Mark: Good morning Carleton. How are you today?

Carleton: Actually pretty good. I'm glad I'm through with radiation and chemotherapy. I am proud of myself that I am still a non-smoker!

Mark: Good for you! *(Here is where we enter into some possibly troublesome information. He got one round of radiation and chemotherapy, but at this stage of the disease, a more aggressive approach is indicated — lung surgery . Why do I feel uncomfortable talking with him about this? Is it about discrimination? Am I afraid as a white man, he'll feel like I'm wanting to "cut him up"? On one hand I need to be aware of any prejudice going on in this matter and I also need to treat him professionally. I am 20 years his junior. Maybe he'll have problems hearing about surgery from someone so much younger than he is. Also, I've disliked smoking all my life, especially since my favorite grandfather died of emphysema. I don't think I am counter transfering but I must be sure not to judge him because he was a smoker. It's a powerful addiction. He deserves the best medical care we can give him.)* Today, we need to discuss the results of your treatments.

Carleton: *(He's awfully young. Just out of residency. Can I trust him?)* Yes, I'd like to hear what you have to say.

Mark: *(Maybe I should just bring up the race and age issue up front.)* But first, can I ask you a question? *(I'll start off with a question about my age first and work into the race issue if it seems appropriate.)*

Carleton nods yes but has a slightly guarded look on his face.

Mark: *(He looks a little guarded.)* I finished my oncology residence a year ago. Some people are concerned that I am so young. Does that bother you?

Carleton laughs with relief.

Carleton: Frankly, yes! *(I might as well be honest with him. I'm glad he brought it up.)*

Mark: That is a concern for some of my patients. Thanks for being honest with me. I graduated top of my class and the clinic gives me very positive feedback as well. If you have any questions, you can ask my supervising physician who is the clinic director.

Carleton: I don't think I will need to do that, but thanks for offering.

Mark: *(So that went well. Now I think I'll ask him about the race issue.)* I have another question.

Carleton looks at him expectantly.

Mark: You are African-American and I am white and sometimes that can cause difficulties in communication. I thought I'd just bring it out in the open and talk with you about it. I wouldn't want any unspoken undertones to confuse the issue of our decision here.

Carleton: What kind of decisions do I have to make?

Mark: Because the chemotherapy and radiation was not as successful as we wanted, lung surgery can give you a better prognosis. This is the very best treatment option for someone at this point in treatment.

Carleton: Well, tell me more about it and then I'd like to think about it and let you know. By the way, thanks for bringing up the race differences. No, it doesn't bother me and I sense it doesn't bother you.

Mark: Sounds good. Now what are your questions about lung surgery?

POINTS TO CONSIDER:

- Mark takes into consideration early on in their appointment various forms of discrimination and prejudice (age and race) as well as any possibility of counter transference.

- He is sensitive to the possibility that age or race might cloud their decision.

- Honest and non-judgmental communication is the best approach when there are questions of potential misunderstanding or prejudice.

- Sensitivity to nonverbal cues is essential in this type of an interview.

• •

If the paper and pen exercise on target groups (See Student Exercise on page 82) has identified some major or even minor stereotypes, it is an indication that you may need to make conscious efforts to see past the stereotypes. As indicated in the exercise, keeping the exemplar of the contradiction to your own stereotypes active in your mind is one way to disarm the automatic stereotypes and serve as a reminder to treat each patient as an individual.

In practice, when health care providers dislike, avoid, or have difficulties with a patient, they need to evaluate if there is a connection with having categorized that person into a target group that automatically triggered certain stereotypes. The problem with this type of labeling is that it leads to self fulfilling expectations. It is a well known phenomenon in social psychology that when human beings expect others to behave in certain ways, the "target persons" respond to those expectations and begin to behave accordingly.[37] This works both positively as well as negatively.[38] When health care providers expect their patients to be like-able, treatable, and manageable, they tend to reinforce those behaviors in their nonverbal behaviors. Unfortunately, the opposite is true also. Their internal prejudices towards a group, which translates into negative expectations of a patient, can produce the expected negative behaviors. An all too common example is when a health care provider treats older patients as foolish and incompetent, and patients fulfill those expectations by acting more helpless than they would if the professional expected them to be a fully functioning human being capable of making good decisions and following treatment regimens. It can become a circular reinforcement loop: i.e. the more the prejudiced providers find that people from a target group fulfill their expectations, the more it will reinforce their prejudice, making it less likely that they will be able to look at patients from that group as individuals. The more they discriminate against patients from specific group(s), the more distrust or distance they will generate from members.

Conclusion

Specific techniques for raising one's level of awareness as a way of dealing with one's own hidden prejudices have been presented. There are several other steps that you as an individual, as well as a professional, can take to counter prejudice and discrimination. One is to consciously seek out opportunities to make contact and interact with minority target groups in your community. You could volunteer to participate in health screenings in the neighborhoods of specific minorities. You could offer to give talks on prevention services at local community centers, AARP meetings, or Weight Watchers Clubs. Such forays into community action not only provide personal satisfaction, but also allow you to experience persons as individuals rather than merely as "all just alike." At the same time, you may also be able to learn more about their values and health concerns.

Such contacts in small groups work in both directions to reduce prejudice. When members of any of the target groups listed above see you volunteer your time, they may relate to you as a positive role model, which will go far to counteract any negative stereotypes they may have had about you as a member of the health care profession, or as a representative of a "privileged" elite. In such informal settings, persons of minority groups with traditions of "historical hostility" may get a chance to meet and like you as an individual. As a consequence, they are more likely to drop their distrust and fear of the health care system or of health care providers. You and your colleagues may benefit from more self disclosure when they need medical care.

You also need to address prejudice and discrimination in the workplace, whether it be in a clinic, hospital, or private practice. Two techniques are recommended. You can role model exemplary behavior, by refraining from joining in joking or gossiping about stereotypes that demean a specific target group. Choosing to tell jokes or indulge in idle gossip about commonly held stereotypes of negative qualities of certain groups is an endorsement of prejudice. Some would defend such jokes as useful for breaking tensions in high stress settings like emergency rooms, or operating rooms, or as a form of harmless venting. While this is undoubtedly true, they also foster a subtle solidarity among those who share the laughter, in the put-down stereotype expressed in the joke. If you wish to influence your colleagues positively you might say, *"Funny, but you know, jokes like that won't help us be less prejudiced."* If you value humor for stress reduction, make an effort to learn some jokes that are free of negative group biases.

You can also become proactive to assure an open and accepting work environment. According to the classic work done by Gordon Allport, "institutional support" is one crucial element in eliminating discrimination.[39] Clearly written office policies following the guidelines laid down for places of employment by the US Equal Employment Opportunities Commission (EEOC), or relevant state statutes are a standard first step. Covered by these guidelines on discrimination are hiring and promotion policies, sexual harassment issues, as well as any acts of discrimination against the public, i.e., patients. However, such policies on the books must be reinforced by strict and consistent implementation. Warnings and sanctions must be quickly applied to staff for any violations. It is equally important that you model exemplary behavior on this issue, whether it is refraining from sexual banter or intervening when conversation in the cafeteria or break room turns into demeaning gossip about a target group, whether that be a racial, or ethnic minority, homosexuals or a disability group. You owe it to yourselves, and you owe it to your patients to strive for health care that is free from any biases as the patient comes into the office, clinic, or hospital, and as you minister to their health needs.

REFERENCES

1. Taylor SE, Peplau LA, Sears DO (2000). *Social Psychology, 10th Ed.* Upper Saddle, NJ: Prentice Hall. 69.
2. De Cremer D, van Vugt M, Sharp J (1999). Effect of collective self-esteem on ingroup evaluations. (Cross-Cultural Notes) *J Social Psychology*, 139, 4:530(3).
3. Cooper-Patrick L, Gallo JJ, at al (1999). Race, gen-

der and partnership in the patient physician relationship, *JAMA*, 282, 6:583-89.

4. Shi L (1999). Experience of primary care by racial and ethnic groups in the United States. *Med Care*, 10:1068-77.

5. Pearlman DN, Rakowski W, Ehrich B, Clark MA (1996). Breast cancer screening practices among black, Hispanic and white women: reassessing differences. *Am J Preventive Medicine*, 12, 5:327-37.

6. Klonoff-Cohen HS, Shaffroth LB, et al (1998). Breast Cancer histology in Caucasians, African Americans Hispanics, Asians and Pacific Islanders. *Ethnic Health*, 3, 3:189-98.

7. Carlisle DM, Leake, BD, Brook RH, Shapiro MF (1996). The effect of race and ethnicity on the use of selected health care procedures: a comparison of south central Los Angeles and the remainder of Los Angeles County, *J Health Care Poor Underserved*, 7, 4:308-22.

8. McNamara KM (1999). Special Issue: racial issues in health care. *J S Carolina Med Assoc*, 95, 3:93-4.

9. Bach PB, Cramer L, Warren JL, Begg CB (1999). Racial Differences in the Treatment of Early-Stage Lung Cancer, *N Engl J Med*, 341.

10. King, TE, Brunetta P (1999). Racial Disparity in Rates of Surgery for Lung Cancer, Editorial. *N Engl J Med*, 341.

11. Sent L, Ballem P, Paluck E, et al (1998). The Asian Women's Health clinic: addressing cultural barriers to preventive health care. *Canadian Med Assoc Journal*, 159,4:350-54.

12. O'Hanlan KA, Cabaj RP, et al (1997). A review of the medical consequences of homophobia with suggestions for resolution, *J Gay Lesbian Med Assoc* 1, 1:25-39.

13. Harrison AE (1996). Primary care of lesbian and gay patients: educating ourselves and our students. *Family Medicine*, 28, 1:10-23.

14. Schwanberg SL (1990). Attitudes towards homosexuality in American health care literature . *J Homosexuality* 19, 3:117.

15. Whatley MH (1992). Images of gays and lesbians in sexuality and health textbooks. *J Homosexuality*, 22, 3-4:197-211.

16. McKee MB, Hayes SF, Axiotis IR (1994). Challenging heterosexism in college health care delivery. *J. American College Health*, 42, 5:2155-16.

17. Gamson J (1998). *Freaks Talk Back: Tabloid Talk shows and Sexual Noncomformity*. Chicago: Univ of Chicago Press.

18. Hennessy R (1994-95). Queer visibility in commodity culture. *Cultural Critique*, 29 (winter):31-75.

19. Adelman M (1990). Stigma, Gay Lifestyles, and Adjustment to Aging: A Study of Later-Life Gay Men and Lesbians. *J Homosexuality*, 20, 3:7.

20. Gibson G, Saunders DE (1994). Gay patients: context for Care. *Canadian Family Physician*, 40:721-25.

21. Table 1 — Oregon: 1999 Youth Risk Behavior Survey, Result Summary For Males & Females (Grades 9 to 12): Harassment Based on Perceived Homosexual Orientation of Individuals: Associations with Depression & Suicide Behaviors. Accessed from http://www.sws.soton.ac.uk/gay-youth-suicide/04-oregon-youth-suicide.htm#table-1

22. Remafedi G (1999). Sexual Orientation and Youth Suicide. *MS-JAMA*, 282:1291-1292. On line at http://www.ama-assn.org/sci-pubs/msjama/articles/vol_282/no_13/jms90031.htm

23. US Department of Health and Human Services (1989). Report of the Secretary's Task Force on Youth Suicide: Prevention and Interventions in Youth Suicide. Vol 3. Rockville, MD: US Dept of Health and Human Services.

24. Jones R (1988). With respect to lesbians. *Nursing Times*, 84, 20:48-49.

25. Council on Scientific Affairs, AMA (1996). Health care needs of gay men and lesbians. *JAMA*, 275, 17:1354-1359.

26. Smith M, Heaton C, Seiver D (1990). Health concerns of Lesbians. *Physician Assistant* (Jan 1990), 81-93.

27. Cogen JC (1997). Prevention of anti-lesbian and gay hate crimes through social change and empowerment in Rosenblum, ED Bond, LA *Preventing Heterosexism and homophobia*, (219-238) Newbury Park: Sage Pub.

28. Butler RN Lewis MI (1982) *Aging and Mental Health: Positive Psychosocial and Biomedical Approaches*. St. Louis: Mosby.

29. Dychtwald K, Flower J (1990) *Age Wave: The Challenge and Opportunities of an Aging America*. New York: Bantam.

30. Penn DL, Martin J (1998). The stigma of severe mental illness: some potential solutions for a recalcitrant problem. *Psychiatric Quarterly*, 69:235-247.

31. Baugham DM (1995). Barriers to diagnosing anxiety disorders in family practice. *American Family Physician*, 52:447-450. Editorial comment on 455–456.

32. Druss BG, Bradford DW, Rosenheck RA, Radford MJ, et al (2000). Mental disorders and use of cardiovascular procedures after myocardial infarction, *JAMA*, 283, 4:506-511.

33. Simon G, Ormel J, VonKorff M, Baralow W (1995). Health Care costs associated with depressive and anxiety disorders in primary care. *Am J Psychiatry*, 152:352-357.

34. Druss BG, Rohrbach RM, Rosenheck RA (1999). Depressive symptomology and health costs in older medical patients. *Am J Psychiatry*, 156:477-479.

35. National Institute on Drug Abuse (1998). *Nicotine Addiction. Research Report Series*. NIH Publication No. 98-4342.

36. Carpenter KM, Hasin DS, Allison DB, Faith MS (2000). Relationships between obesity and DSM-IV major depressive disorder, suicide ideation, and suicide attempts: results from a general population study. *Am J Public Health*, 90:251-257.

37. Jussim L (1989). Teacher expectations: Self fulfilling prophecies, perceptual biases, and accuracy. *J Personality Soc Psychol*, 57:469-480.

38. Darley JM, Fazio RH (1980). Expectancy confirmation processes arising in the social interaction sequence. *American Psychologist*, 35:867-881.

39. Allport GW (1954). *The Nature of Prejudice.* Garden City, NY: Doubleday.

40. Shoda Y, Mischel M, Wright JC (1993). Intuitive Interactionism in person perception: Effects of situational-behavior relations in dispositional judgments. *J Personality Soc Psychol*, 56:41-53.

41. Corbie-Smith G (1999). The continuing legacy of the Tuskegee Syphilis Study: considerations for clinical investigation. *Am J Med Sci*, 1999, 317-358.

CHAPTER 6

Stress Management and Self Care for the Healer

Both short term and long term studies have shown that health care providers are at greater risk for depression, suicide, substance abuse, and divorce than members of other professions.[1] Because self-care and stress management are not generally included in medical training, this chapter addresses this training gap. We examine the external contextual factors as well as the internal personality traits that contribute to stress patterns in health care professions. We offer suggestions for changing the external factors and the personality patterns. Finally, we provide practical guidelines for establishing a personal stress management program.

Overview

Since the 1960s, evidence has been accumulating that the rates for suicide, depression and emotional problems, as well as for substance abuse and divorce are significantly higher among physicians than for other professions.[2] Although relatively little in-depth research has been done on allied health professionals, some of the stressors and risk factors are common to health care settings and the culture.[3] What factors seem to make health care providers statistically more vulnerable to distress than members of other professions? Are there factors in the health care setting that increase vulnerability? Are there internal factors that lead persons with certain traits to choose health care as a profession? What traits put these persons at greater risk? Does the culture and ethic of the health care profession act as a barrier to successfully addressing stress

issues? Do the expectations of patients, colleagues and society make it difficult for them to talk about their concerns? Certainly concern over these questions has sparked renewed interest in how to ameliorate the stress in health care settings and how to help those impaired by it.[4-7] We will now examine these factors in more detail.

PERSONAL FACTORS

Many persons are drawn to the health care professions because they want to help others. However, many of those self-selecting into health care professions may come with psychological vulnerabilities arising out of their individual adjustment to childhood instability or turbulence in adolescence.[8] One groundbreaking longitudinal study first noted that paradoxically physicians were more likely than the control group to show traits of dependency, pessimism, passivity and self-doubt.[9] Another trait thought to be widely shared among health care professionals is perfectionism.[10] While this trait may make for conscientiousness in study habits and patient care, it can also lead to an unforgiving attitude when mistakes occur. Perfectionism is also thought to be a barrier to disclosure to their colleagues. Making medical mistakes was found to cause great distress, but fear of malpractice suits and feeling unable to disclose such mistakes greatly exacerbated stress levels. Other researchers used repeated administrations of the Minnesota Multiphase Personality Inventory (MMPI) to predict symptoms of burnout among 440 physicians.[11] They found that higher burnout rates were significantly correlated with certain personality antecedents recorded in their MMPI before they entered medical training. The MMPI scales most significant were those measuring low self-esteem, feelings of inadequacy, dysphoria and obsessive worry, passivity, social anxiety, and withdrawal from others.

By contrast, a study looking at what made for a successful adjustment among physicians identified several positive traits.[12] The ability to maintain individual identities from the family of origin (individuation) was a strong predictor of psychological well being. Other predictors for good adjustment to the rigors of practicing medicine were the ability to maintain high levels of support from at least one "significant other", and lower levels of practice stress.

THE CULTURE OF MEDICINE

Professionals in health care are exposed to idealized expectations from patients and from society, (including insurance companies, and regulatory and accreditation agencies) and from their colleagues. As one group of researchers put it:

> Physicians are expected to be healers, available to others whenever a crisis or medical need arises, are expected to have unfailing expertise and competence, to be compassionate and concerned, and to provide universally successful care in a cost effective manner.[13]

Institutions within the health care system reinforce these idealized expectations in their training process, clinics, hospitals, collegial relationships, and professional associations. It is understandable therefore that most internalize these expectations as they move from training to practicing professionals. However, no health care professional can consistently live up to such idealized expectations. If reinforced by a perfectionist personality, the effort to live up to such an idealized image can become a barrier to reaching out and getting support. Internalized expectations that they have to be strong and always available and never faltering can foster a denial of personal vulnerability, and fears about revealing mistakes. Health care by its nature contains

unique stresses, such as coping with intense emotions around issues of suffering, fear, sexuality, death, demanding patients and their families, and constant uncertainty about personal limits of medical knowledge.[14] Often these emotional pressures occur in rapid fire sequence. Sometimes the 36-hour on/36-hour off work schedule may exhaust the professional's physical and emotional reserves. It is not surprising that many direct care providers struggle during training and in later years to harden themselves to these emotional and physical demands.

The training process for health care providers itself promotes an unhealthy life style, and emotional distancing.[15] Sleep deprivation during academic training, rotations and residency often produce cognitive impairment and emotional fragility. More importantly, the constant demands of the training process condition the professional to accept the "workaholic standards" of the medical culture, and to take on more work, which may result in the suppression or compartmentalization of their own feelings. Self-neglect becomes common, because long hours and an uncomplaining attitude are rewarded in many practice settings.[16] Health care professionals are noted for not paying attention to their own health. They tend not to seek routine medical care for themselves or their families. In fact, many will prescribe medication for themselves rather than seek out care from another practitioner. Learned self-neglect appears to be one reason. Another is fear of contradicting the idealized image of being strong, by revealing a physical or emotional frailty or failing. A third reason is the issue of trust. While exposed to a lot of confidential and emotional material from their patients, practitioners often find it hard to confide in others.[17] Part of this distrust is the expectations often justified, that they will not receive sympathetic hearing or support from their colleagues (who often have internalized similar idealized expectations of themselves and their profession). Another characteristic of the medical culture — regarding it as "special," reinforces the unwillingness to disclose to a colleague, or to seek emotional support when needed. The respect for their fellow VIP professional may prevent a practitioner from being intrusive in their questioning and less aggressive in their treatment of a colleague. Not wanting to spot signs of emotional distress in a colleague may play a role in not following up on hunches about depression and other symptoms that might lead to subsequent suicides.

• •

PATIENT PROFILE 6.1

I itch all over!

SETTING: Caroline, a 34-year-old married woman, has come in to see Mary for a skin problem. Caroline and Mary went to Physician Assistant school together and were in the same study group. After graduation, they kept in touch, closely at first but later mainly through patient referrals to each other. Mary, who is also married, works in a local clinic with three general practitioners.

Mary walks into the examining room and warmly greets her friend and colleague. They chitchat for a few moments. Then Caroline laughing somewhat nervously says: "Mary, I itch all over. I think I'm allergic to my husband!" They both laugh.

Caroline, (more seriously): I think I have hives. I've watched my diet, eliminated anything I might be allergic to and when George (her husband) and I — " (Breaks down in tears.)

Mary hands her some Kleenex and waits for her to continue. (*I have never seen Caroline cry like this. Something really serious must have happened.*)

Caroline: Well, I feel so embarrassed. There was no one I felt I could talk to. I know most of the psychotherapists in town and just couldn't face any of them. Fish bowl phenomenon, you know. (Deep sigh.) George has been having an affair and he just told me about it. He thinks he wants a separation. Between a knot in my gut and this skin problem, I'm a mess.

Mary: Oh, I'm so sorry, Caroline, it must have been very upsetting to hear about the affair, but

let's take one thing at a time. Tell me about what is going on with your skin.

Caroline: Well, the hives seem to come up out of the blue. The only precipitating factor might be that when George and I start to argue, they pop up, all over. I itch all over. It's awful! Maybe I'm allergic to him!

Mary: And the knot in your stomach?

Caroline: Well, it's probably emotional. The knot in my gut is about here (pointing to the epigastric area). I've been trying to relax but it's hard not knowing what is going to happen to our marriage. Also things at work have been stressful.

Mary: Let's look at what is going on here. First, the knot in your epigastric area. Yes, it could be caused by current stressors in your life. Make a concerted effort to plan your meals and eat balanced meals at regular intervals.

Caroline: OK.

Mary: Next, it does sound like you have hives, and you know they can be stress related. It's most likely connected to your marital problem as well as beginning to be free-floating since you have them "out of the blue". If the reaction is uncomfortable and at a bad time, you could take some Benadryl as needed and see if that reduces the symptoms.

Caroline: Sure.

Mary: The bigger problem is how to approach what is going on in the marriage. What has worked for you in the past when you needed to think something through?

Caroline: Getting away from it all for a couple of days usually helps me clear my mind and figure out what is going on inside of me. Our church has a retreat center open to its members. Maybe I could go there on one of the weekends when I'm not on call.

Mary: Excellent idea! In the meantime, you could take a look at the other stressors in your life and get some help for them.

Caroline: Just talking with you today has helped. Thank you so much. I didn't know where else to turn — who could I trust?

Mary: One way to reduce some of the physical stress is to work out in the mornings or take a brisk walk before going to work.

Caroline: That's a great idea!

Mary: What else can you do to reduce your stressors?

Caroline: Well, George and I need to sit down and really talk about our marriage. Now that the shock of learning about the affair is over, maybe we can talk about our future. I don't want a separation but — (Her voice trails off.)

Mary: Sounds like a good plan. Take care of yourself during this time. Being under so much stress for too long can lay the foundation for more serious physical and emotional problems.

Caroline: Yes, and thank you again. Just talking with you today has relieved a lot of my stress. Can I see you next week?

Mary: Sure, because we need to keep a watch on that knot in your gut and evaluate how your stress management plan is working. Call me if you need to talk before then.

POINTS TO CONSIDER:

- Mary's supportive and professional manner helps Caroline talk about her difficulties.
- Mary also comments about the knot in Caroline's gut and her eating patterns.
- Mary makes a suggestion about Caroline reducing her stress levels through some lifestyle changes.
- Mary supports Caroline's thoughts about how to begin to address the problem in her marriage.
- Reminding Caroline that while under stress, she is vulnerable to additional physical and emotional problems is a good caution.
- Realizing that Caroline feels restricted by the "fish bowl phenomenon", Mary reassures her that Caroline can call her if she needs to talk.

• •

The learned pattern of responding to the need to be available whenever called upon, makes it difficult for many to set appropriate limits. Long hours in medical training are considered to "come with the territory". Reinforced by the idealized expectations, many develop a strong sense of duty and obligation. This makes it difficult to set limits and to say "no" to excessive or unreasonable demands on their time.

Self-denial also plays a part in ignoring stress. The demands of training, rotations, and residency make delayed gratification a normal routine for many health care providers. Many focus on developing task oriented coping skills during training, to the detriment of recreation, relaxation, or even interpersonal and emotional communication. In short, idealized expectations, the culture of medicine, the internalized images and learned behavior patterns all contribute to high levels of stress for health care providers.

What Is Stress?

The early pioneers in stress research focused almost exclusively on the physiological reactions to acute stress events.[18] Hans Selye, a major figure in stress research in the 1950's, defined stress as "the nonspecific response of the body to any demands made upon it."[19] He also stated that the body reacts to stress in three stages: 1) **Alarm Reaction**, 2) **Resistance**, and 3) **Exhaustion**. During the Alarm Reaction, the endocrine system readies the body for **fight or flight**. Physiologically, the blood supply to the outer extremities is increased, while vascular constriction shuts off the blood supply to functions not essential for being ready to flee or fight, such as the digestive tract. During the Resistance Stage, the body adapts and copes with stress in a heightened state of readiness. The Exhaustion Stage commences if the distress in the Resistance Stage continues until the body's reserves are depleted or overwhelmed.

These basic physiological reactions are said to be relics of our distant prehistoric primitive past, when indeed many stressors were life threatening. However, in the modern world, we find ourselves facing environmental and emotional stressors to which the fight or flight response would be inappropriate. For example, when persons suffer a blow to their self-esteem from a personal rejection from a loved one, or a scathing criticism from a supervisor, their physical system may signal an involuntary **internal** stress alarm. However, having been socialized into "proper" behavior, the executive decision making functions of the anterior cingulate cortex usually countermand an **external** stress response. Culturally conditioned beliefs may suppress any outward manifestation with the rational message from the higher brain functions of "Don't show it!" Thus, instead of the historically conditioned response of fight or flight we retain the residue of the suppressed response in a **freeze** reaction. "Freeze" occurs when the body's suppressed readiness for fight or flight produces tensions which are held in various parts of the body, such as the shoulders, neck, back, or stomach. Such tensions tend to be retained in the body if there is no opportunity for release through physical activity or conscious stress reduction and relaxation exercises. The problem rests with the biochemical residues of the stress reaction. In the arousal state, stress hormones are secreted before the higher brain functions can mediate a rational or socially acceptable response.[20] High levels of retained stress hormones and their breakdown products can damage the cellular and systemic levels in the body.[21]

If the involuntary stress response were only temporarily discomforting by causing acceleration of our heart rate and respiration, increased perspiration, and muscle tension, the results would not necessarily be damaging. However, many people do not know how to cope with stress on a day-to-day basis, and thus the effects of stressors can become cumulative and interfere with the body's tendency towards self-repair and maintaining a healthy balance.[22]

PSYCHOSOMATIC DISEASE AS MANIFESTATION OF STRESS

Psychosomatic symptoms or illness are physical manifestations of stress. They stem from the interaction between body and mind. A perfect example is when a person's blood pressure elevates during and after a distressing event. This is a normal reaction to the perception of threat, which induces the physiological changes in the vascular system, i.e., readiness for fight or flight.

Under most circumstances the blood pressure returns to the previous level when the stressful situation is resolved. But if the stress continues, *or* if there is no resolution or expression of the emotions triggered by the stress (i.e., being suppressed), the blood pressure may stay at an elevated level.

Some of the most interesting research has focused on the interaction between stress, emotions and the body's immune system. For example, researchers have established correlations between emotional stress and a reduction in both the number and the efficacy of T-lymphocytes, the body's primary defense against invading pathogens.[23] Persons who have experienced a serious loss, but were unable to express their grief — including anger — were highly susceptible to cancer because the efficiency of the T-lymphocytes was reduced.[24,25] Similarly, it is suspected that various auto-immune diseases may be related to internally created elements of one's personality in the form of perfectionism, need for control, self-sacrificing or self-defeating characteristics.[26]

Returning to the interaction between mind and body, one researcher states "it is the inability to feel in control of stress (helplessness) rather than the stressful event itself" which is most damaging to our immune system.[27] The response to stress affects the body from the cellular to the systemic level including physical coordination, memory, thinking processes, emotional responsiveness, and social skills. Stress can put emotions on a roller coaster ride — unstable, constantly changing, and extreme.

THE ROLE OF APPRAISAL

How we appraise a situation determines whether we consider a stimulus stressful or not in response to the unspoken question, "How do I perceive, comprehend, and interpret the world?" According to brain researcher, John Ratey,[28] perception and evaluation — which produce an **appraisal** — are based on attention and consciousness. Attention in turn has four distinct components that create the brain's ability to monitor the environment: arousal, motor orientation, novelty detection, and reward, and executive organization. As Ratey explains in *A User's Guide to the Brain* (p. 115):

> At the lowest level of monitoring, the brain-stem maintains our vigilance—our general degree of arousal. At the next level, the brain's motor centers allow us to physically orient our bodies so that we can immediately direct our senses to possible new villains or food sources. Then, the limbic system accomplishes both novelty detection and reward. Finally, the cortex—especially the frontal lobes—commands action and reaction and integrates our attention with short- and long-term goals.

This appraisal process may lead one person to find a situation unpleasant and uncomfortable. Another person may appraise the same experience as pleasant, exciting or even exhilarating. Hans Selye calls the first appraisal **distress**, and the second **eustress**. Distress is termed "bad" or unwanted stress, whereas eustress is "good" or desired stress. Although Hans Selye insisted that the physiological stress response to each is similar, it is clear from the descriptions that the outcomes of each can be quite different. Certain life events, like the unexpected death of a loved one, nearly always cause distress. A whole range of other events, like a marriage, the birth of child, or a job promotion, can also produce similar physiological reactions. However, such events while temporarily stressful, also satisfy the hunger for reward by the nucleus accumbens, the principal pleasure center of the brain. Hence, the physiological arousal is generally experienced as eustress.

How each individual appraises a situation depends on a number of factors, some internal and some psychosocial. Some internal or organic factors may be genetic which create neurochemical deficits in the brain.[29] For example, an "anxiety gene" may predispose a person to appraise any unexpected event as distress.[30] On the other hand, persons with genetically low dopamine levels in the pleasure center, may need novel, risk taking and/or challenging situations to satisfy their reward system.[31] In this group we might find persons with Attention Deficit Disorder,[32] and those with addictive behaviors.[33]

Biological predispositions are modified by psychosocial and environmental factors. Early socialization experiences including childhood attachment patterns or traumatic experiences will directly affect a person's appraisal of stress.[34] According to some researchers the emotional response patterns from such early learning experiences become deeply rooted in the limbic system and thus may predispose persons to startle, become anxious or experience panic in response to certain stimuli, as in posttraumatic stress disorder (PTSD). Others without such traumas might welcome the same stimuli. For example, women who have been raped, or who were sexually abused as children, "have been indelibly programmed to be vigilant and fearful." For them male attention might automatically trigger extreme PTSD alarm responses, which other women might regard as pleasantly flattering.[35]

Internal beliefs that derive from the socialization process also play an important role in whether a person is more inclined to appraise situations as distress or eustress. Among distress-producing beliefs are:

1. **I have to be perfect or constantly do something to be accepted and loved.**

2. **I can't say NO or disagree with others because I have to be nice to be liked.**

3. **I have to be in control or else chaos will ensue.**

4. **I have to win otherwise I am a loser.**

Among stress-reducing beliefs are:

1. **I am OK, and others will accept me even if I make mistakes.**

2. **I am entitled to my opinions, and I don't have to agree with everybody in order to be liked.**

3. **Life is fun, or a series of pleasant, curious adventures.**

4. **Problems are challenges that are to be solved cooperatively.**

These contrasting beliefs tend to shape one's personality characteristics. Persons who hold distress-producing beliefs tend to fall into two categories. In the first category are people with Type A Personality, who tend to be workaholics.[36,37] The hostile, cynical sub category of the Type A Personality is especially prone to stress related diseases.[38] In the second group are those who may be quietly anxious, passive-aggressive types, who carry a deadly load of silent resentments.[39] Persons coming out of stable and nurturing environments may automatically form beliefs which ameliorate stress. Some coming from dysfunctional pasts, but who learn **resilience**[40] may develop **hardy personalities** that allow them to make optimistic interpretations of the events in their environment.[41]

There may also be some gender differences in how stress is appraised.[42] For example, many women have been socialized into believing that saying NO to another person's demands on them is being selfish.[43] Many women — especially health care providers — equate fulfilling such demands for serving the needs of others — often with little reward or time for self — with noble sacrificing.[44] Efforts to assert themselves can lead to feelings of guilt which may be stressful. At the same time, the internal orientation towards maintaining social harmony can pressure female health care providers to avoid confrontation and deny the effects of stress in the workplace and at home.[45]

The type of support a person receives from their family can directly affect not only the appraisal, but also the experience of stress. Persons who can confide in their family and receive emotional support from them tend to be able handle external pressures and shocks with less distress. On the other hand, when there is strife or distancing in the family, the person is likely to feel more isolated and hence more distressed. Similarly, how accepted or alienated a person feels from their community can lower or raise their perception and experience of stress in the social sphere of their life.

The amount of social support or lack thereof can be a source of satisfaction or of tensions, frustrations, and disappointments. Being a health care provider is a high-stress occupation. If the degree of trust, cooperation, and camaraderie at work is high, tension is likely to be low. Conversely, stress tends to be high if the work atmosphere is rife with suspicion and rumors, or full of status struggles and distrust.[46]

Further, as reviewed in the chapter "Multiculturalism and Treatment", for members of subcultures, the effort required to learn and to fit into the norms of the dominant culture, and dealing with prejudice and discrimination is often very stressful. For example, health care providers belonging to an ethnic or racial minority may feel they constantly have to disprove negative ethnic or racial stereotypes.[47]

Lastly, your spiritual beliefs and practices and level of involvement in the religious community can influence how you perceive stress as well as how you cope with it. If you are inclined towards the spiritual sphere, personal practices such as prayer or meditation, can make you less vulnerable to stress. On the other hand, for others, religious beliefs about shame, punishment, and worthlessness, may heighten the experience of distress.

Factors making for resilience in children and youth from dysfunctional families

1. At least one stable supportive adult (mentor), usually outside the immediate nuclear family, who becomes a positive role model.

2. High positive expectations from that person and others in their lives.

3. Ongoing opportunities to perform responsible or creative activities and receive positive feedback.

4. Personality and temperament to attract a supportive adult and maintain a good relationship.

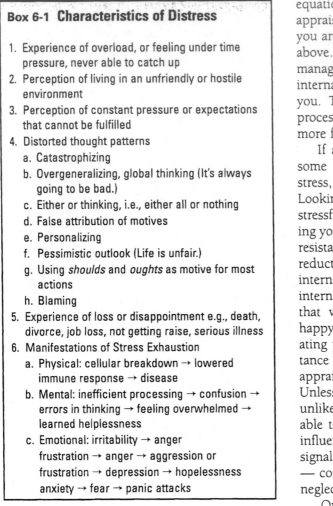

Box 6-1 Characteristics of Distress

1. Experience of overload, or feeling under time pressure, never able to catch up
2. Perception of living in an unfriendly or hostile environment
3. Perception of constant pressure or expectations that cannot be fulfilled
4. Distorted thought patterns
   a. Catastrophizing
   b. Overgeneralizing, global thinking (It's always going to be bad.)
   c. Either or thinking, i.e., either all or nothing
   d. False attribution of motives
   e. Personalizing
   f. Pessimistic outlook (Life is unfair.)
   g. Using *shoulds* and *oughts* as motive for most actions
   h. Blaming
5. Experience of loss or disappointment e.g., death, divorce, job loss, not getting raise, serious illness
6. Manifestations of Stress Exhaustion
   a. Physical: cellular breakdown → lowered immune response → disease
   b. Mental: inefficient processing → confusion → errors in thinking → feeling overwhelmed → learned helplessness
   c. Emotional: irritability → anger frustration → anger → aggression or frustration → depression → hopelessness anxiety → fear → panic attacks

How do these principles of stress apply to you? As we pointed out at the beginning of the chapter, health care workers score "considerably higher than those in the rest of the population" on most instruments measuring stress,[48] therefore, the need to manage stress and balance out the pressures of your life is even more vital.

INTERNAL BARRIERS TO STRESS ASSESSMENT

From this discussion of the various factors affecting the appraisal of stress, it is vital to understand *how* the appraisal of stress is central to the equation of *doing* something about it. When your appraisal process is automatic or unconscious, you are at the mercy of the various factors cited above. Before a person can gain control over and manage their stress, you must find out what your internal messages are about and what distresses you. To accomplish this search, the appraisal process needs to be more conscious, as well as more formal.

If at this point in your reading, you notice some resistance to continuing your study of stress, you should know that this is "normal." Looking at your own stress patterns can be stressful. The most common objection to assessing your own stress is, "I am too busy." If you are resistant to carving out some time for stress reduction activities, you need to look at your internal barriers. You could ask yourself: "What internal messages keep me from doing the things that would allow me to be comfortable and happy with myself? Am I pessimistic about creating positive change?" Be aware that any resistance to committing yourself to change your appraisal patterns, is *part of your stress pattern*. Unless you take this first necessary step, it is unlikely that you will either recognize and/or be able to change the core beliefs and values that influence your appraisal. This could also be a signal to you that you might fall into the pattern — common among health care providers — of neglecting your own well being.

One of the axioms of New Age thinking was "take charge of your life". All too often this is taken to mean that people who know how to completely control their lives are more successful as well as happier. However, we would argue that the ability to adapt to a changing reality is more effective than trying to control reality. The ability to adapt to changing conditions, such as

> One incentive to complete an accurate appraisal is to assure that the limited time you do have to reduce stress, you can use stress reduction methods appropriate to your temperament and style of relaxing most efficiently.

> GOD GRANT ME THE SERENITY TO ACCEPT THE THINGS I CANNOT CHANGE;
>
> COURAGE TO CHANGE THE THINGS I CAN;
>
> AND THE WISDOM TO KNOW THE DIFFERENCE.

medical emergencies, is an especially valuable trait for health care providers. Often time and work pressures in health care environments seem unrelenting. You may need to remind yourself of the concepts in the Serenity Prayer.

Responding effectively to such pressures has more to do with balance than control. Just as athletes must program rest periods to reach peak levels at critical performance times, so health care providers must find their own balance between work and rest. So in terms of finding ways to handle stress, it is far better to consciously determine what blend of coping skills you need than to be at the mercy of unconscious responses to inner messages about "control" or "perfection."

HOLISTIC APPROACH

In our culture we have a tendency to separate or compartmentalize our physical, mental, emotional and spiritual selves. The holistic approach assumes that these aspects of our selves are interrelated and basically inseparable. Addressing each aspect, as well as the interrelationship between them is basic to effective stress management. For the body, this means establishing healthy habits in exercise, nutrition and adequate rest. For health care providers to achieve balance in the mental realm can be a challenge. Most mental stimulation in health care is often one-sided, and mostly cognitive or left brained. For balance, you may need to consciously find time to engage in activities that stimulate the right brain. Artistic endeavors, like painting, playing music, or playing an instrument or singing; body movement such as dance or Tai Chi; participating in theater or acting; or finding a hobby that is non-medical or nonscientific are

suggested. Emotional nourishment usually comes from a sense of connection or interaction with others. Sharing problems, or feeling needed and loved by another, is one way of lowering stress levels. In the spiritual realm, having a sense of purpose or mission in life, and maintaining an attitude of faith and hope can give you the ability to regain balance after losses, disappointments, or stressful work interactions. Spiritual practices can range from attending worship services, to intensely personal practices of regular prayer, meditation, or spiritual retreats. The key to balance is to consciously prioritize incorporating activities from each realm into your life on a regularly scheduled basis. If you have the attitude that you will do such stress reducing activities "when you have time," you are likely to find that you are always too busy to find the time.

Managing Stress

Stress management is generally divided into three categories: 1) **stress release or relaxation**, 2) **coping**, and 3) **problem solving**. With regards to stress release and relaxation, a critical question is "Am I a passive or active relaxer?" Some passive relaxers can walk out the door of the clinic or hospital and leave their stress at the work place. Others let go of their reactions to their stressors quickly by entering easily into a calm, quiet, and comfortable state. Active relaxers need to engage in physical activities before relaxation can occur.

RELAXATION TECHNIQUES

There is a rich collection of self-help books and audiotapes on relaxation and visualization available. Among the techniques for passive relaxation is deep breathing, meditation, listening to special music, a walk in nature, or using guided imagery. One of the most effective passive relaxation techniques is conscious breathing.[49] A time-honored technique is to sit quietly with eyes closed and inhale slowly and deeply and then gently exhale. You may wish to add visual imagery, such as picturing yourself in a favorite place in nature or at the beach.[50] Generally regular practice of such meditative techniques will bring feelings of peace, serenity, or even spiritual ecstasy.[51,52] For others a short catnap, sometimes called a "power nap" is effective. As little as 10-15 minutes of napping can increase mental acuity, and reduce physical tension and irritability. A word of caution: some passive relaxation measures are merely mind numbing. Watching television, playing video games, or surfing the Net, will divert the mind, and slow down one's system until a person is ready to fall asleep, but these semi-passive activities are less likely to refresh or revitalize.

Some people, by virtue of an active temperament, find it hard, if not impossible, to use passive relaxation methods. Instead they need to use active methods of stress release before they can experience relaxation. Physical exercise that allows the body to enter into an aerobic state helps metabolize the stress residues. It has been well established that a regular regimen of working out at a fitness center, jogging, brisk walking, or swimming is effective for stress release, for maintaining a sense of balance and for optimizing physical health.[53,54] A regular practice of various structured exercise programs ranging from highly active martial arts and aerobics classes to the gentler Tai Chi or Yoga, can rid you of distress and recharge you with positive energy. For others, golf, basketball, racquetball, rock climbing, caving, or deep sea diving can be equally effective. Romping with one's children — often but not always aerobic — can recharge you with positive emotional energy. The point is that you need to find out which active stress reduction technique fits your temperament.

A word of caution is to approach such active techniques in a relaxed manner. For example, Type A persons tend to approach physical exercise with a "no pain, no gain" principle and apply the same hard driving perfectionism and competitiveness as they do to their work. Instead of bringing about relaxation, such relentless drive can lead to Selye's Exhaustion Stage in which it is difficult to either give or to receive emotionally.

COPING

Coping is the second major category of stress management. It comes out of the realization that we *cannot* control certain potentially stressful situations like the weather, the traffic, or the number of patients coming into emergency room, but we *can* control our reaction to them. In the coping approach, we change our appraisal of the situation, or come up with strategies to minimize the distressing effects of conditions, events or certain relationships.

Coping in the Health Care Setting

The transition from the classroom to the clinical setting can be accompanied by doubts and fears about role performance, about fitting in, and about the awesome responsibility for making life and death decisions. The long work hours and lack of sleep of clinical rotations can threaten your physical, emotional, mental, and spiritual balance. One coping strategy is to focus on offsetting the physical and psychic drains of this high stress transition. This requires giving a high priority to replenishing yourself with short periods of rest, exercise, light meals, quality "R & R" breaks, and time away from the clinical setting — including weekend escapes. To safeguard your health, you also need to pay attention to your feelings and find ways to express both your excitement and your fears and doubts. One tendency is to suppress such doubts and fears in order to demonstrate that we are made of "the right stuff" in front of our colleagues or supervisors. Remember, everyone goes through this period of emotional anxiety, and giving voice to it is likely to be received with empathy, or even with relief by one's peers who may also be suffering silently.

Seeking support is another crucial coping strategy. Again, this is one that goes against the cultural norm of self-sufficiency. American individualism with its dictum *stand on your own two feet,* may predispose you to believe that you

---

Box 6-2 Stresses Inherent in Health Care[73]

1. Medical Training
   a. Pressure cooker learning: experiencing anxiety about surviving training
   b. Too little time for other interests and needs: social, recreational, spiritual
   c. Baptism through fire: long hours of clinical rotations
   d. Specialization: Postponing the good life to specialize
2. Post training decisions
   a. Debt load from student loans: possibly dictating choice of job
   b. Professional collegiality: support and acceptance
   c. Professional identity: role clarification
   d. Continuing professional development
3. Stressful characteristics of health care
   a. Relating to patients: probing into secretive areas of patient and encountering resistance and fear; personal discomfort around sexuality
   b. Adverse treatment outcomes: accepting "failures", deaths and suffering of patients, lack of acceptance and sympathy from patients and their relatives, threat of litigation
   c. Overwork: on-call night duties, long working hours, stressful postural demands (poor ergonomics), sleep deprivation leading to decisions with possible adverse outcomes for patients
   d. Unpredictability: disrupting family life, interfering with personal relationships and community responsibilities
4. Relating to work place
   a. Administrative matters: paperwork, charting, workload distribution, committee assignments
   b. Managed care: reports, justifications, having decisions second-guessed
   c. Relationships with other professionals, administrators, and staff

---

should *fight* your stress by yourself. While the willingness to look at stress patterns must come from you, fighting your stress alone may leave you feeling isolated and more distressed. Effective coping strategies usually involve some interaction or team effort with others. For example, in the health care setting it has been found that coping skills are best learned as a team, or a support group — even one as small as two people.[55] You can help create an atmosphere with your peers and colleagues to support each other by being good listeners to each other when someone needs to talk or vent about their distress. "Sharing the burden" is useful because it gets the problem out in the open and gives the speaker a chance to hear the problem in his or her own words. Second, the act of being listened to without judgment by caring persons in itself is usually a gratifying experience that reduces stress. While advice giving can be counterproductive, you may wish to brainstorm together on strategies for coping with the stressors in your work environment. In cases of stress related depression, anxiety, or substance abuse, it is recom-

mended that you overcome your tendency to try to resolve it on your own and instead seek professional help.

In addition to having a mutual support group at work, we suggest you create support networks for other areas in your life: social and friendship needs, personal and family needs, emotional and spiritual needs, as well as financial and even legal needs. Ideally, such networks function in layers from more intimate to less personal but more technical realms. Carefully tending to an intimate circle of family or friends will reward you with an emotional safety net of people who will be supportive during rough times. Some find that participating in activities of your spiritual community is calming and reassuring. Being active in community-based organizations will give you a sense of connection, as well as an alternate focus from your work.

Barriers to Coping

As mentioned at the beginning of this chapter, many health care providers who are survivors of dysfunctional families may have difficulty acknowledging stress related problems — whether physical or emotional.[56] Such persons may find it more difficult to cope with personal problems than the changes or pressures at work. Not addressing problems in the personal realm can produce complex and intense emotions ranging from frustration, anger, to depression. As we will discuss in later chapters, a pattern learned in dysfunctional families is to keep personal and family problems a secret. Concerns about airing "dirty linen" protecting privacy, and maintaining a "professional" image often keep health care professionals in denial, and prevents them from seeking peer support. Instead they may adopt one of several negative coping mechanisms. One is to throw themselves deeper into their work. Unfortunately, the escape into workaholism can lead to the neglect of emotional ties to family and friends. In need of emotional support from some source, such persons may turn to sexual liaisons with colleagues or other health care staff, with whom they have close professional contact.

Another negative coping technique is to get a quick pharmacological fix. With easy access to prescription drugs, health care providers may be tempted to self-prescribe. Masking one's problems with drugs or alcohol is not a solution. Impairment due to drug and alcohol addiction is a major occupational risk in health care.[57] Unfortunately, once a person has embarked on the path of using drugs or alcohol to cope with stress, they may be in denial that they have a problem and be unwilling to recognize that they have become dependent. Sometimes alcohol or drug abuse can also lead to inappropriate behavior in their professional life, such as becoming disruptive, acting out sexually, or careless treatment of patients.[58] Impaired health care providers not only put their patients at risk, but also jeopardize their careers, their health, and their relations with significant others.[59] Fortunately, there is confidential help available from professional assistance programs through your professional association.[60] When one becomes a "wounded healer," it becomes essential to take time out to assess one's stress levels, identify the problem area(s), seek appropriate treatment,* and follow through with treatment recommendations.[61]

● ●

PATIENT PROFILE 6.2

MAYBE IT'S TIME TO QUIT

SETTING: *While attending a medical conference, Diego, a 45-year-old physician is having lunch with Frank, a long time friend and colleague. They went through medical school together and completed the same emergency medicine residency. Both are practicing physicians in urban emergency departments. Frank has developed a concern of Diego's use of alcohol, because he believes he could smell alcohol on Diego during the morning meetings. Now at a nearby restaurant, Diego orders 2 Vodka tonics.*

Frank: (*That's his second drink and we've only started lunch. I've watched Diego over the years drink more and more. I wonder if he's an alcoholic. I wonder how he's functioning as a physician.*) Diego, we have known each other for a long time and I'm concerned about something.

Diego, feeling expansive: Sure, buddy. We've been through the mill together. What's on your mind?

Frank: Well, I thought I smelled liquor on your breath this morning at the break and now you've had two drinks with lunch so far. Do you think you have a problem with alcohol?

Diego: (*Turns red in the face and backs away from Frank.*) What business is it of yours how much I drink?

Frank: Look, I am your friend and a colleague. We did go through medical training together, and I am concerned for you. Do you think your drinking is affecting your functioning as an emergency physician? Do you feel guilty about your drinking?

---

*Many centers specialize in assisting health care professionals to assess and reduce stress. A few more well-known ones are: Center for Physician Renewal. Phone: 253-351-8577 E-mail: mdrenew@ aol.com; Center for Professional Well-being. Phone: 919-489-9167. Net address: www.cpwb.org; and The Menninger Clinic 1-800-351-9058.

Diego: Well, what's the harm in relaxing a little. This emergency medicine is getting to me. I sometimes feel I am burning out.

Frank: Yes, it sure is stressful. I can agree with you there. How does the stress mainly hit you?

Diego: I feel wound up inside. Tight. I get home and try and talk with my wife and check in with the kids, but I just can't relax. A couple of drinks helps me unwind.

Frank: I understand, but —

Diego, interrupts Frank: I know, I know. (Sighs — pause, then pensively) Maybe it's time to quit and find other ways to reduce the stress.

Frank: I understand and let's talk some more about this. (*Maybe I can recommend that he seek some help.*)

POINTS TO CONSIDER:

- Frank is alert to the dangers of abusing alcohol and drugs due to the stressors in the medical profession.

- Frank is not put off by Diego's defensive response. Instead with a gentle and caring manner he asks specific questions to get his friend to look objectively at if and how his drinking might be a problem.

- Frank's continued empathy for his friend's situation helps Diego overcome his defensiveness, and be honest with himself and Frank.

• •

How You Can Help

When you become aware that one of your professional colleagues is behaving erratically or makes decisions that can or has put patients at risk, you have a responsibility under your professional code to take action.[62] Although you may feel angry, it is usually more effective if you approach your colleague with compassionate concern. Your aim is to restore your colleague to professional competence.[63] Talk to the colleague directly and share your concern for them. You could objectively describe the pattern of behavior you have observed, and point out the detrimental effects that this has had or could have on patient safety, or on relations with colleagues.

Delicate questioning and empathic listening may help your colleague to acknowledge that they have a problem. Sometimes a colleague may turn to you for help because they trust you and feel you will keep the conversation confidential. Even if you feel uncomfortable or inadequate to the task, you should at least listen empathically and be prepared to do basic counseling with them. Doing so will make it more likely that the colleague/friend may accept a referral for professional help. The next logical step is to urge the person to get professional help. You also need to be prepared if your colleague becomes defensive, denies anything is wrong, and tells you to mind your own business. When that happens you may be tempted to say to yourself, "It's not my responsibility." However, such a brush off does not relieve you of the ethical responsibility to prevent your colleague from harming themselves or their patients.[64] Your next step at this point would be to make one more personal effort, preferably by enlisting one or more colleagues to join in the effort to break through the denial. If that is unsuccessful, you and your colleagues should continue efforts to convince or require the impaired provider, who is in denial, to seek professional help. In a hospital setting you could approach the chief of medical staff with the evidence of your observations, or you might have to report the colleague to the professional association. The various national professional associations can arrange to get the person into treatment. In some instances, a trained counselor from the impaired provider program of the relevant professional association may assemble and ask you to participate in an intervention team to confront and bring the colleague into treatment.[65] It is essential that a professional assessment is made to determine the extent of substance abuse or dependence as well as the level of professional impairment.[66]

PROBLEM SOLVING OR PREVENTION STRATEGIES

A third major strategy for dealing with negative aspects of distress in one's environment is to develop practical problem solving and prevention strategies. You may want to become actively engaged in improving your work environment. This may involve forming or being on committees, which would identify problem areas and propose solutions. For example one such committee might have to consider disciplinary action against an impaired or disruptive colleague. You may resist participating in such activities — such as committee work — because they will add to the demand on your time. However, when you are part of the solution, situations are not as likely to distress you, as when you feel helpless about changing them.

As previously mentioned, one way to keep yourself from being consumed by your profession is to consciously strive to maintain a balance between your personal and professional identity. Time pressures, unpleasant aspects of our work situation may squelch the enjoyment of your profession, or life in general. Operating without relief in a negative stress environment can produce depression and burnout. One way to counteract or prevent this is to take stock by making a list of negative and positive aspects of your professional situation. Such a list can provide you with information to use for making decisions about what you can or cannot change on the pressure side of the ledger, as well as how to improve your professional support networks to alleviate stress. Another technique is to identify your personal and professional capabilities and match them with your professional responsibilities.

• •

PATIENT PROFILE 6.3

IT'S JUST TOO MUCH

SETTING: *Cassie, a 28-year-old single physician assistant, is in her first position at a busy rural health clinic. She has moved to this small town in the hopes of establishing herself as the town's first PA. During the first year, she has learned the various clinic protocols. She sometimes stays late after hours to catch up on her progress notes. Her supervising physician has just asked her, as a*

member of the Quality Assurance team, to organize and conduct a survey of the staff. Cassie fears this request will make it impossible to complete her progress notes. She feels discouraged. She has been questioning her career decision, as well as the move to this small town, feeling isolated and separated from her family and friends. She feels that she has become a paper pusher. She is talking with Dr. Victor Lorey, her supervising physician, about her concerns.

Cassie: I'm sorry to bother you with all of this. I feel like I should handle this myself. (*He must think I am a wimp with these complaints.*)

Dr. Lorey: I know it is hard for you to admit that you are having difficulties, but it is the first step towards finding solutions to the problem.

Cassie: I feel buried in paperwork and too rushed with my patients. It's hard to concentrate on what they are saying. I've been missing things or just plain forgetting them. The other day a woman who had been pregnant, had to remind me that she'd had a miscarriage four months ago. Because I had not reread the chart, the miscarriage had completely slipped my mind. I felt terrible after I had asked her how the baby was coming along.

Dr. Lorey: What you are experiencing is quite common for physician assistants or any health care providers in their first clinical position. Even though this is hard for you now, this is a normal stressor.

Cassie: I tend to be very organized. I can usually achieve all the goals I set for myself. I usually manage my time very well. Now I feel rushed, and it seems that I am always behind.

Dr. Lorey: Feeling rushed is one of the realities of health care, especially these days. Perhaps I need to reassess your job responsibilities and redefine my expectations of you at this time.

Cassie: Oh, alright. (*I wonder what that means?*)

Dr. Lorey: Would you make a list of your responsibilities and your patient load for me to look at?

Cassie: Yes.

Dr. Lorey: In the meantime, let's take you off the Quality Assurance Team until I can get a better grasp of your responsibilities and my expectations.

Cassie: Thank you.

POINTS TO CONSIDER:

- Dr. Lorey reinforces the appropriateness of Cassie talking with him and reminds Cassie that the first step to solving a problem is admitting you have one.

- Dr. Lorey normalizes Cassie's experience, as part of being new in the situation.

- Dr. Lorey takes the next important step and suggests that Cassie's job responsibilities be reassessed so that Dr. Lorey can more realistically redefine his expectations of Cassie.

- Lorey recognizing Cassie's concern about her professional judgment being impacted by the stress, lightens her load by canceling the QA assignment.

• •

A similar list for your personal life can point out strengths and weaknesses in that area. The energy, vitality, and zest derived from one's personal life provide nurturance and resilience that can ameliorate or neutralize the effects of distress in our professional life. On the other side, distress in our intimate relationships will magnify the effects of the stress in our professional life. So we suggest that you review the state of your close relationships, and ponder whether you are giving enough attention to them. It will also help you to list the social activities, hobbies, or situations from which you derive joy, pleasure and contentment. If the list is sparse, you might ask yourself what else you might be able to add to the positive side of the ledger.[67]

The busier your life is, the more important it is to take some time to attend to your inner self. Each of us needs alone time for finishing our thoughts, processing the day's events, as well as for solitary reflection. It can be a time when you can compliment yourself on the intangible gifts and contributions to others during the day. You may find it helpful to review your thoughts and actions by writing in a journal. Internal dialog can also help you to attend to your spiritual needs. Basic existential questions you may wish to review on a regular basis are: ""What is important to me? What can I do to enrich my personal

and spiritual growth? Why am I here? What is my purpose?"

As pointed out above, a number of positive benefits accrue to those who devote some time each day to spiritual practices, such as prayer, contemplation or meditation.[68] There is no longer any doubt of the tangible benefits of regular spiritual practices for our body, mind, emotions, and social relations. On the physiological level, the relaxation response boosts the immune system and increases longevity vs. those who do not have regular spiritual practices.[69] Such practices are also known to sharpen our mental acuity, and decision making. In your social and intimate relations, you are likely to experience a greater capacity to give and receive love. You may also find yourself able to tap into a greater capacity to nourish yourself and others. For example, giving compliments or expressing your appreciation for others being in your life, generally begets a reciprocal flow of positive emotional energy so you can begin to experience the world with optimism and hope.[70] Overall, regular spiritual practices can build resilience and healthy coping with stress.[71]

Similarly humor and laughter are known to be effective in reducing physical and emotional stress. Indeed as the old adage goes "Humor is the Best Medicine."[72] It is a tonic for both you and your patients. Self deprecating humor and laughter can defuse tension and anger and break down fear and embarrassment, and allow you to relate to patients, colleagues, and staff in a more relaxed manner. So, finding the humor in things, laughing at yourself and enjoying a good belly laugh each day can do wonders for your disposition, your relations with others, as well as for the health of your patients.

Conclusion

You cannot eliminate all stress from your life, especially in the profession you have chosen. But conscious attention to how you appraise stress, allows you to make choices about how to react to it. You also can ameliorate the harmful effects of serious, unexpected, or chronic stress situations through improving your coping skills. Part of coping is to program periodic stress reduction and relaxation exercises into your schedule. In addition, you — in concert with others — can problem solve some of the structural or institutional stress conditions in your work setting. Remember, the goal is to thrive rather than merely to survive, to embrace your work, your family and friends.

REFERENCES

1. Council on Scientific Affairs (1987). Results and Implications of the AMA-APA Physician Mortality Project, Stage II. *JAMA,* 257: 2949-2953.
2. Rosenberg HM, Burnett C, Maurer J, et al (1993). Mortality by occupation, industry, and cause of death: 12 reporting states. *Monthly vital Statistics Report, CDC,* 42:1-64.
3. Kerfoot K (1999).The art of leading with grace, *Nursing Economics,* 17, 3:183.
4. Arnetz BB (2001). Psychosocial Challenges Facing Physicians of Today. *Soc Sci Medicine,* 52:205.
5. Firth-Cozens J ((2001). Interventions to improve physicians' well-being and patient care. *Soc Sci & Medicine,* 52, 2:215-22.
6. Mansky PA (1999). Issues in the recovery of physicians from addictive illnesses. *Psychiatr Quarterly,* 70, 2:107-22.
7. Gerrity MS (2001). Interventions to improve physician's well being and patient care: a commentary. *Soc Sci Medicine,* 52, 2:223–5.
8. Miller MN, McGovern KR, Quillen JH (2000). The Painful Truth: Physicians are not Invincible. *South Med J* 93, 10:966-972.
9. Vaillant GE, Sobowale NC, McArthur C (1972). Some psychological vulnerabilities of physicians. *N Engl J Med,* 287:372-375.
10. Christensen JF, Levinson W, Dunn PM (1992). Heart of Darkness: the impact of perceived mistakes on physicians. *J Gen Intern Med,* 7:424-431.
11. McCranie EW, Brandsma JM (1988). Personality Antecedents of Burnout Among Middle-aged Physicians, *Behavioral Med,* 30-36.
12. Weiner EL, Swain GR, Gottlieb M (1998). Predictors of Psychological Well-being Among Physicians, *Family Systems Health,* 16:419-430.
13. Miller MN, McGovern KR, Quillen JH (2000). The Painful Truth: Physicians are not Invincible. *South Med J* 93, 10:967.
14. Duncan DE (1994). Compassion Fatigue, *Hippocrates,* April 1994:35-41.
15. McCue JD (1985). Influence of medical and pre-medical education on important qualities of physicians. *Am J Med,* 78, 6:985-991.
16. Lamberg L (1999). 'If I work hard(er), I will be loved.' Roots of Physician Stress explored. *JAMA,* 282,1:13-14.
17. Stoudemire A, Rhoads JM (1983). When a Doctor Needs a Doctor: Special Considerations for the Physician-Patient, *Ann Internal Med,* 98:654-659.
18. Cannon, WB (1932). *The Wisdom of the Body.* New York: WW Norton.
19. Selye H (1956). *The Stress of Life.* New York: McGraw Hill.
20. Harbuz MS (2000). Stress, Hormones and your Brain. *J Neuroendocrinol,* 12,5:381-382.
21. Sapolsky RM (2000). Stress hormones: good and bad. *Neurobiol Dis,*7,5:540-542.
22. Elenkov IJ, Chrousos GP (1999). Stress, cytokine patterns and susceptibility to disease. *Baillieres Best Pract Res Endocrin Metab,* 13,4:583-595.
23. Herbert TB, Cohen S (1993). Stress and Immunity in humans: a meta-analytic review. *Psychsom Med,* 55:364-379.
24. Simonton OC, Henson RM, Hampton B (1992). *The healing journey.* New York: Bantam Books
25. Schedlowski M, Jacobs R, Stratman G, et al (1993). Changes in natural killer cells during acute psychological stress. *J Clin Immunol,* 13:119-1126.
26. LeShan LL (1994). *Cancer as a Turning Point: a handbook for people with cancer, their families, and health professionals.* New York: Plume.
27. Borysenko J (1981). *Minding the Body, Mending the Mind.* Reading, Mass: Addison Wesley.
28. Ratey JJ (2001). *A User's Guide to the Brain: Perception, Attention and the Four Theaters of the Brain.* New York: Pantheon 111-146.
29. Brunner EJ (1997). Stress and the biology of inequality. *BMJ,* 314:1472-1476.
30. Schmidt NB, Storey J, Greenberg BD, et al (2000). Evaluating Gene X, Psychological Risk Factor Effects in the pathogenesis of Anxiety: A New Model Approach. *J Abnorm Psychol,* 109, 2:308-20.
31. Ebstein RP et al (1996). Dopamine D4 receptor (D4DR) rcon II polymorphism associated with the human personality trait of novelty seeking. *Nat. Genetics,* 12:78-80.

32. Barkley RA (1998). *Attention Deficit Hyperactivity Disorder: A Handbook for Diagnosis and Treatment* (2nd Ed). New York: Guilford Press.

33. Anthenelli RM, Schuckit MA (1997). Determinants and Perpetuators of Substance Abuse: Genetics. In Lowinson JH et al, (Eds) *Substance Abuse: A comprehensive textbook*. (3rd Edition), Baltimore: Williams & Wilkins, p 44.

34. Taylor RE, et al (2000). Attachment Style in Patients with Unexplained Physical Complaints. *Psych Med*, 30, 4: 931-41.

35. Ratey JJ (2001). *A User's Guide to the Brain: Perception, Attention and the Four Theaters of the Brain*. New York: Pantheon 233.

36. Friedman M, Rosemann R (1974). *Type A Behavior and Your Heart*, New York: AA Knopf.

37. Abbott AV, Peters RK (1988). Type A Behavior and Coronary heart Disease: an Update. *Am Fam Physician*, 38,5:105-110.

38. Dembroski TM, MacDougall JM, Costa PT Jr, Grandits GA (1989). Components of hostility as predictors of sudden death and myocardial infarction in the Multiple Risk Factor Intervention Trial. *Psychosom Med*, 51:514-522.

39. Hemingway H, Marmot M (1999). Psychosocial factors in the etiology and prognosis of coronary heart disease: systematic review of prospective cohort studies. *BMJ*, 318:1460-1467.

40. Werner E (1990). Protective factors and individual resilience. In Meisels S, Shonkoff J (Eds.), *Handbook of early childhood intervention* 97-116. New York: Cambridge University Press.

41. Mandleco BL, Craig PL (2000). An Organizational Framework for Conceptualizing Resilience in Children. *J Child Adoles Psychiatric Nursing*, 13, 3:99.

42. Gross EB (1997). Gender differences in physician stress: why the discrepant findings? *Women and Health*, 26, 1-14.

43. Gilligan C (1982). *In a Different Voice*. Cambridge: Harvard Univ Press.

44. Bratt MM, et al (2000). Influence of Stress and Nursing leadership in Job satisfaction of Pediatric Intensive Care Unit Nurses. *Am J Critical Care*. 9, 5:307-17.

45. Frank E, Dingle AD (1999). Self-reported Depression and Suicide Attempts Among U.S. Women Physicians. *Am J Psychiatry;* 156:1887-1894.

46. Holmes SE, Fasser CE (1993). Occasional stress among physician assistants. *J Am Acad Physician Assistant*, 6, 172-177.

47. Post DM, Waddington WH (2000). Stress and coping of the African-American Physician. *J Natl Med Assoc*, 92, 2:70-75.

48. Firth-Cozens J, Payne RL (1999). *Stress in Health Professionals*. Chichester, UK: Wiley.

49. Benson H, Klipper MZ (1975). *The Relaxation Response*. New York: Wm Morrow.

50. Moen L (1990). *Guided Imagery, Volume One* (1992) *Volume Two*. Naples, FL: Unites States Publishing.

51. Gawain S, King L (1986). *Living in the Light: A guide to Personal and Planetary Transformation*. San Rafael, CA: Whatever Publishing Inc.

52. Roth G, Loudon J (1998). *Maps to Ecstasy: A Healing Journey for the Untamed Spirit*. Novato, CA: New World Library.

53. Pescatello LS (2001). Exercising for health: the merits of lifestyle physical activity. *West J Medicine*. 174, 2: 114.

54. Winter RE (1983). *Coping With Executive Stress*. New York: McGraw-Hill.

55. Davis M (1999). Intern discussion groups: a supportive educational experience for junior doctors. *Hospital Medicine*, 60, 6:435-9.

56. Scott KS, Moore KS, Miceli, MP (1997). An exploration of the meaning and consequences of workaholism. *Human Relations*, 50, 3 287:28-32.

57. Gallegos KV, Talbott GD (1997). Physicians and other health professionals. In Lowinson JH, et al Editors *Substance Abuse: A comprehensive textbook*. (3rd Edition), Baltimore: Williams & Wilkins.

58. Lowes R (1998). Taming the disruptive doctor. *Med Econ* 5;75(19):67-8, 73-4, 77-80.

59. Pfifferling JH (1997). Managing the unmanageable: the disruptive physician. *Fam Pract Manag*, 4(10):76-8, 83, 87-92.

60. Corsino BV, Morrow DH, Wallace CJ (1996). Quality improvement and substance abuse: rethinking impaired provider policies. *Am J Medical Quality*, 11, 2:94-99.

61. Scheiber SC, Doyle BB (eds) (1983). *The Impaired Physician*. New York: Plenum Books.

62. Mandell WJ (1994). An approach to the impaired physician. *Physician Executive* 20, 5:7-14.

63. Sotile WM, Sotile MO (1996). The angry physician—Part 2. Managing yourself while managing others. *Physician Exec*, 22(9):39-42.

64. Smith R (1997). All doctors are problem doctors: doctors worldwide must do better with managing problem colleagues. (Editorial) *BMJ*, 314, 7084: 841-842.

65. Talbott GD, Gallegos KV (1990). Intervention with health professionals. *Addict Recovery,* 10, 3:13-16.

66. Rice B (1999). Doctor policing: Too tough? Too easy? Giving rehab programs a new look. *Medical Economics* 76, 9:173-74, 179-180, 185.

67. Rosenfeld MS (1993). *Wellness and Lifestyle Renewal: A Manual for Personal Change.* Bethesda, MD: The American Occupational Therapy Association, Inc.

68. Van Houten P (2001). Meditation and Your Health: The Effects of Meditation on the Human Brain and Behavior, *Share Guide,* 53:30-31.

69. Magarey CJ (1988). Aspects of the psychological management of breast cancer, *Med J of Australia,* 148,5:239-242.

70. Borysenko J (1994). *Fire in the Soul : A New Psychology of Spiritual Optimism.* New York: Warner Books.

71. Borysenko J (1999). *The Power of the Mind to Heal.* Carson, CA: Hay House.

72. Cousins N (1979). *Anatomy of an Illness as Perceived by the Patient.* New York: Norton.

73. Arnetz BB (2001). Psychosocial Challenges facing Physicians of today. *Soc Sci Med,* 52, 2:203-213.

CHAPTER 7

Human Sexuality

Objective discussion between patient or health care providers of health problems related to sexuality can be difficult in part because of the contradictory messages on sexuality in our society, in part because of the discomfort we feel ourselves. We may feel inadequately prepared because in our medical education the topic of human sexuality tends to be dispersed piece meal throughout the curriculum. This chapter brings together the various aspects from cultural influences, the range of expression of sexuality, the intimacy needs of special populations, sexual dysfunctions, to aberrant sexual behaviors. Addressing practice concerns, we ask you to examine your own attitudes, give guidance on using sexual history questionnaires, and suggest treatment and referral options.

American Cultural Messages

A sociologist from another planet studying the contradictory messages in our media and public discourse might conclude that America has an obsessive ambivalence about sex. On one hand, there is the Puritan tradition that says that sex or lust is sinful and dirty. On the other hand, there is the libertine tradition, sometimes called the Playboy philosophy, which extols sex. The two seem at war with each other both in our public life as well as in some individual lives. Conservative religious beliefs tend to paint sex and lust as a "descent into our animal nature." This judgmental attitude about sensuality/sexuality leads many people to have feelings of discomfort, shame or guilt about their own sensual feelings, sexual impulses or erotic longings. The discom-fort makes it difficult for most parents to talk about sex — "the facts of life" — with their children. As experience in many school districts shows, parents, who are themselves uncomfortable teaching their kids about sex, do not want the schools to do it either on the grounds that sex education programs usurp their parental role and would encourage sexual activity. Many parents seem to believe that by not talking about "it," they can somehow prevent or delay the development of sexual feelings and actions in their children. Unfortunately, denial often creates an atmosphere of furtiveness and secrecy about sex in families. The message is "Don't talk about it." In many families successive generations have been uncomfortable addressing their own sexual feelings or problems. One of the consequences of this taboo is that young couples in the throes of sexual arousal, often are unable to talk or negotiate about using protection against pregnancy or disease before they engage in sexual intercourse.[1] They frequently receive misinformation from their peers and develop unrealistic expectations of themselves and of their future sexual activities. As we discuss in the section of sexual dysfunctions, early sexual experiences may set a person up for having subsequent sexual problems.

● ●

PATIENT PROFILE 7.1

WORRIED

SETTING: *George is a 32-year-old male who is in clinic today with the chief complaint of sinus infection. George has been coming to this clinic now for 3 years and has always been seen by the physician assistant, Sam, PA-C.*

Sam: Hello, George, how is that sinus infection?

George: Actually Sam, it is better but I wanted to talk with you about something else. It is a little embarrassing.

Sam: OK. *(Nods reassuringly and waits patiently leaning slightly forward indicating for George to continue.)*

George: You know I have been dating this great little lady for a while now and we've decided to get married. And well, we're getting closer and closer now and we'll probably – you know – do it soon. *(Pauses and checks out Sam's reaction.)*

Sam: Yes – *(Nods and nonverbally encourages George to go on.)*

George: Do you remember when I first started coming here, I told you that I'd mostly had sex with prostitutes during my college years? What I didn't tell you is that I tended to come kind of quickly. I'm worried that this will happen with my fiancee and that I won't be able to satisfy her. Then I wonder if she'll reject me.

Sam: Yes, I remember. George, I'm glad you told me about this. This is called premature ejaculation. It's fairly common in men whose early sexual experiences were rushed. From what you tell me about your college days, your quickie encounters with prostitutes set you up for this.

George: Oh, I didn't know that.

Sam: The good news is that you can get help for this condition. I can refer you to a counselor who specializes in sexual issues. But before we do that I want to rule out any physical or medical reason for your concern. A urine sample from you today will allow us to rule out a urinary tract infection.

POINTS TO CONSIDER:

- Giving verbal and nonverbal encouragement in order to talk in a non-threatening nature is essential when talking about sexual issues.

- Educating George about how he might have developed premature ejaculation reduces the stigma and shame that may be possibly connected with that condition.

- Providing reasons for testing helps George understand possible causes of the problem.

• •

The other side of this confusing picture is the glorification and commercialization of sex in America. The Playboy philosophy objectifies female body parts: breasts, buttocks and genitals. To a lesser extent this is also true about the male "hunk." Orgasm, preferably multiple, seems to be the holy grail of the libertine tradition. Self help articles, books and videos on spicing up our sex life have proliferated. American media and the advertising industry use sex as a potent symbol for selling everything from entertainment to products. Madison Avenue ad writers use our insecurity about being liked or loved as the most potent hook to get us to buy anything from flashy cars to toothpaste. The implied promise is that the possession or use of the proffered material object will make us more sexually attractive or will enhance our potential for intimate relationships.[2] Sex also sells TV shows and movies. Focusing on how TV socializes our children, the Kaiser Family Foundation found that most portrayals showed no clear consequences of the sexual behavior, even though participants never seemed to take precautions against disease or pregnancy.[3]

These two contradictory strains in American culture create considerable tension within our society. Those who accept the Puritan view of sexuality tend to be more judgmental in their attitudes on rape and abortion. They may be more likely to blame a victim of rape for bringing about her misfortune: "The hussy brought it on herself." Similarly, they are likely to have punitive attitudes towards women seeking an abortion: "She should have thought about that before she had sex."[4] Repressive attitudes on sexuality also have major consequences for patterns of individual behavior, as well as for public health. For example, embarrassment and body shame may inhibit both women and men from obtaining routine health checkups, including examination of their reproductive organs that could provide early detection of sexual dysfunction problems, sexually transmitted infections (STIs), and cancer.

Those who embrace the libertine philosophy often refuse to acknowledge that the escalation of graphic detail in the depictions of sex in the media might have negative consequences on children or the erosion of moral values. The notion that only penile-vaginal penetration is "sex" diminishes a whole range of other non-genital actions that satisfy the hunger for touch and affection, such as physical touching, and hugging or holding each other. What concerns most Americans, not only Puritan conservatives, is that the constant exposure to sex on TV, in the movies, and in our advertising makes it difficult for parents to control "the content and taboos of adult life."[5,6] Children at very young ages are exposed to graphic portrayals of sex, making a gradual age appropriate introduction to the subject by parents impossible or irrelevant. Indeed, some parents have difficulties identifying what is age appropriate information.[7,8] With the culture awash in sexually explicit material, parents in many cases feel inadequate to explain sex and values to their children, often leaving kids without guidance and with media induced stereotypes that are risky for their physical and emotional health.[9] Many engage in high risk sexual behavior that presents a danger to themselves as well as to public health. Particularly alarming is the explosive increase in STIs, including HIV infections among adolescents.[10] A major problem appears to be the inability of American adolescents to negotiate about the use of barrier contraceptives prior to engaging in intercourse.[11] Advocates for Youth, a nonprofit organization that works to prevent adolescent pregnancy and STIs and HIV infection, found that the adolescent gonorrhea rate of American adolescents is 25 times higher than in Germany, the adolescent chlamydia rate is 20 times higher than in France, and the syphilis rate 6 times higher than in the Netherlands.[12]

Various conservative groups have promoted sexual abstinence as the answer to "permissive sex education."[13,14] Although the age for first sexual activity for some adolescents keeps falling, surveys also indicate that increasing numbers of adolescents have at least resolved to delay sexual activity.[15] The Teen Abstinence Movement, established in some areas with State funding,[16] is designed to provide peer support to adolescents to resist the pressure to have sex.[17] Abstinence Only programs have found only limited support among adolescents,[18] and are considered unrealistic by sex educators because such programs oppose comprehensive sex education and prohibit making contraceptives available to adolescents in schools.[19] Advocates for Youth and the Sexuality Information and Education Council of the United States (SIECUS) point out that the experience in Europe has shown that comprehensive sex education programs, including counseling on "postponing" sexual intercourse, as well as information on safe sex and health issues do *not* lead to an increase in sexual activity among adolescents (see Box 7-1). In a report touting the benefits of sex education, the US Surgeon General called for a multipronged effort to promote safe sex among those most prone to be sexually active.[20] Largely as a result of better education, condom use by American adolescents is up significantly, leading to a decline in the adolescent pregnancy rate.[21]

Discovering and treating STIs early is a vital public health function you can perform. Among adolescents as well as adult singles, the incidence of sexual activity with multiple partners is still high and so are the attendant rates of STIs.[22] But

---

Box 7-1 Characteristics of Sex Education Programs Evaluated to be Effective[70]

- Exploration of personal values and feelings
- Information about advantages of postponing sexual intercourse
- Information on safe sex and pregnancy prevention
- Skill building regarding peer pressure
- Focus on active learning through experiential activities
- Acknowledgment of social and media influence on behavior
- Age appropriate information and activities
- Developmentally appropriate information and activities
- Culturally appropriate messages
- Training for those implementing programs

because talking about sex is an awkward subject, youthful patients will seldom volunteer information about problems related to their sexual activity or behavior. STIs, especially HIV, present an increasing danger to individual and public health the longer they go undetected and untreated. Various professional organizations, as well as the Centers for Disease Control and Prevention (CDC) say that it is imperative that health care providers include routine questions about sexual activity in all medical histories, even with patients as young as 10-12 years old. The Chlamydia Project sponsored by the CDC, has demonstrated that intensive screening efforts in family planning clinics and HMOs for STIs, can bring about significant reductions in STIs and pelvic inflammatory disease in young women.[23] You may also be able to offer life changing or life saving education and guidance to those who are infected and for those who will be their future partners.[24] When treating adolescent males, you may also need to counter the view that only sissies use condoms, which is based on exaggerated views of masculinity. ("If you use a condom, you're a faggot.")[25]

Range of Sexuality

Human sexuality encompasses the sexual knowledge, beliefs, attitudes, values, and behaviors of individuals. Religion or culture tries, with varying success, to define the "appropriate" norms of human sexual behavior. Yet, sexual activity is such an intensely private matter that such norms have only limited success. Little was known about the wide range of sexual behaviors until the ground breaking survey research done by Alfred Kinsey and his associates beginning in the 1940s.[26,27] The prevalence statistics about a number of sexual practices cited in the Kinsey research opened the question about what is "normal." The findings also attracted vehement opposition because they ran counter to the religious and cultural taboos of the time. Nonetheless, despite partisan questioning of his methodology,[28] most of Kinsey's research has been validated by subsequent studies.[29]

The first introduction to sexual experience for most young people is masturbation, or sexual self-stimulation. Conservative religious leaders still regard masturbation as sinful or shameful. Much of the public feels it is a topic that should not be talked about. Even the medical profession has a curious history of falsely attributing various physical and mental debilities to masturbation.[30] Sex educators, on the other hand, are proposing it as a safe and healthy alternative to intercourse.[31] It provides a way to gratify sexual desire without entering into a relationship for which an adolescent or single adult may not be emotionally ready.[32] Masturbation usually continues throughout life, and men and women report using it during marriage. It is a safe way for persons without a partner to stay in touch with their sexuality and to release sexual tensions. However, feelings of guilt and shame persist, and you are likely to encounter patients who are reluctant to admit to it.[33] The health care provider can normalize masturbation so that it can be a healthy alternative to partner sex.

The portrayals of uncommitted sex in the media notwithstanding, the societal norm is still sex within marriage. With lots of "how to" information available even in the more traditional magazines, such as: *Reader's Digest, Good Housekeeping,* and *Modern Maturity,* more married couples appear to be willing to experiment with wider ranges of sexual practices than before. The greater accessibility and reliability of contraceptives has freed many couples from the fears of unwanted pregnancy, thus increasing enjoyment. Many women have been supported by the feminist movement to accept and enjoy their sexuality.

At the same time, it is evident that norms about sex outside of marriage have undergone significant changes since the Sexual Revolution of the late 1960s. Sex before marriage now seems to be accepted practice, as is living together and having sex without marriage. Weaker commitment to marriage is blamed for the higher divorce rate among couples that had cohabited prior to marriage than among couples who had not.[34] Of public health concern is that more people are having sex with successive partners. It is said that with the long dormancy period of HIV, the sexual histories of both partners dating back ten years is relevant. Men and women having multiple sex partners ought to have regular HIV testing. In practice this is seldom done. The fear of death through AIDS may have tempered promiscuity in both heterosexual and homosexual persons, however, it seems not to have prompted higher rates of *consistent* condom use against the transmission of disease.[35]

GAY, LESBIAN, BISEXUAL AND TRANSGENDERED SEXUALITY

Human sexual attraction and activity is not confined to persons of the opposite sex. Figure 7-1 illustrates a continuum of sexual attraction and of life style from purely heterosexual to purely homosexual. Where along the continuum each person falls may be determined by biological imperatives, i.e., genetics or prenatal hormonal programming in the womb. Since 1981, research evidence has been steadily accumulating that the bodies and brains of homosexual males and females differ subtly in structure and function from their heterosexual counterparts. Most of the evidence points to the role of elevated androgen levels in the womb, or a hypersensitivity of the fetus to androgens in creating these differences.

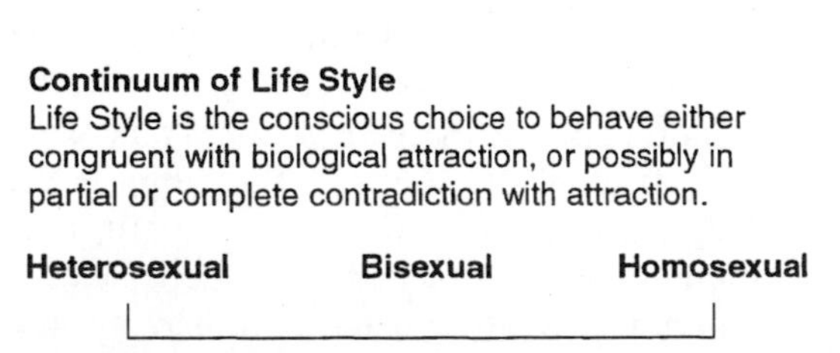

There is also evidence of an impact on a specific area in the fetal brain associated with determining sexual attraction.[36,37] Thus, elevations or fluctuations in androgen levels in the womb at critical periods of fetal development appear to play a major role in the biological determination of homosexual or bisexual orientation.[38] Paradoxically, elevated androgen levels may be responsible for "hard wiring" the brain for same sex attraction in both males and females. The explanation is that the effect of androgen exposure in masculinizing the fetus may not be monotonic.[39] In other words, too much androgen (or hypersensitivity due to a genetically elevated number of androgen receptors)[40], while having a masculinizing effect on physical development,[41,42] may push the sex attraction programming back to the default, or female value.[43]

The exact ratios of prenatal programming along the heterosexual to homosexual continuum are difficult to determine because humans have the ability to override the programming.[44] Thus, we have some persons who for psychosocial reasons choose to behave contrary to their biological programming. For example, some women who were sexually abused as children or who were raped as adults, may choose to opt for a lesbian life style because of strong feelings of antipathy, and distrust towards men.* On the other hand, fear of social disapproval or non-acceptance, forces many persons who are programmed for homosexual attraction to choose a heterosexual life style. Some may also openly live the "socially approved" heterosexual life style while secretly having homosexual experiences or relationships. Those with a bisexual programming are attracted to both the same and opposite

Continuum of Sexual Attraction
Attraction based on internal biological 'programming.'

Heterosexual	Bisexual	Homosexual
(Attracted only to opposite sex)	(Attracted to either sex)	(Attracted only to same sex)

Continuum of Life Style
Life Style is the conscious choice to behave either congruent with biological attraction, or possibly in partial or complete contradiction with attraction.

Heterosexual	Bisexual	Homosexual

Figure 7-1 Range of sexuality.

*An exception are "LUGs" (lesbian until graduation). These are young college women who want to avoid the complications of heterosexual relationships, both from the standpoint of distracting them from their studies, and the fear of pregnancy and STIs. Instead they have lesbian relationships with room mates or female friends. After graduation they give up the homosexual life style, find a husband and raise families. Rimer S (1993) Campus Lesbians Step into Unfamiliar Light. *New York Times*, June 5, p 6.

gender relationships. However, few have an openly bisexual life style.

Living the life style contrary to the biological programming is often experienced as uncomfortable, or even stressful by the person. Determining their gender orientation is an especially difficult issue for children and adolescents. Some, but not all children, whose brain structures were wired for same sex (or bisexual) attraction are likely to behave in ways not in line with socially approved stereotypes for their anatomic gender, as evidenced by their choice of toys, or activities which may attract labels like tomboy, sissy, or fag.[45] As they enter puberty and start to explore their sexuality, they may experience confusion and inner turmoil as well as more intense social disapproval.[46] The internal struggle for self acceptance and acceptance by others of their gender orientation produces high rates of depression, attempted and successful suicide, as well as elevated rates of substance abuse and chemical dependency, prostitution, and running away among such conflicted adolescents.[47] Faced with societal and/or family disapproval and hostility, some may keep their orientation hidden. Others may go through the difficult process of coming out.

A small percentage of girls and boys believe their body is the "wrong sex." Some may pursue becoming a transgendered person throughout their lifetime.[48] The psychiatric community labels this experience as Gender Identity Disorder. It is characterized as a "strong and persistent cross-gender identification (not merely a desire for any perceived cultural advantages of being the other sex)" and a persistent "discomfort with his or her sex, or a sense of inappropriateness in the gender role of that sex."[49] This can occur in children as well as adolescents and adults. Two professional advocacy groups have established protocols for transgendering (male to female or female to male). Most health care professions follow the *Standards of Care for Gender Dysphoric Persons* presented by the Harry Benjamin International Gender Dysphoria Association. Some practitioners feel that the Benjamin Standards are too specific and rigid.[50] In

---

COMING OUT — A process by which an individual, in the face of societal stigma, moves from denial to acknowledging his/her sexual orientation. Successful resolution leads to acceptance of him/herself in that life style. This usually involves integrating that acceptance into all spheres of life, i.e., social, vocational, familial. A second major step after internal acceptance is to confront the issue of disclosure to the external world. It may be only partial, to trusted friends and coworkers; or complete, including identifying him/herself publicly and/or participating in activities to promote public acceptance of gay rights.

---

the wake of dissatisfaction, the International Conference on Transgender Law and Employment Policy adopted the *Health Law Standards of Care for Transsexualism.*[51]

Sexual History

Human sexual behavior is quite diverse, even before looking at paraphilias (aberrant sexual behaviors). We also know that there is a gender difference in the meaning of sexual activity or intercourse. Women tend to view the sexual act more as an act of giving and an expression of intimacy in the context of relationship, connectedness, warmth and security. For men, emotional considerations, while not unimportant, tend to be secondary to satisfying a biological urge, and achieving a tension release through orgasm. For those men who were socialized into traditional beliefs of male superiority, the sex act may be seen in the context of conquest, domination and control. Internalized cultural expectations that men "should" be ready to instantly respond and satisfy their partner can create performance anxiety that can turn into secondary impotence. As you will find in your practice, there are many exceptions on both sides. Each individual, whether man or woman, approaches sexuality from their own unique perspective.

Hence, the need for sexual history questions as part of your medical history. SIECUS has proposed that at minimum health care providers should ask the following questions:

1. **Tell me about your earliest sexual experience.**

2. **Briefly, give me a history of your sexual experiences to date.**

3. **Have they been with men, women, or both?**

4. **Did you agree to these experiences?**

5. **How does condom use or contraception fit into your sexual behaviors?**

6. **Does your partner actively support your use of condoms or contraception?**

7. **How likely is it that you will have more than one sexual partner?**

8. **Do you have any questions or concerns that you would like to discuss about your sexual response or your relationship?**[52]

BARRIERS TO TAKING SEXUAL HISTORY

Some health care providers like to believe that a sexual history is something separate from a medical history. However, it needs to be an integral part of the complete medical interview. When patients are reluctant to raise sexual concerns or problems some providers conclude, "if the patient doesn't bring it up, it's none of my business." They may be concerned that the patient might perceive them as prying, or as having a prurient interest in their sex life. Even when the short questionnaire indicates a possible sexual problem, health care providers often will not ask critical follow up questions due to their own discomfort around sexuality. Some may worry that they will lose face if they become aroused, flustered, embarrassed while taking a sexual history or when they need to follow up on items and physically examine breasts or genitalia. An easy way to rationalize inaction is to blame time constraints and avoid taking a sexual history as part of the medical history. The best approach is to be

well prepared in advance and desensitize yourself to the impact of revelations of sexual problems and issues. This also includes being familiar with and not getting flustered when patients, not familiar with the clinical terms for genitalia, use slang terms and graphic descriptions of sexual activities.

INCLUSIVENESS

Sexual orientation is a highly charged emotional issue for many patients.[53] Fear of disapproval often prevents patients with a non-heterosexual orientation from seeking help for many gender related health problems.[54] Hidden prejudices and misunderstandings can also complicate the health care provider's relationship with their patient.[55] It is important that health care providers have a clear sense of their own sexuality, so that they may know how to cope with transference and countertransference issues that could lead to problems. We also recommend that you honestly examine any internal messages of disapproval, moral judgment and/or homophobia you may have towards gay, lesbian, bisexual, or transgendered persons. As a health care provider, you are asked to overcome your prejudices when you treat patients of any sexual orientation or with any sexual problems. In your office or clinic setting, the same anti-discrimination principles that apply for race or other minority groups, should also be strictly enforced for persons of different sexual orientation. If you have evidence that there is prejudice among your colleagues and staff, we suggest you be proactive in countering any negativity or hostility towards patients who are not heterosexual.

Most patient information forms or medical history questionnaires contain questions relating to sexual functioning. Often these questions are more specific for women. In general, such forms also tend to assume heterosexual orientation. Thus, if the answer to the question "Are you sex-

---

HOMOPHOBIA — a negative attitude or fear of homosexuality or homosexuals.

ually active?" is affirmative, and the response on use of contraceptives is negative, an automatic conclusion based on heterosexist assumptions might be that the woman (or man) does not care about pregnancy. Heterosexist biases in the language of such questionnaires are now recognized to be serious barriers to the health care of gays, lesbians, or bisexuals. They fear that if they came out to their health care provider, they will be treated in a rejecting manner. A medical history questionnaire that uses inclusive language is one signal that lessens the fear of discrimination.[56] For example, instead of the typical "what type" question on contraceptives which assumes heterosexuality, the question could be "Do you have a need for birth control?" Similarly, the question "Are you homosexual?" is more threatening than "Are your partners men, women or both?" Asking such questions in a non-biased manner gives the patient with a gay, lesbian or bisexual lifestyle permission to confide in their health care provider about their health concerns. Although most professional health care associations now mandate the use of inclusive language, there is still a lag in practice. When you practice in a clinical setting, you need to assure that the medical or sexual history questionnaires conform to these standards of inclusivity. A more detailed Sexual History Questionnaire can be reviewed in Box 7-2.

ADOLESCENTS

Health care providers also have to use caution and sensitivity when taking a history from adolescents. Similarly "inclusive" language should be used to allow adolescents with gay, lesbian or bisexual leanings to identify themselves without fear. However, even this line of questioning must be approached delicately because some adoles-

cents might take offense if they think that you "suspect" them of being homosexual.[57]

In the year 2000 the average age of initial intercourse was 16.[58] However, adolescent sexual behaviors have become more varied. For example, oral or anal sex is seen by some girls as a way to "protect" their virginity. A game played at some teen parties is "sex train." Played like musical chairs, a group of adolescent in couples will have anal sex until the music stops, at which point every one changes partners.[59] Another trend is for "good friends" to share their sex partners with each other. Given some of the non-coital behaviors mentioned above, clinicians should routinely question patients as young as 11 or 12 about their sexual behaviors. Young patients either may be too embarrassed to talk about their sexual activities, or may be fearful that what they reveal will get back to their parents. Thus, it may be necessary to use an indirect approach, and to assure confidentiality (within legal limits). Good openers for establishing confidential rapport would be "Are you dating, or going with someone? A boy or a girl?" When asked with friendly interest, it is more likely that the young patient will offer information about the relationship as well as what they are doing to express love for each other. If the person does not volunteer the information, you can then follow up with either an indirect or direct question depending on the degree of openness of your young patient. Whether or not to use the adolescent's own language instead of clinical terminology depends on your judgment of the patient's comfort level with clinical terms, as well as your own ability to use the colloquial terms. Some questions might be, "In what ways do you satisfy each other's sexual needs?" This can be followed

---

HETEROSEXISM — the attitude or belief that a heterosexual relationship is preferable to all others; it implies discrimination against those practicing other forms of sexuality.

Sexual Behaviors[71]

Masturbation, kissing, holding hands, touching, caressing, massage, oral, vaginal, or anal intercourse. These behaviors may take place with a partner of the same or opposite gender.

Box 7-2 Sexual History

Guidelines For Obtaining A Sexual History

1 — Introduce the sexual history with a transitional statement alerting the patient to the topic and the reason for inquiring. At the same time the patient will be giving you permission to talk about sexual matters.

2 — Set level of specificity. Some questions for women in childbearing age would be irrelevant to post menopausal women.

3 — Convey respect and empathy for patient and his/her concern or problem.

3 — Establish comfortable and effective language system.

4 — Begin with less threatening questions and move gradually toward higher risk material.

5 — Assume the patient has done everything when asking for information (e.g., "When did you begin to..." rather than "Have you ever...".

6 — Avoid "why" questions. Instead ask "what" or "how" questions.

7 — Avoid asking leading questions or suggesting answers. If suggestions are necessary to elicit responses from the patient, present a continuum or range of options.

8 — Watch for, and tactfully label, any inconsistencies in patient's account. These inconsistencies, conscious or unconscious, may point to important material.

9 — Bring closure and summarize to let the patient know that he/she has been heard and understood.

10 — Minimize intrusive recording procedures.

Sexual History Questionnaire

These questions can be part of a routine social history. They are designed to avoid a heterosexist bias.

ALL PATIENTS:

Are you married, partnered or single?

Who is important to you in your life? Is there a significant other in your life?

Who is your emergency contact?

Are you having sex with anyone?

Do you have male or female partners? or both?

Do you practice safe sex with (all of) your partners? What is your method? How?

Do you need birth control?

Have you ever had sex while using drugs or drinking?

Have you ever been abused or raped?

Have you ever exchanged (had) sex for money or drugs?

ADOLESCENTS:

Do you go out or go steady with someone? boy? girl?

Do you have a boyfriend or girlfriend? Have a crush on someone?

Do you ever make out? Pet?

Have you gone all the way? done it? Have you had oral sex with anyone?

Did you want to? Did you not want to?

Did you feel forced? Have you ever been abused or raped?

Have you had sex with boys, girls or both?

Do you know about safe sex? How do you practice safe sex? What is your method? How?

Is there anything you would like to know about gender, sex, intercourse, reproduction, safe sex?

ALL:

Do you have anyone to talk to about sex?

Do you have anyone to talk to about your feelings about sex?

Do you ever not feel safe?

Has anyone ever forced you/ does anyone ever force you to have sex when you do not want to? touched your body when/where you do not did not want them to?

---

up by specific question about mutual masturbation, oral sex, anal sex, and sexual intercourse. If the adolescent answers affirmatively to any of the above questions, you need to find out what they know about safe sex and/or if they are practicing safe sex. If the indication is that they are ignorant or have faulty information about contraception or safe sex, you can make a short detour in your history taking and explain some key facts, and/or jot down a reminder to do so later.

Another concern especially with girls is to find out if sex was forced or possibly abusive. With adolescents there are a number of situations leading to involuntary sex: heavy peer pressure, fear of rejection, incapacity due to intoxication, or date rape. Such encounters can leave deep emotional scars. Adolescents who have had involuntary or forced sex may feel regret, guilt, shame and/or confusion. They may blame themselves for "causing" it. They may also have held in their feelings because they were not sure in whom they could confide or feared they would be ridiculed if they did share what happened. If you sense that you are the first person in whom they may be confiding, listen with empathy as much as you can. If it seems too complicated, you may wish to encourage the adolescent to talk with their parents or a counselor. Indeed, you may want to explore with them their relationship with their parents, and how free they feel discussing with them their own feelings about sexual activity, or a bad experience they have had. While you have an obligation to maintain confidentiality, you can encourage the adolescent to either tell their parent(s), or ask permission for you to share the information with the parent that the adolescent designates. In either case, you should in a separate conference with the parent(s) encourage them to open a dialog with their adolescent about sexuality, relationships, and feelings. Since adolescents are minors, any evidence of sexual abuse, rape or statutory rape creates a legal obligation for mandatory reporting. In complicated cases, we suggest bringing in a designated expert on child or sexual abuse. (See Chapter Eleven).

Special Populations

OLDER PERSONS

In the context of human sexuality, it also necessary to look at the needs of special populations. For example, sex and intimacy needs of older persons are sometimes ignored or forgotten by health care providers. Sexual feelings and the need for intimacy continue throughout one's life course development. Most older couples enjoy sex and intimacy.[60] In fact, freed from time and performance pressures and fears of becoming pregnant, many report greater enjoyment of sexual intimacy than in their younger years. The journey to orgasm is less rushed, as sexual arousal tends to be slower for both. A major barrier to intimacy for many older persons is lack of partner and opportunity. With the pattern of men dying younger, there are a lot of older women without partners. Sexual inactivity of widowed post-menopausal women may accelerate the normal thinning of vaginal walls and the decrease in lubrication normal for that age. When such women resume sexual activity without some preparation or precautions, they may experience discomfort, pain or even injury. Similarly, male widowers who remarry after some time of sexual inactivity may experience paralyzing performance anxiety, known as "widower's syndrome."

CHRONIC ILLNESS AND SEXUALITY

Health care providers also may not realize that a chronic illness, which makes sexual intimacy impossible, may leave the healthy partner seriously depressed. Another common problem arises when ignorance or fear of hurting the "recovering" partner may prevent both partners from resuming sexual activity after a serious illness or operation. Some couples who are unable to negotiate about these taboo difficulties, will forego sexual activities altogether. They may be unwilling to reveal these issues to their health care provider unless prompted with sensitivity and empathic understanding. We suggest that you routinely ask all your recovering patients, no matter what their age, about sexual activity and sexual functioning. Indeed you can perform a valuable service of reassurance and education. One technique that normalizes the situation is to say: "Many patients who have had this same surgery or have this same diagnosis usually experience some difficulty in resuming their sexual relationship with their partner. Is this a problem now?" You can let those who are coming from a period of no sexual activity know that their apprehension is normal, that sexual functioning can be restored in most cases. With patience, leisurely foreplay and lubrication, in the form of a water-soluble jelly, most couples can resume sexual activity after periods of inactivity, or within relatively short intervals after a serious illness, such as a heart attack or bypass surgery.[61]

THE DISABLED

The sexual and emotional intimacy needs of physically or mentally disabled persons also tend to be overlooked or ignored both by society and the health care professions. For example, we may see a quadriplegic as an object of sympathy or even pity, but not as someone who might have sexual desires and needs. As a consequence of this "labeling," many disabled persons feel unwanted and without sex appeal.[62] Health care providers need to be especially careful not to ignore sex and intimacy issues with disabled persons. Routine questions about sexual activity should be included in the medical history. Responses should be explored with great sensitivity. In some instances, follow up questions may unearth situations where your patient was sexually abused by someone taking advantage of the disability or mental impairment. In that case, you need to activate a similar protocol as for child sexual abuse and notify Adult Protective Services.

• •

PATIENT PROFILE 7.2

GIVEN UP

SETTING: *Carolyn is a 33-year-old female who has recently married. She became a paraplegic during her early adolescence as a result of an auto accident. She is in the clinic today to see Dr. Coats, who has been her primary care physician for the past five years. Carolyn's presenting concern today is that sexual intercourse is painful.*

Dr. Coats: Good morning, Carolyn. I see you've been married for three months now, I remember you had been concerned about having sexual intercourse. How is it going?

Carolyn: Sex is still really painful. It hasn't gotten any easier and we have sort of given up on having sex. It's hard on him and I'm worried he'll leave me.

Dr. Coats: Describe to me what happens.

Carolyn: Everything is OK when we are kissing and hugging and I feel ready for him but then when he begins to enter me, it hurts. There's a burning sensation during and afterwards and then I feel badly and start to cry and he's really nice saying it's OK and that he loves me anyway, but I know he is worried about me.

Dr. Coats: You say "burning." Can you describe that some more?

Carolyn: It comes and goes but mainly I just feel pain and tenderness down there.

Dr. Coats: I'm glad you told me about this problem. I can understand that it would be upsetting to you. Of course we need to consult with your neurologist to rule out any involvement from your previous injury.

Carolyn: Yes, I was wondering about that too.

Dr. Coats: However, I would like to have urine sample taken to rule out a urinary tract infection.

POINTS TO CONSIDER:

• Since Carolyn clearly states the reason for seeing Dr. Coats, Dr. Coats starts asking appropriate questions immediately.

• Including contact with Carolyn's neurologist is essential.

• Recommending that Carolyn give a urine sample is the first and most logical step to take.

• •

INSTITUTIONALIZED PERSONS

Health care providers also need to be aware of the sex and intimacy needs of persons in long term care facilities, psychiatric hospitals, or rehabilitation centers. In general, staff and family members have difficulty accepting that residents in these settings would have sexual feelings and would want to express them. A major barrier to expressing these needs in institutional settings is the lack of privacy. For example, it is not uncommon for a staff member, who comes upon a resident who is masturbating in bed, to berate the person. For someone who may already be feeling guilty about masturbation, morally judgmental comments, like "That's evil and disgusting" can be devastating to self-esteem and emotional well being. Staff may need to be educated that the right of patients to fulfill their sexual needs through autoerotic activities in private, should be respected. Similarly, residents who fulfill each other's need for touch and intimacy through hand holding, stroking, or holding each other should not be teased or discouraged, as long as they meet minimum decency standards and both parties are consenting. Sex and intimacy are basic human needs that do not stop when persons are institutionalized.

SITUATIONAL HOMOSEXUALITY

Persons in contained environments, like prisons or submarine-amphibians, also have major barriers to the normal expression of sex and intimacy needs. These same gender environments usually produce what is termed "situational homosexual conduct." Persons deprived of access to opposite gender outlets for the expression of sexual intimacy needs are likely to turn to same sex partners for gratification. While engaging in same sex practices these persons consider themselves as heterosexual.

In prisons, sex is a power and control issue where the strong exact sexual services from the weak, often in a violent and sadistic fashion.[63,64] On board ships, or submarines, same sex gratification may occur due to prolonged isolation. It is generally consensual, infrequent, but furtive and hidden. Ships that go into port at regular intervals generally have less situational homosexuality because sailors have access to females, mostly prostitutes. "Real" homosexuals are despised and can be at severe risk for physical harm in the military. As a health care provider, you may encounter victims of either forced sex or of harassment.

Sexual Dysfunctions

In the course of a lifetime, most persons of either gender are likely to experience temporary interference with their sexual functioning. In fact, a national survey found that 43% of women surveyed and 30% of men suffer from some sexual dysfunction.[65] High levels of stress, illness, and the side effects of certain medications are obvious causes for sexual dysfunction. Less obvious are emotional factors like depression, emotional distancing, or poor communication skills in a relationship. Sometimes patients in talking about their psychosocial pressures may indirectly hint about problems in the area of personal intimacy. At that point it would be appropriate for you to directly question how the stress has affected their sexual functioning and performance. You can explore whether health problems or possible side effects of medications might be affecting sexual functioning of either the patient or their partner. Many of these factors are transient and can often be remedied, either medically, through education, or referral (see below).

Some sexual dysfunctions are more permanent. They may be rooted in organic factors or in severe physical or emotional traumas. At one end of the spectrum are disorders that lower the capacity for sexual function. **Hypoactive Sexual Desire** (aka asexuality) can occur in either gender for various reasons. It is characterized by persistent or recurring lack of desire for sexual activity that is not caused by medication or substance abuse. On the organic side, low hormonal levels may cause temporary or life long asexuality. Depression — during or after a serious illness, post partum, or from other psychosocial causes — can significantly lower sex drive or interest in sex. On the psychological level, there may be various childhood traumas that can cause asexuality. For example, ultraconservative religious upbringing in which any display of child or adolescent sexuality was condemned can lead to a complete repression of sexual feeling. Similarly, childhood sexual abuse can turn a person away from any hint of sexual feelings. For adults, excessive demands, or marital rape by their partner may trigger a shut down of sexual desires. The last three can also cause **Sexual Aversion Disorder**. This condition is usually accompanied by feelings of disgust, fear, or anxiety about the sexual act, or genital secretions or smells. When this aversion is generalized to all sexual stimuli, even being touched during a medical examination can cause fear, anxiety, or even panic. A patient flinching or moving away from physical contact during an examination, may indicate past sexual trauma. In such cases you need to tell the patient in advance of touching them or using an instrument like a speculum. It may help to warm the instruments and your hands. But a patient with a history of sexual trauma or possibly even bad experience during a previous examination, may be unable to relax despite verbal reassurances. She may constrict her muscles, pull away, or adduct her thighs. In such cases a follow-up sexual history should be taken after the patient has dressed and is seated in your office.

At the opposite end of the continuum from extreme hyposexual desire or aversion is **sexual addiction**. This is a compulsive drive for frequent sex, often indiscriminately with any partner. Formerly known as satyriasis in men and nymphomania in women, it is now regarded as an addictive disorder. As with other addictions, it can be as disruptive to normal functioning. It should be treated as an addiction, rather than as either a sexual dysfunction or a moral failing. (See Chapter 9 on Addictions.)

A common sexual dysfunction for men is **premature ejaculation.** This is when ejaculation occurs either before penetration, or within 30-60 seconds of penetration followed by loss of erection. Certain early experiences may condition the male to have a rapid ejaculatory response. This often occurs if the first sexual encounters took place furtively and/or under time pressures, like in a back seat of a car, or with a prostitute. (See Patient Profile 7-1.) Also an early history of heavy petting and ejaculation without penetration — often with clothes on — may condition the man to have a rapid ejaculatory response. Premature ejaculation may cause serious rela-

tionship problems. If the wife or partner is unable to release their sexual tension through intercourse with a partner impaired by this dysfunction, they may feel resentment and may withdraw from all intimate contact, or seek other partners.

Ejaculatory incompetence, aka Male Orgasmic Disorder, is the inability to reach orgasm during intravaginal containment. Some psychosocial factors linked to this disorder are strong religious beliefs, guilt over having been involved in incest, or early experiences of having been abused sexually. Similarly having been caught "in the act" of masturbating or having sex and being severely punished or shamed for it can also bring about ejaculatory incompetence.

Primary impotence, aka Lifelong Male Erectile Disorder, is diagnosed when a man either has never been able to achieve and maintain erection sufficient for coital connection, or when he can achieve erection but always loses it upon attempted penetration. Among the organic causes of this disorder are diabetes mellitus, multiple sclerosis, renal failure, peripheral neuropathy, peripheral vascular disease, spinal cord injury, or injury of the autonomic nervous system through surgery or radiation. Primary impotence often is accompanied by feelings of anxiety and fear when approaching sexual intercourse. Psychosocial reasons can also include: having had an incestuous relationship with one's mother, extreme religiosity, or having been severely punished as a child for expression of sexual feelings or behaviors.

Secondary Impotence, aka Acquired Erectile Disorder, is a pattern of some coital success but then occasional to permanent erectile failure, or losing one's erection shortly before or after penetration. This is not an uncommon condition for many men. Psychosocial causes are fatigue, stress, cultural demand for performance, and anxiety and fear about previous loss of erections. Extreme dominance by the partner may also produce impotence. In addition, excessive alcohol and/or drug intake, and certain medications (anti-hypertensives, antidepressants, neuroleptics) can inhibit arousal or performance.

Female sexual dysfunctions include Orgasmic Disorder, Vaginismus and Dyspareunia. In order for a condition to

"be diagnosed as sexual dysfunction, an identified sexual problem must be causing the woman personal distress or interpersonal difficulties and must meet specific criteria. Although a woman may exhibit the defining criteria, if she does not have personal or relationship difficulties as a result, the sexual dysfunction can not be diagnosed."[66]

Orgasmic Disorder is characterized by a persistent or recurrent delay or absence of orgasm following normal to high level of sexual excitement. As with Male Orgasmic Disorder there are two types: Acquired and Lifelong. Precipitating psychosocial factors include childhood sexual trauma or abuse, previous abortions, severe religious upbringing or a severe sense of personal inadequacy. Organic factors can also include female genital mutilation. Sexual dysfunction due to a systemic medical condition, substance abuse or medications such as antidepressants must also be ruled out. It is often marked by distress or interpersonal difficulty in relationships.

Vaginismus is the spasming of the perivaginal muscles upon stimulation in order to avoid penetration. In some cases, sexual responsiveness, vasocongestion and orgasm may occur with clitoral stimulation, however the muscles cramp thereby stopping penile penetration. Identification of any contributing medical cause for the spasms, such as a history of repetitive catheterization, can help the patient accept the condition. This condition can also be viewed as an unconscious nonverbal protest against sexual relations, since it is usually linked with psychological fear and pain, sexual trauma, or negative attitudes about sex learned in childhood. One standard treatment is a program of gradual desensitization supported by marital therapy with a behavioral orientation. Also instruction in self-dilation where a lubricated finger or test tubes graduated in size (Hegar dilators) are inserted gradually with the concomitant utilization of relaxation imagery generally help reduce spasming.

Dyspareunia is genital pain associated with sexual penetration. Among physical causes are bruising or irritation to the hymenal ring, scar tissue from either gang rapes, abortions, or third or fourth degree episiotomy extension tears. Other conditions contributing to pain may be endometriosis, pelvic inflammatory disease, pelvic or vulvar pathology, infections, age-related atrophic changes, allergic reactions to contraceptive foams and jellies, or a prolapsed uterus pressing on the bladder and within the vagina. Psychosocial stress could include relational difficulties (resentments) with the partner, fatigue, and illness. Not being aroused physiologically due to inadequate foreplay is also a frequent cause in both orgasmic disorder and dyspareunia. Post-menopausal women may lose vaginal elasticity and the ability to lubricate adequately. Some antihistamines and other cold medications can also inhibit adequate lubrication.

PARAPHILIAS — ABERRANT SEXUAL BEHAVIOR

Sexual behaviors that fall far outside the norm are known as paraphilias. They are characterized by recurrent, intense, sexually arousing fantasies, urges or behaviors generally involving non-human objects, the inflicting suffering or humiliation upon oneself or others, including children or other non-consenting persons. They are usually committed by a small percentage of the population, are usually concealed by their participants, and they are generally considered addictive because they are insistently and involuntarily repetitive. No single theoretical explanation fits all cases of paraphilias, although generally psychosocial and biological factors are thought to interact to produce these behaviors.[67] The function of a general practice health care provider is to help identify such behaviors and to convince patients addicted to such behaviors that they need professional help. This is especially important if the behavior is seriously self-harming or possibly even life threatening. The following descriptions are for the most common sexual paraphilias. Less common are: necrophilia, zoophilia, and klismaphilia. Pornography addiction will be covered in the chapter on Addictions.

Fetishism is the sexual use of objects by men of women's underwear, or by women of men's underwear or sweaty athletic wear, such as jock straps or training clothes. The object is usually required for erection or tumescence. Generally masturbation is involved while holding, sniffing, rubbing or pressing the object against one's body. **Frotteurism** is the touching or rubbing of one's body and/or genitals against a non-consenting person's body or genitals. It is usually done in crowded places like subways or buses.

Pedophilia is perhaps the most disturbing of the paraphilias because of the psychological damage to the child victims. Pedophilia is identified as sexual activity with a pre-pubescent child (13 years or younger). It can include a range of behaviors from exposing themselves, masturbating in their presence, touching and fondling or forcing the child to touch or fondle them, to cunnilingus, fellatio, and penetration of various orifices with the perpetrator's penis, finger, tongue, or foreign objects. In 90% of cases, the pedophile is someone whom the child knows.[68] Effective treatment for pedophiles (other than incarceration) is rare. However, some pedophiles have submitted to voluntary castration to eliminate the compulsion to molest children. Most states under Megan's law require sex offenders released from prison to register with local police. A national listing of sex offenders is maintained. Should pedophiles come to your attention either from a perpetrator (highly unlikely) or from a child victim, you have a duty to report this to the local Child Protective Services Agency. (See Chapter 11 on Child Maltreatment for further details.)

Sexual masochism and sadism involves consenting or non-consenting partners engaged in mutually harmful behavior. Masochism is being humiliated, beaten, bound or otherwise made to suffer. Sadism is to inflict suffering on a person. These acts are real, they are not simulated. It may involve the use of restraints, blindfolding, paddling, spanking, whipping, pinching, beating, burning, the use of electric shocks, rape, cutting, stabbing, strangulation, torture,

mutilation or killing. A particularly egregious part of this subculture is the use of "snuff" films or videos in which the victim, usually a child, is actually killed on camera. The disorder is addictive and can increase over time.

Hypoxyphilia is a severe form of sexual masochism and sadism in which sexual thrills come from oxygen deprivation through chest compression, nooses, ligatures, plastic bags or chemical inhalants. This paraphilia can cause death or serious brain damage. Despite these dangers, those who engage in hypoxyphilia claim the legal right to do so because they report that it leads to "spiritual or transcendent" experiences.

Transvestic fetishism is cross-dressing which usually involves heterosexual males. It can originate with or lead to gender discomfort or the experimentation with homosexual experiences. **Voyeurism** is the observing of unsuspecting individuals, usually strangers who are in the process of disrobing, are naked or are engaged in sexual activity. The proverbial "Peeping Tom" usually masturbates either while watching the individual or later while recalling the episode. **Telephone scatologia** or obscene phone calls usually originate from persons who have inadequate social skills and who are either threatened or bored by the prospect of maintaining a normal relationship. **Necrophilia** is the sexual arousal or sexual activity in the presence of or with a corpse. **Zoophilia** (aka bestiality) is committing sexual acts with animals. **Klismaphilia** is sexual arousal from having enemas.

Treatment and Referral

SEXUALLY TRANSMITTED INFECTIONS

In many instances, it is a relatively simple matter to identify and treat infections of sexual organs. However fear and embarrassment often prevents people from seeking medical treatment until it causes major discomfort. Some infections, often unrelated to sexual activity, such as a bladder infection or vulvovaginal candidiasis, simply need to be treated medically. But with most sexually transmitted infections, the health care provider has a public health responsibility to address the sexual behaviors of the patient. Treatment of STIs, solely with antibiotics is incomplete, without getting some information on the behaviors responsible for the sexually transmitted infections. As you question your patients about their knowledge or use of safe sex practices, you may encounter knowledge, but inconsistent use, abysmal ignorance, strange misconceptions, or illusions of "It can't happen to me." In cases of HIV, specific protocols for testing, counseling, education, and mandatory reporting requirements need to be followed.

One crucial educational function is to point out how certain behaviors put the patient at risk for STIs in the first place. A second function of a health care provider is to educate patients on how to protect themselves and their partners in the future by practicing "safe sex." In this role of educator, you need to pay attention to your choice of words, tone of voice and body language, lest you come across as moralizing and judgmental. Maintaining a neutral tone of voice and suppressing reactions of shock or disapproval, will keep the patient listening. A special caution for educating adolescents: sex education is a hot issue for some parents, who seem to believe that giving information to their children will encourage sexual activity. Therefore it is advisable to let parents know that you plan to give the adolescent some basic health information regarding sexuality, and ask if they have any objections. Also you need to remember that adolescents will not share this personal and sexual information freely with you until trust and rapport have been established. This may take multiple visits. However, with a clinic presentation of a sexual concern or problem, the focus of the history must be on their sexual activity, practice and level of knowledge.

SEXUAL DYSFUNCTIONS

The role of educator is also important in many instances of sexual dysfunction. For example, a male patient who learns from you that his impotence or hyposexual desire is organically caused or due to the side effects of prescription drugs, may experience a sense of relief from his feelings of failure. Such knowledge may be equally important to the patient's sexual partner who may have built up feelings of frustration and estrangement. A number of sexual dysfunctions are in fact caused by performance anxiety arising out of the cultural pressures discussed earlier. In some of these cases, a small dose of "Sex Education 101" about the way stress and expectations can interfere with performance, about differences in arousal patterns between men and women and about the need for patience and openness with each other, can be more helpful than you might imagine. For some dysfunctions such as may occur after a long lapse in sexual functioning, as in widower's syndrome, giving patients information might be sufficient for them to teach themselves to reach normal functioning again. In general, informing an "afflicted" patient that stress or performance anxiety induced temporary loss of sexual desire or functioning is common or "normal" in most relationships, can be reassuring by itself.

Of course, many sexual dysfunctions are not resolved so easily. For example, when you have indications that the dysfunction might be due to underlying emotional trauma, it is best to refer that patient to a mental health professional with an expertise in sexual dysfunctions. Similarly, if you perceive that poor relations in a couple may have produced the sexual dysfunction (usually impotence or frigidity), you would refer them for relationship counseling. For other situations you

---

When to Refer

Long standing dysfunctions

Multiple dysfunctions

Current or past abuse

Psychological disorder or acute psychological event

Unknown etiology

No response to medical treatment

may need to convince the patient that referral to a certified sex counselor would be the best route to normal functioning. For example, **sensate focus** techniques pioneered by Masters and Johnson are very specific and involve both partners. These techniques and the professional counseling that goes along with them are best done under the guidance of certified sex counselors or even in a special clinic setting.[69]

PARAPHILIAS

Paraphilias, as stated above are compulsive addictions. Persons engage in them secretly, often with guilt or shame, knowing that these practices are outside the norms of standard behavior. They seldom reveal them to either health or mental health practitioners. Sometimes you will hear about them through a non-consenting partner or spouse. You might ask about paraphilias "Why should I know about these unusual practices?" Although it is unlikely that you will treat many patients with paraphilias, if you are not prepared, you might not only be flustered, but your management of such a patient might be less than effective and professional. When you have such a case, it is important to stay neutral in your response. Avoiding a judgmental attitude is much more likely to get the patient to accept suggestions for treatment. As a first step you could educate the patient on the fact that the paraphilia is an addiction, and that one characteristic of addictions is that they are generally progressive, and thus are likely to interfere with their daily functioning more and more. If the patient accepts this view of the paraphilia as an addiction, you would then suggest to them the need for treatment. If they are willing, you could refer them to either a specialist or psychiatric clinic for treatment. Treatment approaches vary widely and need to be tailored to each individual. They range from behavior modification techniques, such as desensitization, classical conditioning, and aversion therapy to social learning techniques, which focus on improving interpersonal skills for normal relationships; and biological solutions, ranging from hormone treatment to chemical or surgical castration in efforts to suppress not only the aberrant behavior but also sexual drive and responsiveness.

Conclusion

This chapter has looked at various perspectives of human sexuality. Sexuality is an abstract word encumbered with many individual and cultural meanings. For many people dealing with their sexuality is a difficult emotional issue, fraught with moral strictures. Those individual attitudes, as influenced by cultural expectations, directly affect sexual functioning. Hence, when you encounter patients with "sexual" problems, it is rarely a straightforward physical problem that can be treated simply through the application of your medical training. Your overt reaction to a finding evidence of risky sexual behavior, is a key to getting further information. When you show empathy, concern and a non-judgmental attitude, a patient is more likely to listen and cooperate. This allows you to combine the role of health care provider with that of educator. When you provide accurate information to your patients, it can have a powerful positive effect on their emotions and their behavior. In instances of high-risk behavior, sexual identity crisis, dysfunctions or temporary loss of sexual competence, due to a wide variety of organic or psychosocial factors such information delivered in a neutral manner, can disarm internal negative messages, provide hope and reassurance, and motivate patients to change behavior and attitudes.

● ●

PATIENT PROFILE 7.3

NEVER BEEN TESTED

SETTING: *Bob is a 58-year-old divorced male, steel mill worker, and heavy cigarette smoker of 2 packs a day for the past 15 years. He returns to the office today to learn about the results of his lung biopsy. For the past eight years, Bob has* *received his primary health care from Tracy, the physician assistant in the HMO.*

Tracy: Hello Bob. You will be happy to hear that the lung biopsy proved to be a benign lesion.

Bob: Whew, was I worried! What could cause something like that?

Tracy: There are many reasons, Bob. But in your case, the heavy smoking and pneumonia, which you had twice in the last year.

Bob: I just got to quit smoking. (Big sigh.) Tracy, there's something else I wanted to ask you about that is kind of related. Years ago I was treated for gonorrhea. Since then I have learned that one of my partners was bisexual. I've never been tested for HIV. Do you think I should be tested for HIV?

Tracy: That's probably a good idea.

Bob: OK. Do you think the pneumonia I had is the same type that people with AIDS get?

Tracy: Yes, that's possible. One step at a time here. I will give you a brochure on Smoking Cessation Programs in the area so that when you are ready to quit, you have the information.

POINTS TO CONSIDER:

- Bob expresses concern of other possible health problems. Tracy responds with support.

- Preventative medicine is being applied here. Tracy gives Bob a brochure on Smoking Cessation Programs.

• •

In order for you to be able to react professionally when presented with unusual situations or sexual behaviors by your patients, you need to clarify and understand your own attitudes towards the wide range of expressing sexuality. As discussed previously, transference or countertransference are inevitable as patients are attracted to their health care provider or vice versa. Understanding the dynamics of this attraction, being able to recognize it when it occurs, and taking immediate steps to disarm or neutralize it, is essential to avoiding boundary violations that could lead to professional misconduct.

REFERENCES

1. Committee on Adolescence (2001) Condom Use by Adolescents, *Pediatrics*, 107, 6:1463.
2. Kilbourne J. (2000) *Deadly Persuasion: Why Women and Girls Must Fight the Addictive Power of Advertising.* New York: Free Press.
3. Kunkel D, Cope KM, Farinola et al (1999) Sex on TV: A Biennial Report to the Kaiser Family Foundation. *Univ California, Kaiser Family Foundation Report # 1452*, Feb 1999.
4. Chamberlain P, Hardisty J (2000) Reproducing Patriarchy: Reproductive Rights Under Siege. *The Public Eye Magazine*, 14, 1, Summer 2000.
5. Stossel S (1997) The Man Who Counts the Killings, *Atlantic Monthly*, May 1997, 86-104.
6. Kunkel D, Cope KM, Biely E (1999) Sexual Messages on Televisions: Comparing Findings from Three Studies. *J Sex Research*, 36, 3:230-236.
7. Johnson, TC (1999) *Understanding Your Child's Sexual Behavior: What's Natural and Healthy* Oakland CA: New Harbinger Publications, Inc.
8. Haffner, DW (editor) (1995) *Facing Facts: Sexual Health for America's Adolescents.* National Commission on Adolescent Health. New York: Sexuality Information and Education Council of the United States (SIECUS).
9. Word LM, Rivdeneyra R (1999) Contributions of Entertainment Television to Adolescents' Sexual Attitudes and Expectations: The Role of Viewing Amount versus Viewer Involvement. *J Sex Research*, 36, 3:237-249.
10. Joint United Nations Programme on HIV/AIDS (UNAIDS). *Report on the Global HIV/AIDS Epidemic.* Geneva, Switzerland: UNAIDS, 2000.
11. The National Campaign to Prevent Teen Pregnancy (2000) The Cautious Generation: Teens Tell Us About Sex, Virginity, and "The Talk," The National Campaign to Prevent Teen Pregnancy, Washington, DC.
12. Alford S, Feijoo A (1999) European Approaches to Adolescent Sexual Behavior and Responsibility, Washington, DC: Advocates for Youth (Monograph).
13. Piccione JJ, Scholle RA (1995)*Combating Illegitimacy and Counseling Teen Abstinence: A Key Component of Welfare Reform.* (Backgrounder #1051). The Heritage Foundation, August 31, 1995.
14. SIECUS (1999) Opponents of Comprehensive Sexuality Education. *Fact Sheet.* Washington, DC: Sexuality Information and Education Council of the United States (SIECUS).

15. Santelli JS, Lindberg LD et al (2000) Adolescent Sexual Behavior: Estimates and Trends From Four Nationally Representative Surveys. *Family Planning Perspectives* 32, 4, July/August 2000, 156-165, 194.

16. Press Release by Governor George E. Pataki announcing 38 grants worth more than $5.6 million to community-based organizations for teaching teenagers "the benefits of abstinence." Sept 25, 1998.

17. Wilson J (2000) Program pushes teen sex abstinence, Message not just aimed at virgins. *Jacksonville Times Union.* May 27, 2000.

18. Garrison J (2001) Abstinence-Based Sex Ed is Failing, Teens Say. *Los Angeles Times*, Sept 30, 2001, B7.

19. Advocates for Youth & Sexuality Information and Education Council of the United States (SIECUS). Poll on America's Attitudes toward Sexuality Education. Conducted by Hickman-Brown Research for Advocates and SIECUS between February 23 and March 3, 1999. Washington, DC: Hickman-Brown, 1999.

20. Satcher, D (2001) Evidence Based Intervention Models,. In *Surgeon General's Call To Action to Promote Sexual Health and Responsible Sexual Behavior.* Accessed on Internet on October 3, 2001 at www.surgeongeneral.gov/library/sexualhealth/call.pdf

21. Ventura SJ, Mosher WD, Curtin SC. et al (2001) Trends in Pregnancy Rates for the United States, 1976-97: An Update. Nat Vital Statistics Report, 49,4:1120. Accessed on Internet October 3, 2001 at www.cdc.gov/nchs/data/nvsr/nvsr49/nvsr49_04.pdf

22. IOM, Committee on Prevention and Control of Sexually Transmitted Diseases, *The Hidden Epidemic,* Washington, DC: National Academy Press, 1997.

23. CDC. (2000) Youth Risk Behavior Surveillance: US 1999. Preview at web site: www.cdc.gov/mmwr/preview/mmwrhtml/ss4905a1.html

24. SIECUS (1999) Making The Connection: Sexuality and Reproductive Health. A brochure for Health Care Providers. New York: SIECUS.

25. Stoltenberg J (2000) Of Microbes and Manhood, *MS Magazine,* Aug/Sept 2000, 60-63.

26. Kinsey AC, Pomeroy W, Martin CE (1948) *Sexual Behavior in the Human Male.* Philadelphia: Saunders.

27. Kinsey, AC et al (1953) *Sexual Behavior in the Human Female.* Philadelphia: Saunders.

28. Jones JH (1997) *Alfred C. Kinsey A Public/Private Life.* New York: WW Norton.

29. Gathorne-Hardy J (2000) *Sex the Measure of All Things: A Life of Alfred C. Kinsey.* Indiana Univ Press.

30. Bynum B (2001) Discarded diagnoses: Onanism. *Lancet,* 358, 9286:1020.

31. Rosenthal S (1997) Jocelyn Elders is the master of her domain. *US News & World Report,* 123, 17:65.

32. Papalia DE, Olds SW (2001) *Child Development. 8th Ed.* New York: McGraw Hill.

33. Halpern JT, Udrey JT, Suchindra C, Campbell B (2000) Adolescent Males' Willingness to Report Masturbation. *J Sex Research,* 37, 4: 327.

34. Whyte, MK Choosing Mates — The American Way. *Society,* March-April 1992:71-77.

35. Committee on Adolescence (2001) Condom Use by Adolescents, *Pediatrics,* 107,6:1463.

36. LeVay S (1991) A Differences in hypothalamic structure between heterosexual and homosexual men *Science.* 25 3:1034-1037.

37. Swaab DF, Hofman MA (1990) An enlarged suprachiasmatic nucleus in homosexual men. *Brain Research* 537: 141-148.

38. Herman RA, Jones B Mann DR, Wallen K (2002) Timing of prenatal androgen exposure: Anatomical and endocrine effects on juvenile and female rhesus monkeys. *Hormones and Behavior.* (in press).

39. McFadden D, Pasanen EG (2000) Comparison of auditory evoked potentials in heterosexual, homosexual. and bisexual males and females. *J Research in Otolaryngology.* Available online prior to publication at http://link.springer-ny.com/link/service/journals/10162/contents/00/100008/paper/

40. Hamer DH (1999) Genetics and male sexual orientation. *Science* 285:803a.1.

41. Bogart AF, Hershberger S (1999) The relation between sexual orientation and penile size. *Arch Sex Behav* 28:213-221.

42. Williams TJ, Pepitone ME, et al (2000) Finger length ratios and sexual orientation. *Nature* 404:455-456.

43. Herman RA, Jones B Mann DR, Wallen K (2002) Timing of prenatal androgen exposure: Anatomical and endocrine effects on juvenile and female rhesus monkeys. *Hormones and Behavior.* (in press).

44. Wegesin DJ (1998) A neuropsychologic profile of homosexual and heterosexual men and women. *Arch. Sex Behavior* 27:91-108.

45. Schneider M (2000) Sissies and Tomboys: Gender Nonconformity and Homosexual Childhood. (Review) *J Sex Research,* 37, 3:298.

46. Ryan C, Futterman (2001) Social and Develop-

mental Challenges of Lesbian, Gay and Bisexual Youth. In Lesbian, Gay, Bisexual, Transgendered, and Questioning Youth. *SIECUS Report* 29,4:5-19. New York: SIECUS.

47. Gibson P (1989) Gay male and lesbian youth suicide. In Feinleib MR (ed), *Report of the Secretary's Task Force on Prevention and Intervention in Youth Suicide.* DHHS: Public Health Service, 3:110-142.

48. Bartlett NH, Vasey PL, Bukowski WM (2000) Is Gender Identity Disorder in Children a Mental Disorder? *Sex Roles,* 38:753.

49. APA (1994). DSM-IV, p. 537. APA: Washington, DC.

50. *Alternative Sexuality Resources* (1990) Harry Benjamin Standards of Care for Gender Dysphoric Persons, revised draft , found at web address: www.altsex.org/transgender/benjamin.html

51. *Alternative Sexuality Resources* (1993) Health Law Standards of Care for Transsexualism, found at www.altsex.org/transgender/healthlaw.html

52. SIECUS (1999) Making the Connection: Sexuality and Reproductive Health. A brochure for Health Care Providers. New York: SIECUS.

53. Simkin RJ (1998) *Not all your Patients are Straight.* CMAJ, 159,4:370-378.

54. Smith M, Heaton C, Seiver D (1990) Health concerns of Lesbians, *Physician Assistant,* Jan 1990.

55. Allen JE (1999) Invisible Women (Report on discrimination by health care provider against lesbian resulting both in trauma for patient and lawsuit against clinician) *Los Angeles Times,* June 21, 1999, S-1, S-8.

56. Stevens PE, Tatum NO, and White JC (1996) "Optimal care for lesbian patients," *Patient Care,* March 15, 121-140.

57. Ryan C, Futterman D, Stine, K (1998) Helping our Hidden Youth," *Am J Nursing,* 98 (12), 37-41.

58. Santelli JS, Lindberg LD et al (2000) Adolescent Sexual Behavior: Estimates and Trends From Four Nationally Representative Surveys. *Family Planning Perspectives* 32, 4, July/August 2000, 156-165,194.

59. Interview with Sharon Smith, HIV Case Manager, Region IV, West Virginia, on November 7, 2001.

60. Butler RN, Lewis MI (1993) *Love and Sex After 60.* New York: Ballantine, Random House.

61. American Heart Association (2001) Sexual Activity and Heart Disease or Stroke. (AHA Fact Sheet). Accessed on Nov 2, 2001 at www.americanheart .org/Heart_and_Stroke_A_Z_Guide/sex.html

62. SIECUS (2001) Sexuality of Persons with Disabilities, (SIECUS Position Statement) Sexuality Education for People with Disabilities, *SIECUS Report,* 29, 3:2.

63. Scarce M (1997) *Male on Male Rape: The Hidden Toll of Stigma and Shame.* New York: Insight Books.

64. Struckman-Johnson C (1991). "Male Victims of Acquaintance Rape." In A Parrot and L Bechhofer (Eds.), *Acquaintance Rape.* New York: Wiley.

65. Laumann EO, Paik A, Rosen RC (1999) Sexual Dysfunction in the United States: Prevalence and Predictors, *JAMA,* 281:6, 537-544.

66. Smith MA, Shimp LA (2000) *Women's Health Care.* New York, McGraw-Hill, 148-149.

67. Sarason IG, Sarason BR (1999) *Abnormal Psychology: The Problem of Maladaptive Behavior* (9th Ed).Upper Saddle River, NJ: Prentice Hall.

68. Hyde, JS (1994) *Understanding Human Sexuality.* New York: McGraw-Hill.

69. Masters WH, Johnson VE (1970) *Human Sexual Inadequacy.* Boston: Little Brown.

70. Hoffman A (1997) Programs at a Glance: Effective, Comprehensive Sexuality Education, Advocates for Youth, website: www.advocatesforyouth.org/PAG/EFFECTIVE.HTM

71. Haffner, DW (editor) (1995) *Facing Facts: Sexual Health for America's Adolescents.* National Commission on Adolescent Health. New York: Sexuality Information and Education Council of the United States (SIECUS).

CHAPTER 8

Care Giving and End-of-Life Issues

In this chapter we examine caring for elderly patients, end-of-life care, and death and dying. We discuss how the culturally conditioned denial of aging impacts our attitude towards health care as well as preparing for death. We look at the stresses of the burden of caregiving for an aging parent incapacitated by either a sudden or gradual loss of functionality. We will examine the difficulties of making decisions related to various care options as well as on end-of-life care, including the issue of advance directives. We explore how children and adolescents cope with death and how the death of a child or an adolescent impacts adult parents. We suggest guidelines how health care providers can appropriately respond in such situations.

●

PATIENT PROFILE 8.1

I THOUGHT WE HAD MORE TIME TOGETHER

SETTING: Martin, a 64-year-old married male, comes in with the presenting problem of "I am worrying all the time now and my blood pressure is up." He is being treated by Dr. Romney, a specialist in geriatric medicine who works closely with the local hospice. Lindy, Martin's wife of 38 years, has pancreatic cancer. Dr. Romney has treated Martin for high blood pressure and Lindy for arthritis for the past 7 years.

Dr. Romney: Hello Martin. How can I help you?

Martin: My blood pressure is up and I am worrying all the time now.

Dr. Romney: First, let's take your blood pressure. We might need to adjust your medication. What are you worrying about?

Martin: It's Lindy. I just can't get over how fast she is going down. (Martin's eyes well up with tears and he starts to cry. Dr. Romney leans forward and hands him a box of tissues.)

Dr. Romney: Yes, that type of cancer usually progresses quickly. It is a shock to see someone you love change so drastically. Now, tell me what you are worried about.

Martin: Everything! The children. The grandchildren. Money. The house. What to do about the house. It is so big and after she's gone, I'll just rattle around in it. If I sell it, where would I go?

Dr. Romney: Let's take one thing at a time. You are really jumping ahead of yourself. Can you take the time you have together and enjoy each other's company?

Martin: We do, but I just worry about how hard it'll be on her when the pain starts increasing.

Dr. Romney: I am sure you have a lot of questions and they can pile up on you and cause excessive worrying. I know one way to get some of these questions answered. Maybe you need to talk with her oncologist and see if it's time to bring hospice into the picture. Remember we talked about it when she was diagnosed?

Martin: Yeah, (big sigh), I guess it is time. Time. I thought we had more time together.

POINTS TO CONSIDER:

- Dr. Romney takes Martin's blood pressure first then asks him what is worrying him.

- Because of Dr. Romney's experience with hospice, he knows that quiet, unobtrusive but authentic comfort is the best thing for Martin.

- Continued gentle questioning is important to getting a full picture of Martin's worries as well as finding out if there is anything out of the ordinary burdening Martin.

- Reminding Martin of their discussion about hospice focuses Martin's worries into an action plan.

• •

Aging, and Death and Dying in American Culture

American culture is youth and beauty oriented. The cosmetics industry thrives on fear of aging. The aim of advertising appears to be to create dependency on beauty aids that enhance, or maintain our youth.[1] An illusion is created that we can stay forever young. We are also a culture that denies death. Most families avoid talking about death or dying.[2] They also tend not to plan for their own demise.[3] When a life threatening crisis occurs either unexpectedly or even with advance warning, many will have left no instructions for the survivors on how to handle the difficult decisions surrounding the end of life. Among the decisions often left to those remaining behind are those concerning health care in the final stage of life when a person may no longer have the capacity for making decisions.[4] Similarly how to dispose of the bodily remains — often not discussed — falls as a burden on the survivors.[5]

There is also an ambivalence about aging in our society. We cannot ignore the demographic reality that American society as a whole is aging rapidly. In some areas of the country, persons over 65 already make up over one quarter of the population.[6] The bulk of baby boomers, now in middle age, will join the over 65 generation starting in 2012.[7] The rapid increase of persons entering old age and the prospects of millions more joining them soon has spawned commercial enterprises catering to this segment of the population. They range from retirement communities, leisure travel, financial investments, private companies which provide care management, anti-aging cosmetics, vitamins, food supplements, health foods, to pharmaceuticals

enhancing sexual vigor. Good looking older men and women are depicted as being in glowing health, engaged in "fun" activities. Advertisers flatter this generally healthy segment of recent retirees by picturing the retirement years as the Golden Years of enjoyment of life. For those older persons in declining health, there are personal care homes, home health care, and long term care facilities. Politicians of both major parties cater to the primary interests of this segment of older persons: Social Security and Medicare benefits.

But there is also a dark side to American attitudes on aging. The flip side of the American obsession with sex, youth and beauty are the negative stereotypes of aging.[8] They are replete with such unflattering adjectives as useless, crotchety, crabby, forgetful, rigid.[9] One of the most powerful messages is that the older person is superfluous. These messages are driven home when people retire. Although most Americans look forward to retirement, many are not prepared for the sense of feeling disconnected from their colleagues at work, or the absence of the work routine that comes with the change in status. In a society that highly values personal productivity, being retired can lead to a self-image of "I am no longer useful." Second, our culture has a way of devaluing the wisdom of older persons as out of step or irrelevant. Some adult children keep their parents at arms length, and sometimes give nonverbal messages of not taking them seriously.[10] A third message often conveyed is that the older person is no longer physically or mentally competent. Adult children or even total strangers will often try to discourage an older person from doing a task that they feel the person should no longer be doing. Often this is done irrespective of the physical or mental capacities of the older person. Older persons usually resent being discounted or being treated like a child. In fact, Robert Butler first identified this pattern of treating them as if they were incompetent as the **childrenization** of older persons.[11]

Whether an older person internalizes these negative stereotypes depends on several variables. Being married or in a couple relationship can create mutually supportive positive images which provide some protection. Being widowed makes one more vulnerable to these negative messages. Another variable is activity level. The more physically and mentally active or involved the individual is, the more positively they will see themselves. Conversely, some persons with poor social skills, or those with low fixed incomes, or those "trapped" in high crime neighborhoods may become isolated in their own homes. Such persons are likely to feel fearful, helpless and either depressed or anxious, or both.[12] The state of one's health is another variable. In general, the healthier the individual is, the less likely they will see themselves as useless or incompetent. On the other hand, those who are experiencing chronic or increasing health problems are more vulnerable to internalizing negative stereotypes. In line with labeling theory, some older persons "buy into" the negative labels and even start acting them out. We may see that the large cohort of generally healthy baby boomers growing old now will reject such labels. At the same time they are likely to resist or deny that they are aging until declines in physical functioning force them to make accommodations. Indeed one of the developmental tasks for the older person is to accept the aging process as a normal part of this stage of life.

Developmental Tasks of Aging, Loss and Facing Death

In Chapter 3, the discussion of life course development ended with the family facing the challenges and crises of midlife. In this chapter we conclude our review of human development by looking at the tasks of late life. Erik Erikson calls the final challenge or crisis of adult development **integrity versus despair.**[13] During this final developmental stage, the older person confronts the need to accept their lives — as they have lived it — in order to be able to accept their approaching death. According to Erikson, the struggle is to achieve a sense of integrity, of the coherence and wholeness of life, rather than to

give in to despair or regrets over mistakes made or things left undone. The final virtue of this stage is wisdom. Wisdom includes accepting the imperfections in one's self and others. This applies to the life one has lived, the roads not taken, recognizing that one's parents did the best they could and are worthy of love, and living with the losses that accompany aging. Those who do not achieve acceptance are overwhelmed by regret and despair realizing that there is not enough time to take other roads to life satisfaction and integrity.

One of the challenges of this life stage is the reorganization of the family after the death of the original parents. The task of taking on the role of leadership and sustaining ancestral continuity through the perpetuation of family traditions and history now falls on the adult children who may be in their 50s or 60s. They are the ones called upon to give advice and possibly financial assistance to their own adult children. Or in the case where their adult children consist of working couples, they may take on providing day care for their grandchildren.* Such intergenerational transitions are seldom negotiated easily, even if the death came with advance warning after a long illness. For some who naively believed that their parents would always be there for them, the demands of this transition, i.e., to be the new heads of the family can be emotionally difficult. The adult children may be experiencing complicated bereavement and unrelenting grief at the loss of their parents. Several researchers describe that the loss of parents can leave persons feeling orphaned. Some may regress and feel childlike, needy, vulnerable, and confused.[14] This state can "instantly strip away decades of confidence" each time the bereaved adult child confronts the sense of abandonment.[15] Losing a parent often drastically shifts the roles of the adult children, and therefore the family dynamic usually is also

---

*Over 5 million children are cared for daily by grandparents. US Census Bureau (1999) *Coresident Grandparents and Grandchildren* Report (P23-198) available from http://www.census.gov/population/www/socdemo/grandparents.html

altered. One or more of the family members may be uncomfortable, unable or unwilling to accept their new leadership role. Sometimes these "orphaned" adult children turn to each other for solace. At other times, old sibling rivalries will emerge and they may squabble. For example, if one adult child was the principal care giver for some time before the parent's death, there may be strong feelings between the surviving siblings, as well as bitter struggles over who deserves what from the inheritance.[16] Because the transition after the death of the last original parent may be so stressful, the health care provider needs to be alert to the psychosomatic symptoms of this distress. Foremost among these is unrelenting grief that in extreme cases may turn into major depression. You may need to refer such a person for counseling or to a grief support group.

Another major developmental task for many is adjustment to retirement. Those who retire often experience an identity crisis. This is especially true if the retirement was either forced or mandatory. The lack of having a purposeful endeavor, and the changes in physical habits that accompany the transition from work life to retirement can be disorienting, especially for men. Economic and health status are crucial factors in how persons negotiate this transition. Those with comfortable means and in good health tend to enjoy their retirement.[17] Those retirees with marginal financial means or poor health tend to worry more, experience more depression, engage in obsessive compulsive behaviors, and display psychosomatic symptoms which have no organic cause.[18] Some studies have shown that 36 months after retirement is a critical period for life threatening health crises.[19]

THE LOSSES OF OLD AGE

Older persons face multiple losses. Many losses are incremental. This is often true in the realm of physical health. As people move from their 50s into the 60s or even early 70s, changes in physical functioning may be very gradual. However for the "old-old," those over 80, there may be rapid declines. For them, this is a time of multiple losses. Crippling degenerative conditions can affect every aspect of physical functioning and daily living. The decline in the five senses — sight, hearing, smell, taste and touch have physical, emotional, and social consequences. The loss of hearing and/or sight can cut off the older person from the outside world. They may miss out or misunderstand crucial care instructions from a health care provider or other care givers. Since hearing loss often comes on gradually, many persons are either unaware, or pretend that it is not a problem. Refusal to get hearing aids for reasons of pride are common, but low income persons may also be inhibited by cost reasons. An aging parent who does not acknowledge or take responsibility for their hearing loss can be very irritating to adult children or care givers. It can lead to misunderstandings, estrangement, and withdrawal from contact. The loss of sight also limits the older person's ability to be out in the world. Often it means no longer being able to drive, which takes away their independence.

The loss of smell and taste reduces their enjoyment of food and can lead to reduced appetite. The loss of the sense of touch can be dangerous to their safety. When a person is no longer sensitive to temperature or pain, serious injury may result from burns, exposure to cold or from bumping into furniture. Various age related physiological changes and diseases can limit mobility and affect the sense of balance. Arthritis, diabetes or other debilitating conditions can also severely limit mobility. All these physical losses can lead to increasing isolation and depression. Some older persons become prisoners in their own homes.

Another serious isolating factor is the loss of cognitive functioning. **Dementia** has many known causes: metabolic-toxic, structural, and infections. These classifications include diagnoses of folic acid deficiency, Alzheimer's disease, Huntington's chorea, Parkinson's disease, brain tumor, and viral meningitis. Traditionally, dementia is classified as Alzheimer's or non-Alzheimer's type. The most common diagnosis of the non-Alzheimer's dementia is multi-infarct dementia that is associated with cerebrovascular disease. Other causes can be: strokes, vascular insufficiency, head trauma, chronic alcoholism or various progressive degenerative diseases of the brain. For some dementias, the debilitating effects may be overcome through physical and speech therapy. However, loss of cognitive function can result in affective and behavioral disturbances. Health care providers must remember that dementia is sometimes reversible, a condition sometimes called **pseudo dementia**. The cause may be depression, polypharmacy and drug interactions, or hypothyroidism. In the case of isolated persons living alone, inadequate nutrition and lack of social stimulation also need to be investigated as possible causes for dementia. When the picture of dementia is correctly diagnosed as pseudo dementia, the appropriate treatment may completely reverse the dementia.

Another set of losses occurs in the social realm. Men die earlier and widows may no longer feel welcome by other couples. The deaths of their peers further reduces their social contacts. When a number of close friends die over a short period of time, they may experience what is known as grief overload. Such multiple bereavements with inadequate time to grieve or adjust to each loss can lead to chronic depression.[20] (See below for further discussion of grief and mourning.) Sometimes transformations of their immediate neighborhood from one of safety and comfort to one full of unfamiliar people or possibly crime may further limit their social support system, as well as making them fearful to venture out into the world. With television as the window on the world for most homebound elderly, the constant reporting on violent crime, as well as the general violence in TV programming, reinforces fears that the world outside is dangerous. They become prisoners in their own homes.[21]

PLANNING CARE

Just reading through the above list of possible losses can be depressing. Not all older persons experience these losses as problems. Many take the various losses in stride as part of growing old. Others stoutly deny that they have any problems. It is often the latter that may make it difficult for you to plan effective treatment. They may ignore your suggestions that they have routine checkups, or have procedures that are highly recommended for persons over 50 years of age, i.e., colorectal screening, prostate testing, bone scans, mammograms and pap smears. In some extreme cases of denial, they may be scornful of your health assessment, and dismissive of your treatment recommendations. If you understand that for some of these persons denial is a desperate effort to maintain normalcy, and not to give in to frustration and despair, then you can avoid taking their resentful attitude towards you as a personal affront. They may be angry with you because you are the messenger of bad news. So, patience and understanding of their anxiety, coupled with firm insistence on realistic discussion of the medical facts is indicated. In cases where older patients distrust you, either because you are new, "too young," or because they may have had previous bad experiences with health care providers, it may be useful to address the trust issue. (See Box 8-1.)

At the other end of the spectrum, you will encounter some lonely older persons who are starved for attention. Their visit to the health care provider's office becomes their opportunity for social contact and emotional release. They may want to talk about every little pain or body irregularity. It will help you to be patient if you realize that social isolation produces the obsessive ruminations that can turn any pain or irregularity in body function into a major concern. Empathically legitimizing the concern or fears underlying their stated symptoms may reduce their need for attention and reduce the symptoms. ("I can see how the gas and constipation have made you uncomfortable, and how you are worried about it.") Downplaying or ignoring the symptoms is likely to produce an exaggeration of them. In general, the health care provider needs to guard against giving verbal or nonverbal signals that are likely to be perceived as dismissive or condescending. The phrase "Well, that's to be

---

BOX 8-1 Dealing with Distrust

1. Watch for opportunities to empathize with the person who expresses distrust and then bring up your concerns in an empathic manner.

   "It sounds like you are worried about getting the best care. Have some experiences in the past with health care providers left you disappointed?"

2. Focus on the patient (or care giver) and learn more about them.

   If a patient — "Dealing with this health care problem has been rough on you. Can you tell me how this has been affecting you?"

   If a care giver — "How has it been for you trying to care for your husband?"

4. Ask what would help the patient or care giver to trust you.

"From what you have told me, and how it has been for you, I can see how you might find it hard to trust me or other health care providers. What could I do to have you trust me more?"

5. If there is fear and distrust about being treated by other providers (in an HMO or in the hospital) in your absence, you need to reassure them that this is a team effort.

   "I can see how it might be difficult for you to deal with someone different every time you come in. I assure you that we communicate about your situation. My goal is to see you get the best medical care. Will that work for you?"

(Adapted from Platt FW, Gordon GH (1999) Dealing with Distrust of Doctor's Care. In *Field Guide to the Difficult Patient Interview,* Baltimore: Lippincott, Williams & Wilkins.)

---

expected at your age," often uttered with good intention, is neither educational nor reassuring to the patient. Explaining the degenerative processes involved in a specific condition after empathizing with their feelings is more appropriate. The health care provider must make a careful assessment of the elderly patient to determine if the expressed concerns are indeed part of the normal aging process or the signs and symptoms of a new or progressing disease process.

Transference and countertransference

The health care provider also needs to guard against transference and countertransference with their older patients. In a situation where you are significantly younger than your older patients, you may find that some patients will relate to you as if you were their son or daughter. In positive transference you may be able to use these warm feelings towards you to obtain treatment compliance. But you also need to be aware that an older patient may not reveal serious problems to you, because they feel that they don't want to impose on you. ("You're so busy, I didn't want you to worry about *my* problems.") In negative transference, you need to stay alert for antagonistic, or dismissive responses to your

statements or treatment regimen. In some cases, the older patient may make efforts to control the situation and tell *you* what to do. It is important to be aware of both positive and negative transference. If it interferes with your efforts to provide good care then it needs to be addressed directly. In the case of negative transference, you may wish to use the steps suggested for a dialog with the distrustful patient.

You also need to be alert for countertransference. If you find yourself being either overly solicitous, or impatient and dismissive, it is likely that you are dealing with countertransference issues. Again the caution here is to bring such reactions to conscious awareness rather than to let such feelings dominate your interaction with the patient and interfere with optimal care.

Assessing Care Needs

The earnest hope of most people is that they stay healthy and independent into high old age. As pointed out above, loss of health can be very gradual or very sudden. **A crisis of care** can develop with or without warning. A heart attack, a stroke, a fractured hip from a fall at home, or an auto accident can produce an unexpected crisis of care. A crisis of care that develops over time is often more difficult to assess. This is when there is a gradual deterioration in health from arthritis, emphysema, loss of sight or other degenerative conditions. Similarly, onset of dementia is often marked by incremental increases of episodes of disorientation, memory loss, or loss of cognitive function. In such situations, the older person and the family may not wish to acknowledge that "minor incidents" are part of a pattern of deteriorating health or functioning. It is usually only after falls or accidents, or wandering away and getting lost that the family will face up to the care dilemma. Such a crisis generally calls into question the person's ability either to live alone, or even with other family members such as the spouse or adult children.

One effective method for assessing how much help is needed is to convene an **interdisciplinary team meeting**. Ideally such a meeting would be attended by the medical health care provider(s), rehabilitation specialists (physical or speech therapists), a social worker, and of course, members of the family. The assessment should include a comprehensive geriatric assessment of functional ability, physical health, psychological health and socioenvironmental factors. It is intended to determine the elderly patient's ability to perform the **activities of daily living (ADLs)** and the **instrumental activities of daily living (IADLs)**. The ADLs include the self care activities that people must accomplish to survive without help. Patients unable to perform these activities usually require caregiver support for 12-24 hours per day. The IADLs include performing heavy housework, going on errands, managing finances, and using the telephone to summon help or arrange appointments — activities required if the person is to remain independent in a house or apartment.

In addition, an assessment of the social support system is usually made by a social worker. This is especially important if the patient insists on returning to living alone at home, of if there are no nearby relatives who can (or are willing) to move in temporarily with the older person.

Activities of Daily Living (ADLs)

- Preparing meals
- Managing special diets (salt free, or diabetic)
- Dressing
- Bathing and toileting
- Managing medications regimens (multiple medications at different times of day)
- Climbing stairs (ambulation in general)

Questions to be asked are: Are there friends and neighbors who will assist with meal preparation or other daily living tasks? If not, is the patient eligible for home health care, or for chore services through the local agencies (e.g., the Committee on Aging)? In cases where a period of institutional rehabilitation is indicated, the task is to find a facility that is close enough as to be accessible to relatives. Finally, the assessment should also include a review of the financial resources of the older patient. It is essential to determine if the patient has enough money for ordinary living costs, medical co-pay costs, and medications. Many older persons with extremely limited incomes can afford either food or medicine, but often not both. For reasons of pride or shame, discussing financial resources can be a touchy issue. Many older persons are not aware of the various government assistance programs for which they might be eligible. The social worker should be relied on for information and as the referral specialist to access applicable community resources and government programs. In general, the health care team should fully support the social worker's efforts to help the patient and the family to make post hospitalization or post treatment care arrangements.

THE FAMILY CONFERENCE

Most older persons want to return to their own home after a hospitalization for any sudden debilitating crisis. Whether this is realistic depends on such crucial variables as how much assistance in daily living the patient needs, and how it will be provided. When it becomes clear from the interdisciplinary assessment that the patient is unlikely to be able to perform enough ADLs or IADLs to resume independent functioning, the discharge coordinator or social worker should convene a **family conference**.[22] To prepare for such a conference, the health care provider needs to coordinate closely with the social worker to clarify the requirements for medical, nursing, and rehabilitative care. They also need to determine how much care can be provided by home health under existing Medicare regulations. The family needs to have this information so its members can decide who is willing and able to contribute what and how much of the care in terms of time and/or finances. The patient's personal physician, or the most knowledgeable member of the health team, should attend the family conference to authoritatively present the "medical" facts. This would include an assessment of the patient's medical condition, the degree of functionality, the prognosis on the patient's ability to regain normal functioning, and the requirements for rehabilitative care. If mentally competent, it is essential that the patient be included in the conference and the decision making. As an incentive for such participation, Medicare will reimburse for such an interdisciplinary family meeting for after-care planning if the patient is present. The patient's presence may also avoid recriminations and non-cooperation by the patient later on.

If impaired physical or mental functioning calls for round the clock care, the options for in-home care are limited to the availability of a family member, like the spouse, or the affordability of a hired nurse or sitter, possibly augmented by home health care. Alternatively a family member — typically a daughter or daughter-in-law — could take the patient into their home. Because such a move may turn out to be permanent, it needs to be considered by the whole family. Although it may be convenient and save time to make a quick decision to take in the older person, it is not good in the long run to have one person shoulder the entire burden of decision making and caring for the patients by themselves. Caring for an aging, ailing parent in one's own home can become an all-consuming task. It can seriously strain the relationship of the caregiver with their spouse and children, who are likely to feel neglected. Another stressor is that the ailing elderly patient often directs their frustrations and anger over the loss of freedom and physical capacities at the caregiver. The dynamics of such stresses can lead to resentment by the caregiver to the point of wanting to get back at the "ungrateful" patient. This can lead to elder abuse. For all of these reasons, it is critical that the rest of the family be involved and be asked to make specific commitments of time, energy and/or money to contribute to the care. Clear commitments should also be recorded as to who is willing to give respite relief to the designated caregiver.[23]

One answer to this kind of stress on caregivers is for the family members or the individuals needing care to engage the services of a geriatric care manager.[24] This is a relatively new type of professional — either a nurse or a social worker — who helps plan and organize care for disabled elderly people.[†] They can often help families chose the right level of care, arrange the kind of the services that are available, like Meals on Wheels, or home health care. They can do what busy or distant family members may have difficulty doing. They can oversee that the various medical and non-medical needs are being met. This may include arranging and accompanying the patient to medical appointments, presenting relevant information to the health care provider, acting as an advocate, asking questions, and recording the treatment recommendations. Depending on the degree of trust placed in them by the family or the individuals needing care, they may also be empowered to attend to the legal, financial, emotional, and spiritual needs.

---

†For consumer information on geriatric care managers contact www.aarp.org/confacts/health/caresource.html. To locate care managers in a specific geographic area contact www.caremanager.org

For a variety of reasons — ranging from inadequate finances or housing, family estrangement to geographic distance — in-home care often cannot be arranged. Or the person may be so disabled by a stroke or dementia that they require a level of care beyond the capabilities of relatives. Alternatives are personal care homes or long term care facilities. The primary question in many such situations is: how will such care be paid for? Under federal mandate, all states have enacted **Estate Recovery laws.**[25] These acts generally require that financial assets such as bank accounts, investments, IRA's, annuities, as well as property other than their own home, be liquidated or **"spent down"** before the person becomes eligible for Medicaid to pay for long-term care. Their tangible estate — usually a home — is exempt while the patient is alive. However, the state may require that it be sold after the patient's death. All or part of the proceeds of the sale are used to reimburse the state for the cost of long-term care. There are various exclusions — such as if the surviving spouse, or disabled children live in the house — as well as for family farms. Sheltering such assets by transferring them to the adult children shortly before the patient needs to be placed in a long term care facility is no longer possible because there is now a five year **look back** period in most states. This means that assets transferred within five years of the person's needing long term care are not exempt from estate recovery. These legal requirements may come as an unpleasant surprise to the adult children of the person needing long term care. The prospect of losing their inheritance often prompts a decision by the family to assume the care burden themselves. In such cases it is essential that the health care team arrange for adequate home health nursing care and special equipment needs.

Care of the Dying Persons

Chronic care for an older person can often turn into end-of-life care, however the demarcation between chronic and end-of-life care is seldom clear. Unfortunately, in many instances a **conspiracy of silence** prevents any discussion about death, or the patient's wishes about the type and amount of care efforts to be made around the time of death. This conspiracy includes not only the care givers and the extended family, but members of the helping professions. A person facing death who raises the issue of their last wishes or of dying, may be faced by a chorus of denial from relatives and other care givers. Responses like: "You'll outlive us all." "Stop talking that way" are designed to silence the patient and feed the denial that the person is dying. Aborting a discussion about dying due to the discomfort felt by the family or care givers closes off a golden opportunity for both patient and family members to do preparatory grief. For example, sharing reminiscences and laughter allows both the patient and family members to attain closure, and to begin accepting the impending death.[26] Equally important, denial prevents a discussion of end-of-life planning. The dying person may wish to tell their loved ones what kind of terminal care they want, or do not want, where and how they want their bodily remains disposed of, and how they want to be memorialized.

ADVANCE DIRECTIVES

Mandated by the federal Patient Self Determination Act of 1990, **advance directives** are designed to communicate the person's wishes about what kind of medical interventions they wish to have *in case they are mentally disabled and cannot comprehend the nature and significance of health care decisions or are unable to communicate their wishes.* Such plans should be recorded in written instruments. There are generally two types: the **living will** and the **health proxy**, more commonly known as **Medical Power of Attorney**. The living will is designed for end-of-life situations, such as when the health care team agrees that there is little hope for recovery or when the patient is in a vegetative state. It expresses the patient's desire about whether they want life sustaining interventions towards the end. Some patients may specify that they do not want their natural dying process to be reversed or prolonged. Thus, their living will may state "Do Not Resuscitate" (DNR). It may also include specific instructions to refuse treatment that will prolong life, or to refuse specific interventions such as dialysis, respirators, or feeding tubes.

The Medical Power of Attorney, also known in some states as **Durable Power of Attorney for Health Care**, names a surrogate decision maker (and a back-up) whom the patient trusts to make decisions for them in case they are unable to make those decisions themselves. In order to be valid, either or both, of these documents need to be signed and completed *while the patient is still mentally competent.* They also need to be made available to the health care team. Unfortunately there are several problems with advance directives. For example, the SUPPORT Study, a large, multiyear research-and-demonstration project found that in many end-of-life crisis situations neither family nor health care providers think about or pay attention to advance directives.[27] Another problem is that in many instances neither the relatives nor the health care providers know if directives exist or where they might be. Support has been gathering for the effort of the National Funeral Consumer Alliance to standardize where persons put their advance directives.[‡] They suggest families place them in the freezer section of the refrigerator inside a plastic container envelope. A magnetized sticker on the outside of the refrigerator can be used to remind family, and or caregivers, or EMTs to locate the directives and take them to the emergency room when needed.

If advance directives are not in place before a person becomes incompetent, most states also provide for the emergency appointment of a **health care surrogate**. Generally, the attending physician makes such an appointment on the spot in crisis situations when an incapacitated patient cannot give permission for necessary treatment procedures. Most states list a hierarchy of eligible persons according to the closeness of the relationship to the incapacitated patient. In reality what often happens in emergency situations is that the caregiver who brought the patient to the hospital is asked to become that surrogate, at least temporarily. When — as often is the case — the relative or care provider had no prior discussion with the patient about such contingencies, that person may be taking on the daunting task to give or withhold permission for care decisions affecting the patient's viability and quality of life.

Role of Health Care Provider in Advance Planning

It is in the direct interest of the health care provider to be involved in helping the patient to complete advance directives. Box 8-2 provides a sample format for leading a patient through the decision making process about their wishes for end of life care. Since the family care giver(s) also need to be informed, they should be included in such a dialog when possible. Routine or non-emergency office or clinic visits can provide the opportunity for the health care provider to allay common myths and fears about such instruments. One misconception is that a living will could be used to deny an older person standard medical treatment for curable medical problems. Another is that a medical power of attorney would take away the patient's power to make medical care decisions, and give it to the surrogate decision makers as soon as they sign the advance directives. Such misconceptions can create strong resistance by patients who are reluctant to give up their "independence," as well as by potential surrogates who fear being responsible for every health care decision for the patient. You can explain to all parties that any advance directive comes into force *only* if or when the patient becomes incompetent to make such decisions themselves, either because they cannot understand or comprehend the nature of the decision to be made or they are unable to communicate about it. They also remain in force only until the patient recovers sufficiently to be able to make

---

‡Local member branches of the Funeral Consumer Alliance can be obtained via E-mail at famsa@ funerals.org or on the web at http://www.funerals.org/

BOX 8-2 Discussing Advance Directives

This is a model for opening up the topic and then discussing the patient's specific wishes for end of life care decisions.

"Other patients have indicated circumstances in which they would not want to have CPR or to be placed on life support. Would you like to talk to me about these things so that we will be able to respect your wishes in the future, in the event you become too sick to tell me yourself?" If the patient says, "yes," proceed as follows. "First let me briefly summarize your current medical condition and tell you about how well CPR would work for someone who has your medical problems...."

Now if it is OK, let me ask you some questions:

–In your present condition...

–If your cancer spreads and you are expected to live only a few more months...

–If you develop permanent brain damage so that you cannot remember who or where you are and are unable to recognize your family or care for yourself...

–If you become permanently unconscious (this has been called a vegetative state) so that you never wake up...

...would you want CPR?

...would you want to be put on a breathing machine?

...would you want to go into the intensive care unit?

...would you want to receive tube feedings?

...would you want dialysis?

(Adapted from *WVNEC Newsletter* 5:4, Fall 1995. Morgantown: West Virginia.)

their own decisions again. Situations in which a patient can temporarily lose their ability to make or communicate decisions would be cases of stroke, head trauma, or pseudo dementia. However, in cases of a vegetative coma or advanced dementia (Alzheimer's), such powers could remain in force until the person dies.

Taking a few moments to explain and give reassurances about how and when advance directives come into play can open up a dialog between you, the patient, and the family care giver about the kinds of decisions to be made. For example, you can explain that resuscitation (CPR) tends to have a high success rate (50-90%), when a healthy heart arrests due to electrocution, vascular incident, suffocation, drowning, drug overdose, or anesthetic complication during surgery.[28] However, studies have shown that in cases where physical organs have been deteriorating to the point of pulmonary arrest or heart failure, survival rates to hospital discharge for this invasive procedure are only between 3-5%.[29]

You can also clear up misconceptions about feeding tubes or hydration. When curative care has become futile, the emphasis shifts to palliative care. This usually centers around pain management, hydration and respirative assistance.[30] The patient, care giver, and family members need assurances that the patient's suffering will be kept to a minimum. Families often get anxious about decisions on whether or not feeding tubes should be part of that care. Patients and family often see the choice as being between being fed or starving to death.[31] You can educate the patient and care givers that a gastronomy tube provides only liquid nutrition and none of the pleasures associated with food. Second, you can point out that most persons in a vegetative state or with severe dementia who stop eating, do not indicate they are uncomfortable.[32] Self reports from terminal cancer patients, who are lucid, suggest that they experience analgesia and even euphoria when they stop eating,[33] whereas eating or taking nutrition often increases pain, leads to vomiting and causes general discomfort from gas, constipation, or toxic wastes that the kidneys cannot clear. In fact, patients in terminal conditions may resist and resent forcible attempts to feed them. In practice, the decision to place a gastronomy tube in a terminal patient is often made to satisfy the emotional needs of family members who may not be ready accept that their loved one is dying. Unfortunately once a patient is intubated, making the decision to remove it — aside from procedural hurdles — is usually emotionally even more difficult. Taking a few moments to quietly explain the possible negative effects of feeding a terminal patient may help the family to reconsider.

HOSPICE CARE

Hospice is one kind of palliative care that allows terminally ill patients to be cared for at home. It is provided by nurses and physicians who are specially trained in pain management and other end-of-life palliative care procedures, including emotional support for patient and family.[34] Under federal Medicare reimbursement guidelines, hospice care is available when patient, family and/or the health care team conclude that curative efforts are no longer productive, and when it is estimated that the patient has six months or less to live. (If the patient outlives the 6 months, Medicare certification can be renewed.) Hospice care would seem to be a logical choice for the care of most terminally ill patients. However, it is not as widely used as it could be for two major reasons. One is that the health care professionals, who are trained to save lives and "win the battle" against disease, are frequently unwilling to call an end to curative efforts. Second, doctors are reluctant to pronounce — and many patients are unwilling to accept — the six months "death sentence." Generally, an interdisciplinary care conference can help clarify the situation for all concerned — patient, care giver, and family. It also distributes the decision, so that the health care provider does not carry the sole responsibility for the terminal prognosis.

Once a decision has been made to end curative efforts, **supportive or palliative care** may be the only realistic goal. From that point on, the health care provider has two important responsibilities to allow a dying patient. The first is to manage pain and suffering as effectively as possible. The second is to allow the patient and family to maintain control over the process of dying as much as is feasible. What the dying person may need most is a good intuitive listener who will help them think clearly and make good decisions about choosing options in a complex

health care system.[35] At this time, helping a patient and/or family find meaning in the experience of dying is often more important than adhering to medical routines or surgically correcting physiological abnormalities that are causing distress and discomfort.[36] The enlightened health care provider can also educate the patient and family that these goals can usually best be achieved with hospice care at home rather than having the patient spend their final days, weeks, or months in a hospital setting or a long-term care facility. Being at home rather than in an impersonal institutional setting allows the patient to feel in charge of their dying process. Although hospice care is emotionally taxing on the patient's family, spending this time with the dying loved one is usually also experienced as an intense and rewarding growth experience for the patient and the family. Often trained hospice staff will be able to facilitate open communication so that by the time death arrives, the patient and the care giving family have successfully completed most or all of the stages of grief.

We should add that as part of good supportive care, the patient facing death also needs to be touched by the care givers. In the bustle to fulfill medical, personal hygiene and comfort needs, health care professionals, as well as family members, may forget about the patient's need to be reassured through words, hugs and loving touch. Sometimes when there is disfigurement or the person is dying of AIDS, caregivers may recoil from touching or holding the person. Loving concern can do much to overcome such fears and can be experienced by both the caregiver and the patient as a rewarding experience.

POST DEATH ARRANGEMENTS

After a person dies, the survivors are left with the task of making arrangements for the disposal of the body and/or for a funeral or memorial service. Frequently, the attitude of denial discussed above precludes an open discussion of final arrangements. This puts a tremendous emotional strain on the survivors, which makes them vulnerable to exploitation over funeral arrangements.[37] Here too, a health care provider can play an educational role. First, you can facilitate a discussion between an elderly patient and the care giving relative — before the need arises — by asking what kind of instructions they wish for the burial or disposal of their body. Although you will find that in most cases, few if any, arrangements have been made, your direct question and your positive expectations can trigger a discussion. On a follow up visit, you could ask again what kind, or if any arrangements have been made. Second, you could briefly outline the different options for final arrangements.

The traditional funeral option may put a family of modest means in financial difficulties. A typical funeral package which usually includes embalming, preparing the body for "viewing," a casket, a vault, a burial plot and other "extras" can easily cost $5,000 to $10,000 (Year 2001), but may run into much more.[38] Cremation is a less expensive way of disposing of the body, although if arranged through a funeral home, the cost may still exceed $3,000. Some persons have cultural or faith-based objections to having their dead body incinerated. A third option is to join a consumer group interested in arranging low cost funerals. For example, the National Funeral Consumer Alliance strives to provide "meaningful, dignified, affordable funerals" or means to dispose of the body. Other options include organ donation and body donation. Many states now provide a process by which persons can specify on their driver's license that they wish to be organ donors. If the death was sudden and unexpected, some families find solace in knowing that after death their loved one can "live on" by contributing organs that might give life or sight to someone in dire need. Similarly, people can make arrangements to donate their bodies for medical education and research. Most medical education schools with gross anatomy laboratories have needs for cadavers, and will make arrangements with individuals or families. Your role in such discussion is to get the patient and family to think about the options, hopefully to make decisions ahead of need. The aim is to reduce the emotional and possibly financial stress on the survivors, but also to give reassurance to the patient that their wishes will be respected.

Impact of Death: bereavement, grief, and mourning

The health care provider needs to be alert to the effects of bereavement on their patients. Grief itself is a normal reaction to death or loss. As we adapt to the loss of a loved one, we undergo a complex process of grieving and mourning. The five stages of grief first identified by Elisabeth Kübler-Ross (see Box 8-3) are not linear, but rather wave like or cyclical. Each cycle is initiated by another reminder or confrontation of the reality or finality of the loss. Each time the survivor(s) realize that the deceased is no longer there to share confidences, and experiences, they feel bereaved and they mourn the loss. However, such repeated confrontations also are necessary

---

BOX 8-3 Stages of Grief

The five stages of the grief process identified by Elisabeth Kübler Ross are:

1. *Shock or denial* — emotionally or mentally has not accepted the death. Often will find self expecting the deceased to still be there.
2. *Bargaining or guilt* — retrospectively bargaining for the life of the loved one who died, often accompanied by regret or guilt for things left unsaid or not done.
3. *Anger* — the survivor may be angry at the deceased for abandoning them. They may be angry with God for "taking" the loved one. They may be angry with themselves for not having done enough to "prevent" the death. Or their anger may be directed at the health care providers "who didn't do enough."
4. *Depression* — sadness and depression may blanket the survivor.
5. *Acceptance or resolution* — the survivor accepts the death and moves on with life, no longer preoccupied with any of the preceding stages.

(Kübler-Ross E (1997) *On Death and Dying.* New York: Macmillan.)

for the process of reorientation during which the survivor incorporates the death into an altered schema of self and the world.[39] In general, with sufficient time and social support, the mourning process will allow the survivor(s) to resume normal functioning.[40]

• •

PATIENT PROFILE 8.2

FOOD JUST DOESN'T INTEREST ME!

SETTING: *Carlos, a 59-year-old male, is here today to see his physician assistant because he cannot get to sleep at night and wonders if he has insomnia. Molly, the physician assistant, has been in the family practice for one year and does not know Carlos very well but has read in his chart that his father, who lived with him and his wife, has recently died from a massive CVA.*

Molly: *(I see here that Carlos' father just died. I wonder how he's taking it.)* Hello Carlos. I am sorry to hear about your father. Sometimes that means things really change in families. How are you doing with everything that's been going on?

Carlos: Not well. I have difficulty getting to sleep at night and then when I do, I don't rest well. I wake up tired.

Molly: How's your appetite?

Carlos: Not good. Food just doesn't interest me! It's hard on my wife. She is a great cook.

Moly: Have you noticed any change in your energy levels?

Carlos: What energy? Everything seems so demanding and draining on me.

Molly: Are you still doing the things that you used to enjoy? Golf? Bridge?

Carlos: I have let all that go. It seems hard to care about anything now.

Molly: Sometimes when a parent dies, it can be pretty hard on us. You have three important signs of depression. Your sleep and appetite are disturbed and your energy level is low. Sometimes an anti-depressant can help in situations like this. Would you be willing to take a medication that can help you?

POINTS TO CONSIDER:

• Molly reviews Carlos' chart before she enters the examination room.

• Supporting comments regarding the father's death express empathy. The death of a loved one is a major stressor and requires an inquiry to patient's adjustment and acceptance. It is important to explore the grieving process which Carlos is experiencing.

• Molly questions Carlos regarding possible depression and recommends an anti-depressant. (For more information on depression see Chapter 12 Patients with Mental Disorders.)

• •

How the grief process progresses depends on such factors such as type of death, personality characteristics as well psychosocial support.[41] The timing and nature of the death(s) can complicate or prevent the completion of the grief process. For example, we mentioned above that when a number of loved ones die in short succession — as often happens to older persons when their same age friends die — the survivors may experience **grief overload**. This is when there is not sufficient time to move through the grief stages after each loss before being faced with the next death. Generally, it is marked by depression, and in extreme cases a sense of hopelessness and paralysis. The manner in which a person died can also complicate mourning. If the death was violent or gruesome it can produce **traumatic grief** in the survivor.[42] This is marked by symptoms similar to post traumatic stress disorder (PTSD). Survivors may report anxiety, being jumpy, or having intrusive memories and flashbacks about the death, or the deceased. They may exhibit excessive bitterness and resentment against the world in general, or possibly the medical establishment if they believe that not enough was done to save their loved one. Similarly, ambiguity around a death, such as a disappearance, or a soldier missing in action, or when a body is never recovered after a disaster also produces complicated grief. Not seeing the physical remains of the presumed deceased often prevents the survivor from being able to reach the final stage of the grief process: resolution or acceptance.

In cases where there was forewarning of death, survivor(s) may feel guilty for not having "done enough" to prevent the person from dying. For instance, the surviving spouse of a heart attack victim may believe that if only they had insisted that their partner had seen a doctor sooner, they would still be alive.[43] Death by suicide is particularly hard on surviving family members. For years afterwards, those left behind are pained by internal recriminations about what they "should" have done to prevent the suicide. Suicide also carries with it a social stigma which may be attached to the family. The manner of suicide may also affect how the suicide is viewed in the community.[44] If alcohol or drugs were involved, the family may feel shunned by the community's moral judgment. The family's increased isolation may lead to additional doubts, depression, anger and alienation in their community. The survivors may find themselves outside the natural loop of support and concern. The shock of the suicide and the discomfort by the community makes the developmental tasks after death very difficult for the family. Because the suicide greatly complicates the already difficult grief process, it is essential that the family health care providers offer additional support and help, and be alert to stress induced disease conditions. Due to the stigma of suicide, a family may want to enlist the health care provider in a conspiracy of silence, possibly requesting that he list a different cause of death.

In summary, each individual's personal make up and resilience to planned and unplanned shocks and changes in life also affects their response to death. Among the individual variables in the reaction to death are the person's history of previous losses, any existing psychiatric disorders, as well as the relationship of dependency to the deceased. The personal frame of reference for grieving is also directly related to the core beliefs and values which are absorbed from the psychosocial environment, such as family, peers and culture. Whatever the background,

the process of confronting and adapting to the reality of death can be quite stressful to the bereaved. Box 8-4 lists the multitude of physical, emotional, cognitive, behavioral symptoms that may be signs of grief. In most people proceeding through the grief process, these symptoms are transient, and will lessen or disappear altogether over time. Generally, if the bereaved moves through different stages of grief and arrives at the stage of acceptance, most of the symptoms of grief will disappear after about six to twelve months.

However, not all persons are able to move through the process in a healthy fashion. In such cases the symptoms listed in Box 8-4 may persist and worsen with time. For example, in families where the topic of death or dying is never discussed, there may be a communication shut down after the death of a family member. Fear of disapproval may inhibit family members from expressing their feelings of grief and sadness. Such a negative atmosphere denies family members the mutual support necessary for readjustment and acceptance of the loss.[45] Suppressed grief can become maladaptive in several ways. The pent up emotional energy of masked or distorted grief can produce a number of dysfunctional behavior patterns, ranging from escapist behaviors, like addictions, to very hostile behaviors. However, in others, denied grief may turn into chronic depression. When unrequited grief and depression interferes with normal functioning over a long period of time, it becomes pathological. In a worst case situation, the person will psychosomatize serious illnesses, or become mentally unstable.[46]

PERCEPTIONS OF DEATH AT DIFFERENT STAGES

Impact of Death on Children

Children respond quite differently to death than adults, and their reactions vary according to their developmental stage.[47] Very young children before the age of five have little understanding of the essential meaning of death. They live in the present and do not understand the passage of

Box 8-4 Symptoms of Grief

Physical	Emotional	Cognitive	Behavioral
Back, neck or muscle pain	Shock, numbness	Disbelief, denial "not really dead, just gone."	Depressive behaviors: sleep disturbances
Headaches	Apathy, anhedonia	Confusion, disorientation	social withdrawal
Feelings of weakness or fatigue	Loneliness	Memory, concentration problems	decreased sexual desire appetite change (more or less)
Tightness in chest	Sadness, sorrow, despair	Absentmindedness	
Difficulty in breathing deeply "like a band around my chest"	Yearning, pining "I feel like crying all the time."	Difficulty making decisions "It's like I am in a fog."	Sighing, crying, weepiness Clinging, difficulty with separations, especially in children
Restlessness/ hyperactivity "I feel wired."	Helplessness, hopelessness "I feel overwhelmed."	Ruminating, obsessing "Why?"	
Chills, sweats	Anger, irritability, hostility	Retrospective bargaining imagining how death could have been prevented	Angry or hostile behaviors
Sleep disruption	Anxiety, agitation		Argumentative
Startle response	Mood swings "emotional roller coaster" "I feel like I am going crazy."	Visions, dreams, nightmares about the deceased or death "Sometimes she appears to me."	"Acting out" by children Truancy, school phobia Self endangering risk taking
Tightness in stomach area "like knot in my gut"			
Diarrhea/Constipation	Self reproach, regret guilt "If only I had... he'd still be alive."	Worrying about "getting right with God"	Increased sexual activity
Weight loss			Increased use of alcohol, drugs
Dry mouth	Relief, peace, calm	Change in core beliefs "World no longer safe."	Looking for the deceased
Higher susceptibility to infections	Perceptions of "presence" "Sometimes I feel her with me."	Awareness of own mortality	Carrying objects of the deceased
Psychosomatization of various aches, illnesses		Sense of unreality, depersonalization	Visiting or staying in places linked to the deceased
		Loss of sense of direction	Telling, retelling story of death
		Sense of meaninglessness "What's the use."	Idealizing the deceased

(Adapted from Jordan JR (2001) *Grief counseling & clinical practice: what therapists need to know.* The Family Loss Project: Sherborn, MA.)

time, therefore they do not understand that death is permanent. They may think that death is reversible or temporary. Because children view themselves as the center of their universe, they may engage in a form of **magical thinking.** One form of magical thinking is when the child believes that they caused or were responsible for the death of their loved one because of a behavior ("I was a bad boy."), a negative emotion ("I was mad at him") , or an omission ("I didn't kiss him good night."). A young child may even believe that God took the loved one away as a punishment for those "bad" behaviors. Being observant and really listening to a child at this time is key to assessing the extent of guilt or any misplaced sense of responsibility for the death.[48] See Box 8-5.

How a child's initial experience with death is handled may set a pattern of response to death later in life. Talking to a child about the death of a loved one is not easy. Sometimes a distressed parent will ask their health care provider how to explain death to their child. Your role here is as an educator of a parent who may be distraught

---

BOX 8-5 Physical and behavioral symptoms of grief in young children

- Increased crying
- Temporary regression of behaviors (bed wetting or bathroom accidents, thumb sucking, excessive clinging)
- Become withdrawn, talk less
- Engage in minor misbehavior
- Stomach or headaches
- Complain of feeling tired or feeling real sad
- Confusion about household routines and schedules that are altered
- Worries about who will care for the dead person, who will feed them, where they live when they are dead, will they be loved by anyone, where they are.

---

and fearful about saying the wrong things to the child. Child bereavement specialist Wolfelt suggests some guidelines which apply no matter what belief system one adheres to.[49] You can pass these on to parents, or give some of these reassurances directly to the child. Box 8-6 contains some of the Do's and Don'ts of talking with a young child about death. In general, the guiding principle for dealing with young children is to be honest, but short on words and long on hugs.

Older children up to the age of 9 or 10 years do have some understanding about the finality of death and may develop curiosity about death. They may need a further clarification of what death is and is not. They may worry intensely about what happens after death. Some may fear that one death means that another one is sure to follow. Or they may have fears that they may die. They may want to stay at home from school fearing that another loved one will die if they are at school. They may develop a fear of the dark, and may want to sleep with the parents or older siblings. Usually a child in that age group is affected by the disruptions in family routines more than anything else. They may be sad because the person is no longer there to meet their own needs, e.g., baby-sitting, sharing of chores, or reading to them at bedtime. They may be unsettled by other changes in scheduling, like who does what. Their school performance may suffer. The child needs to be assured that grief is a natural and necessary process to go through and resolve. The family may also need to be reminded that grief is an important developmental task for *all* its members.[50] In cases of loss of a loved one it is comforting for younger children if the parents can maintain as much of the normal daily routine as possible.

BOX 8-6 Do's and Don'ts in Talking with Children about Death

Do...

...explain that death is inevitable for all living things.

...ask them how they feel about the loss of the loved one.

...reassure that feelings of sadness, anger, fear are OK.

...assure that the death of the loved one was not their fault.

...be honest though brief about what the cause of death was.

...assure child that you and others will be around for a long time.

...model appropriate grieving for children, including crying.

...allow children to be part of planning for ritual or memorial services.

...be alert to their feelings, give hugs, and other reassurances.

...allow child to act out grief in fantasy play or drawings.

Don't...

...use euphemisms to shield child from the reality of death.

...say that deceased went to sleep, on a trip.

...overwhelm child with complicated explanations.

...scold the child for grief related feelings or behaviors.

...say person died because child was bad.

● ●

PATIENT PROFILE 8.3

HAVING ACCIDENTS

SETTING: Marion, a 30-year-old married female with a 4-year-old son, Sammy, has come in to talk with her physician assistant, Peter. Her father, Sammy's grandfather, with whom Sammy was close died 2 months ago. Peter has been treating Marion for 6 years now at a local health clinic with 5 physicians. The presenting problem is that Marion wants to talk with Peter about Sammy.

Peter: Good morning Marion. So you want to talk with me about Sammy?

Marion: You remember that my father, and Sammy's grandfather passed away 2 months ago. You know how close Sammy and his Grandpa were! He is missing his Grandpa a lot. I miss him too. We all do. *(She tears up but continues.)* Almost daily he is asking "why this and why that" and wonders about things. I want to give him the right answers and help him but I don't think I am doing any good.

Peter: What makes you believe that?

Marion: Well he has started to wet the bed several times a week and having "accidents" at Day Care. I don't know what to do any more. I need your help.

Peter: Certainly. I can help you and Sammy, but first tell me at what age Sammy was toilet trained, day and night?

Marion proceeds to give Peter the details he requested.

Peter: It sounds like he is taking his grandfather's death fairly hard and is regressing some. What have you told him about his grandfather dying?

Marion: I told him Grandpa was dead and wouldn't come back and that it wasn't his fault. I gave him some old pictures of Pa and we have started telling stories about the kinds of things they liked to do together.

Peter: That is great. I am sure that is helping him. You can also tell him if he has any questions he should ask you or your husband.

Marion: Oh, we've done that, but I just don't feel like he's getting it.

Peter: When they are four years old, they often are more confused by the change in people's schedules than anything. He is most likely missing his grandfather for those special times together. What else has changed since your father died?

Marion: Our routines mainly.

Peter: Can you give me an example?

Marion: Mealtimes. We catch meals when we can and sometimes I just throw something quick together.

Peter: It is important to reestablish some routines so Sammy feels safer. He might be feeling scared because of all the changes. Also here is the name of a book about children and grief. It might give you some more ideas. I think our local hospice has copies for parents. Begin to limit Sammy's intake of liquids in the evening. Also ask the Day Care staff to remind Sammy on the hour to go to the bathroom. The accidents should decrease gradually.

Marion: Thank you, Peter.

POINTS TO CONSIDER:

- Peter identifies that Sammy might be regressing some and questions Marion further about what has been said about his grandfather dying. He lets Marion talk while he listens.

- Peter acknowledges that he will help Marion and Sammy.

- Peter reminds Marion that keeping an open dialog with Sammy is essential.

- Peter explores the developmental stages of Sammy explaining how children's perception and understanding of death differ from adults.

- Peter reiterates the importance of maintaining routines with children when a loved one has died.

- Peter offers additional help in the form of a reference on children and grief.

● ●

Impact of Death on Adolescents

Adolescents are undergoing many developmental changes in physical, mental, emotional, and social spheres. Because of the rapid fluctuations in emotions, hormones, and social relations, the impact of someone close to them dying can be exaggerated.[51] The death of a close person in their lives may trigger feelings of helplessness. They may feel intense sadness and depression. Or they may develop intense anger and rage at the dead person, the doctors, you, their family, the world, or God. They may act out and "not be themselves." They may also experience severe remorse about the last negative encounter they had with the dead person. They may also begin to have fears about their own death. If an adolescent has never had anyone die in their life before, the shock of the fact of one's own mortality may be severe. Parents and health care providers need to watch for signs of withdrawal, drastic changes in behavior, depression, and anxiety. If the loved one has been very ill for a long time, the adolescent may feel a sense of relief but may feel guilty for feeling that way. Helping the bereaved adolescent to accept all of their feelings will facilitate the grief process for them. For example, explaining the stages of grief may serve as a road map for navigating through their emotional turmoil. Reassurance, "being there," and honesty is the best approach with adolescents.[52] You need to be alert to the above issues and encourage the parent(s) to keep the home situation as stable as is possible under the circumstances.[53]

Suicide of one of their friends makes the bargaining phase of grieving especially intense for adolescents. Friends of the deceased often had some sense that they were troubled. This may set them up to wonder obsessively what they should have done to prevent it.[54] Parents, teachers and health care providers need to watch out for signs of depression occurring among friends of the deceased. When there are one or more fatal tragedies or suicides in a school, special grief counselors are often called in to assist the student population in their grief process and to prevent "copy cat" suicides. Some schools also hold special memorials. Letting students plan and be part of such a service is therapeutic for all involved.

Parents Losing a Child

Parents who have lost a child may come to their regular health care provider, and talk about their loss, sometimes over an extended period of time. This requires extra attention and empathy. In the early stages of grief, a quiet and substantial presence is often the best approach. You must be very careful not to judge their feelings or behaviors. It is easy to get impatient with a person if you think they "should get over it." Being accepting and supportive is the best attitude to take in this situation. Often grieving parents will benefit from talking with other parents who have lost children. A referral to one of several self-help groups is considered the best option here.[¶]

Provider Response to Death and Dying

An ancient — some would say sacred — obligation for health care providers is to alleviate human suffering, particularly when death is imminent. Yet, all too often providers will offer heroic procedures to terminal patients that in all likelihood will not prolong life, but may instead generate additional suffering.[55] Paul Rousseau, a palliative care specialist, calls such strategies "misdirected efforts to provide hope to patients and assuage physicians' impotency over a disease process."[56] He discusses four fundamental assumptions why many providers have difficulty admitting or honestly addressing the terminal nature of their patients' disease progression. These are: 1) inference of failure, 2) self confrontation of mortality, 3) time constraints and economic disincentives, and 4) the paucity of education and role models. The first assumption suggests that health care providers infer that when a patient dies, the disease has "persevered

---

¶One national support group for bereaved parents is Compassionate Friends. Phone: 630-990-0010.

and subjugated" their own curative abilities.[57] Rather than admit this "failure", providers may wish to believe that it is more beneficent to continue aggressive treatments such as chemotherapy and radiation therapy, rather than confront the perceived futility of restorative or curative therapies. The problem is that such strategies are likely to instill a false sense of hope in the patient and their family. They can weaken the relationship between the family and the health care provider when such therapies fail to produce a cure, and reduce the patient's quality of life before death. It also deprives the patient and the family of opportunities to prepare for death. Initiating instead a candid discussion about impending death and about the futility of aggressive therapies, may be emotionally difficult initially.[58] However, honest and direct communication is likely to enhance the relationship of trust between provider, the patient, as well as the family. When such honesty is coupled with assurances of standing by the patient to oversee the management of pain and suffering, the patient and the family can devote time to end-of-life emotional and spiritual issues such as reconciling relationships, granting and receiving forgiveness, and to making arrangements for death and funeral planning.[59]

The second assumption implies that avoidance of confrontation of their own mortality may adversely affect the provider's ability to care for dying patients. Being in the here-and-now world of constant activity, busy providers rarely contemplate that their own demise could come about any time through an accident or sudden illness. A dying patient may be an unpleasant and discomforting reminder of their own finite existence. This discomfort may provoke ordering more aggressive therapies which deny the reality of the incurable and inevitably terminal illness. This avoidant approach tends to make the provider emotionally unavailable which leads to the patient feeling abandoned.

The third assumption suggests that the time constraints and economic disincentives of the managed care system may actually encourage poor palliative care. Financial reimbursement for heroic measures are much more lucrative than for palliative care. The time constraints in capitated managed care organizations with their emphasis on high patient volume may discourage the more time consuming nature of attending to palliative care and the dying patient.

Rousseau suggests that the fourth assumption — inadequate education on palliative care —may lead to less than adequate end-of-life care. He suggests that providers "who lack applicable education and skills may reflexively distance themselves from patients, augmenting the fear, trepidation, and uncertainty surrounding the dying process."[60] When providers distance themselves, it can create resentment on the part of the surviving family. This is especially true if the provider(s) or health care team have led the family to believe that the aggressive therapies they had recommended would allow their loved one to survive. Whereas a realistic discussion of the imminence of death would have allowed the family to focus on preparatory grief work, the false hope placed in heroic curative efforts which proved futile may turn into frustration, anger, and the desire to get back at the provider, possibly through a malpractice suit.[61]

BEING THERE FOR THE DYING PATIENT

R. MacLeod noted that many health care providers still appear to believe the old axiom that "professional detachment facilitates good clinical care," whereas emotional caring will cloud decision making on good medical care.[62] MacLeod cites Dr. Francis Peabody who said that "the secret of the care of the patient is in caring for the patient." Edmund Pellegrino, a noted ethicist defined caring as a moral obligation to promote the good of the patient.[63] An integral part of caring is empathy, which one medical educator succinctly described to his students as "It *could* be you." (i.e., the provider could easily be the patient).[64]

The patient with a terminal illness is often enveloped in fear, vulnerability, isolation, and loneliness. Knowing and having empathy for the patient in this state is prerequisite for understanding the patient's needs and concerns. Such empathic understanding will allow the provider and patient to work together for quality end-of-life care.

Role of Emotions

Part of good end-of-life care is attending to the various needs of the dying patient. Specialists in geriatric medicine and palliative care recognize that the management of symptoms and the integration of medical support services are insufficient by themselves in providing for the needs of a dying patient.[65] One palliative care specialist suggests the qualities of openness, responsiveness, and fidelity as conditions for developing "authentic relationships" between the provider and the terminally ill patient.[66] Openness is listening and paying attention to the patient's needs and concerns; be they physical, emotional, or spiritual. Responsiveness is being able to acknowledge those needs empathically. Fidelity is seen as the "justified expectations" that are part of the provider patient relationship. One such expectation is that the provider stand by the patient in difficult times. Within the context of such an authentic relationship, the expression of emotions is entirely appropriate.[67] As pointed out in Chapter 4 (Communication Skills), sharing your own sadness, or sympathizing with a patient's frustration or even anger generally is quite effective in helping the patient cope with their emotions. Normalizing the expression of emotions is especially important in end-of-life situations when so many fear and anxiety producing issues exist.

Spiritual Concerns and Needs

Equally important to attending to the emotional needs is to be responsive to the spiritual needs of patients. Spiritual issues, such as questions about death and the meaning of their own lives, arise naturally in the dying process.[68] There is mounting evidence that the role of religious struggle may be a predictor of mortality among medically ill elderly patients.[69] According to some surveys, most dying patients want their health care provider to address their spiritual concerns.[70] Many providers are uneasy about venturing into the realm of religion and spirituality.[71] In the absence of training and experience in addressing the spiritual needs of patients, the concern is of being accused either of religious-medical quackery, or possibly of proselytizing.[72] However, those with the most experience in caring for the needs of the terminally ill, have always attended to the spiritual needs of their patients.[73] They are convinced that helping patients to address and possibly resolve their spiritual concerns and worries is essential to their overall well being, precisely at the time when medical interventions have lost their curative, even life sustaining values.

The model for addressing spiritual needs in any end-of-life situation presented by Sulmasy comes out of the hospice practice. (See Box 8 7.) The first step is to pay attention and acknowledge the verbal and nonverbal clues given by the patient. They may be in the form of a plaintive query, "Why is God doing this to me?" Or it might be the rosary beads or a Bible on the bedside table. Using simple communications techniques, you can acknowledge that you heard the patient or noticed the evidence of spiritual involvement. You can "break the ice" with such simple statements as "It sounds as if you are really questioning why God is doing this to you." or "Is that a rosary?" "Are you reading the Bible?" A more direct invitation to the patient to bring up his religious concerns would be to say, "It sounds as if your illness is putting a strain on your relationship with God." Or in the case of the rosary beads or the Bible, you could follow up with "What part does prayer or religion play in your life?"

How well you can handle questions of spirituality is also affected by countertransference issues. For example, your own need to "stay in control" may make it difficult to help a religious person to accept turning control over to God as death approaches. Such a personal need for control may also make it difficult for you to learn any spiritual lessons that the dying patient can teach you. For these reasons, it is important for you to take inventory of your own spiritual beliefs and

> ## BOX 8-7 Responding to patient clues about spiritual concerns
>
> - **Acknowledge** Do not ignore the clues, whether verbal or nonverbal, but acknowledge that you have noticed the spiritual concern. For example, simply ask, "Is that the Koran you're reading?"
> - **Respond** Extend an invitation for the patient to "open up" and share more spontaneously. It may be necessary to ask explicitly — for example, "Would you like to speak more with me or a chaplain about your spiritual concerns?"
> - **Listen** Avoid the temptation to provide answers, even if the patient is of your own religious background. By listening respectfully and attentively you can best achieve the task of eliciting spiritual concerns.
> - **Refer** Having elicited the patient's spiritual concerns and having reassured the patient that these are "safe" topics for discussion in the context of the physician-patient relationship, make arrangements for referral if important issues remain unresolved after a brief discussion. Appropriate referrals include suggesting that the patient pursue the matter further with his or her clergy or make a referral to the hospital's pastoral or spiritual care department.

(Adapted from Sulmasy DP (2001) Addressing the religious and spiritual needs of dying patients *West J Med,* Oct; 175 (4): 254.)

values, so you can be conscious of how they might affect your delivery of end-of-life care.

Conclusion

As our population ages, geriatric medicine will become increasingly more important. Training to serve our rapidly aging population needs to keep up with the vast demographic shift foreseen for the next two decades. This chapter serves to acquaint you with the issues surrounding death and dying and end-of-life care encountered in regular health care as well as with geriatric patients. In keeping with the theme of this book, we have endeavored to illuminate these complex issues from the psychosocial perspective. Our

aim is to let the reader understand the cultural, emotional, and often financial difficulties of the family, the care giver and the patient as they struggle with these issues. In the section on death and dying, we have included a discussion of the impact of death on children, adolescents as well as on adult family members. The loss of a loved one can be so traumatic on some survivors that the level of functioning of individuals can change dramatically for the worse. Our goal in this discussion is to alert the health care providers to signs in the survivors of extreme grief reactions that could turn into psychological dysfunction and/or physical illness. The task of the attending professional health care providers becomes more difficult when these issues are not addressed. This is why we emphasize the health care provider's role as educator and facilitator. It is in your direct interest to help the family break through the barriers of discomfort and denial, and to get them to talk about these essential issues. Open dialog and informed planning and decision making in the care of an elderly or dying person will reduce the stress on both patient and family. Jointly creating specific goals will also simplify care of the patient's medical needs, as well as give clear direction to decisions about life sustaining efforts in end of life situations.

REFERENCES

1. Kilbourne J (2000) *Deadly Persuasion: Why Women and Girls Must Fight the Addictive Power of Advertising.* New York: Free Press.
2. Field JM, Cassel CK (Eds.) (1997) A Profile of Death and Dying in America. In *Approaching Death: Improving Care at the End of Life,* Institute of Medicine. Washington, DC: National Academy Press.
3. Mitford J (1998) *The American Way of Death Revisited.* New York: Alfred Knopf.
4. SUPPORT Principal Investigators (1995) A Controlled Trial to Improve Care for Seriously Ill Hospitalized Patients: The Study to Understand Prognoses and Preferences for Outcomes and Risks of Treatments (SUPPORT), *JAMA* 274:1591-1598.
5. Morgan E (1999) *Dealing Creatively with Death: A Manual of Death Education and Simple Burial.*

(14th Ed). Hinesburg, VT: Upper Access Books.

6. US Census Bureau (2000) Table: Total Number of Persons Age 65 and over, 1900-2050. *Decennial Census Data and Projections.* http://www.agingstats.gov/

7. Peterson PG (1999) *Gray Dawn: How the Coming Age Wave will Transform America and the World.* New York: Times Books.

8. Birren JE, Schaie KW (Eds.) (1985) *Handbook on the Psychology of Aging.* 2nd ed. New York: Van Nostrand.

9. Dychtwald K, Flower J (1999) *Age Wave: How the Most Important Trend of Our Time Will Change Our Future.* New York: Bantam Books.

10. Pipher M (1999) *Another Country: Navigating the Emotional Terrain of our Elders.* New York: Riverhead Books.

11. Butler RN (1975) *Why Survive? Being Old in America.* New York: Harper and Row.

12. Mulsant BH et al. (1996) Comorbid anxiety disorders in late-life depression. *Anxiety* 2(5):242-247.

13. Erikson EH (1985) *The Life Cycle Completed.* New York: Norton.

14. Brooks J (1999) *Midlife Orphan: Facing Life's Changes Now That Your Parents Are Gone.* New York: Penguin.

15. Levy A (1999) *The Orphaned Adult: Understanding and Coping With Grief and Change After the Death of Our Parents.* Cambridge, MA: Perseus Press.

16. Wold LF, Anderson C (1998) *Family Realities: Helping Aging Parents, Closing the Family Home, Dividing Family Possessions, Putting Affairs in Order.* New York: Harmony House.

17. Schick FL (1986) *Statistical Handbook on Aging Americans.* Phoenix AZ: Oryz.

18. Bosse R, et al (1987) Mental Health Differences Among Retirees and Workers: Findings from the Normative Aging Study. *Psychology and Aging,* 214:383-389.

19. Birren JE, Schaie KW (Eds.) (1985) *Handbook on the Psychology of Aging.* 2nd ed. New York: Van Nostrand.

20. Miller K (1998) Prevalence of depression in healthy elderly persons. *Am Family Physician,* 57, 9:2238-40.

21. Bazargan M (1994) The effects of health, environmental, and socio-psychological variables on fear of crime and its consequences among urban black elderly individuals. *Int J Aging & Hum Dev* 38 (2):99-115.

22. Silverstone B, Hyman HK (1989) *You and Your Aging Parent: a Family Guide to Emotional, Physical, and Financial Problems.* 3rd ed. New York: Pantheon Books.

23. Berman C (1997) *Caring for Yourself While Caring for Your Aging Parents: How to Help, How to Survive.* New York: Henry Holt.

24. Greider L (2001) Care managers emerge as a new force in helping. *AARP Bulletin.* 42, 11:9.

25. Cantwell JR (1995) *Reforming Medicaid.* US House Committee on the Budget Policy Report No. 197NCPA Washington: US Government Printing Office.

26. Klein A (1998) *Courage To Laugh: Humor, Hope and Healing in the face of Death .* New York: Penguin Putnam.

27. Lynn J (1997) Unexpected Returns: Insights from SUPPORT. Robert Wood Johnson Foundation accessed at http://www.rwjf.org/app/rw_publications_and_links/publicationsPdfs/library/oldhealth/cha8.htm

28. Weinstein BD, Moss AH (1995) Is there a Right to CPR. *WVNEC Newsletter,* 4:2, 1-2. Morgantown, WV: WVU Press.

29. Moss AH (1995) Outcomes of CPR in Nursing Home Residents. *WVNEC Newsletter,* 4:3, 5.

30. Foley KM, Gelband H (Eds.) (2001) *Improving Palliative Care for Cancer: Summary and Recommendations.* Institute of Medicine. Washington, DC: National Academy Press.

31. Morrison RS (2000) Planning and providing care at the end of life. *Hospital Practice,* Oct 15, 2000, 61-68.

32. Morrison RS, Siu AL (2000) Survival in end stage dementia following acute illness. *JAMA,* 284, 47.

33. Cleeland CS et al. (1994) Pain and its treatment in outpatients with metastatic cancer. *N Engl J Med* 330, 592.

34. National Hospice Organization (1998) *Hospice Care: A Physician's Guide* Arlington, VA: National Hospice Organization.

35. Pipher M (1999) *Another Country: Navigating the Emotional Terrain of our Elders.* New York: Riverhead Books.

36. Merck & Co (1995) *Merck Manual of Geriatrics,* 2nd ed. Whitehouse Station, NJ: Merck Laboratories Pub.

37. Carlson L (1998) *Caring for the Dead: Your Final Act of Love.* Hinesburg, VT: Upper Access Books.

38. Memorial Society of the Greenbrier Valley (2001) Survey of Burial Costs. Lewisburg, WV.

39. Neimeyer RA (2000) *Meaning, Reconstruction and*

the Experience of Loss. Wash. DC: American Psychological Association.

40. Attig T (1996) *How We Grieve: Relearning the World*. New York: Oxford University Press.

41. Stroebe MS, Stroebe W, Hansson RO (2001) *Handbook of Bereavement: Theory, Research, and Intervention*. New York: Cambridge University Press.

42. Jacobs S (1999) *Traumatic Grief: Diagnosis, Treatment and Prevention*. Philadelphia: Brunner/Mazel.

43. Rosenbloom D, Williams MB (1999) *Life After Trauma: A Workbook for Healing*. New York: Guilford Press.

44. Sprang G, McNeil J (1995) *The Many Faces of Bereavement: The Nature and Treatment of Natural, Traumatic, and Stigmatized Grief*. New York: Brunner/Mazel.

45. Doka K (1989) *Disenfranchised Grief: Recognizing Hidden Sorrow*. New York: Lexington.

46. Jacobs S (1993) *Pathologic Grief: Maladaptation to Loss*. Wash, DC: American Psychological Association.

47. Johnson J (1999) *Keys to Helping Children Deal with Death and Grief*. Hauppauge, NY: Barron's Educational Series, Inc.

48. Worden WJ (2001) *Children and Grief: When a Parent Dies*. New York: Guilford Press.

49. Wolfelt A (1994) *Helping Children Cope with Grief*. Bristol, PA: Accelerated Development.

50. Greenlee, S (1992) *When Someone Dies*. Atlanta, GA: Peachtree Publishers.

51. Webb NB (2002) *Helping Bereaved Children: A Handbook for Practitioners*. (2nd Ed). New York: Guilford Pub.

52. Grollman EA (1993) *Straight Talk About Death for Teenagers: How to Cope with Losing Someone You Love*. Boston: Beacon Press.

53. Bode J (1993) *Death Is Hard To Live With: Teenagers Talk about How They Cope with Loss*. New York: Delacorte Press.

54. Kuklin S (1994) *After a Suicide: Young People Speak up*. New York: GP Putnam & Sons.

55. Rousseau PC (2001) Caring for the Dying: why is it so hard for physicians. *West J Med*, 175: 284-285.

56. Rousseau PC (2000) Truth telling and the older adult. *Clin Geriatrics*, 8: 32-35.

57. Mount, BM (1986) Dealing with our losses. *J Clinical Oncology* 4: 1127-1134.

58. Platt FW, Gordon GH (1999) End of Life discussions. In *Field Guide to the Difficult Patient Interview*, Baltimore: Lippincott, Williams & Wilkins. 130-138.

59. Sulmasy DP (2001) At wit's end: dignity, forgive-ness, and the care of the dying. *J Gen Intern Med*, 16:335-338.

60. Rousseau PC (2001) The fear of death and the physician's responsibility to care for the dying. *J Hospice & Palliative Care*, 18, 4: 224-226.

61. Rousseau PC (2001) Caring for the Dying: Why is it so hard for physicians? *West. J Medicine*, 175:284.

62. MacLeod R (2000) Learning to care: A medical perspective. *Palliative Medicine*, 14:209-214.

63. Pellegrino ED (1985) The caring ethic: The relationship of physician to patient. In Bishop AH, Scudder JR (eds): *Caring, Coping, Nurse, Physician Relationships*. Birmingham: Univ of Alabama Press.

64. Spiro HM (1992) What is empathy and can it be taught? *Annals Internal Med* 116:843-846.

65. Gazelle G (2001) A good death: Not just an abstract concept. *J Clin Oncology*, 19:917-918.

66. Abratt RP (2001) A "good death" revisited in the context of doctor-patient relationships. *J Clin Oncology*, 19:3999.

67. Benner P (1997) A dialogue between virtue ethics and care ethics. In Thomasma DC (ed) *The Influence of Edmund D. Pellegrino's Philosophy of Medicine*. Dordreent, Netherlands: Kluwer Academic Publishers.

68. Sulmasy DP (2000). Healing the dying: spiritual issues in the care of the dying patient. In: Kissel J, Thomasma DC, eds. *The Health Professional as Friend and Healer*. Washington, DC: Georgetown University Press; 188-197.

69. Pargament KI, Koenig HG, Tarakeshwar N, Hahn J (2001) Religious struggle as a predictor of mortality among medically ill elderly patients: A two-year longitudinal study *Archives of Internal Medicine*, 161:1881-1885.

70. Daaleman TP, Nease DE (1994) Patient attitudes regarding physician inquiry into spiritual and religious issues. *J Fam Pract* 39:564-568.

71. Kristeller JL, Zumbrun CS, Schilling RF (1999) "I would if I could": how oncologists and oncology nurses address spiritual distress in cancer patients. *Psychooncology*, 8:451-458.

72. Sloan RP, Bagiella E, VandeCreek L et al. (2000) Should physicians prescribe religious activities? *N Engl J Med*, 342:1913-1916.

73. Daaleman TP, VandeCreek L (2000) Placing religion and spirituality in end-of-life care. *JAMA*; 284:2514-2517.

CHAPTER 9

Chemical and Behavioral Addictions

The goals of this chapter are to give you an understanding of differences and commonalities in the etiology of substance and behavioral addictions, to inform you about the various types of substance and behavioral addictions, to tell you how you can screen for them, to alert you to how they can cause medical problems and complicate other medical conditions which interact negatively with treatment, and finally to give you recommendations for referral and treatment.

Under diagnosing substance abuse or dependence as well as behavioral addictions appears to be a major problem in primary care. According to a 1999 survey of primary care doctors, 9 out of 10 (94%) primary care physicians failed to accurately identify substance abuse when presented with early symptoms of alcohol abuse in an adult patient.[1] The survey also revealed that 41% of pediatricians failed to diagnose illegal drug abuse when presented with a classic description of a drug-abusing adolescent patient. In many instances, even when such problem behaviors are identified, health care providers are often unclear on how to address them with their patients and then treat them.

Definitions and Etiology

The literature on addictions often depicts a continuum that goes from occasional use, abuse, compulsive use, to chemical or behavioral dependency. The DSM-IV eschews the word addiction in favor of dependence, described as a "cluster of cognitive, behavioral, and physiological symptoms that lead the individual to continue use of the substance despite significant substance-related problems."[2] In this text, the term **addiction** is used interchangeably with dependency to indicate the compulsive nature of the drug taking behavior. Dependency or addiction generally is marked by two other characteristics: **tolerance** and **withdrawal**. The DSM-IV defines tolerance as "the need for greatly increased amounts of the substance to achieve intoxication or the desired effect or a markedly diminished effect with continued use of the same amount of the substance." Withdrawal is characterized as "a maladaptive behavioral change, with physiological and cognitive concomitants, that occurs when blood and tissue concentrations of a substance decline in an individual who had maintained prolonged heavy use of the substance." **Craving** is defined as the "strong subjective drive to use the substance...likely to be experienced by most (if not all) individuals with Substance Dependence." (DSM-IV: p 176; Table 9-1.)

There are two types of addiction: chemical and behavioral. As indicated above, substance addictions center on compulsively ingesting or inhaling chemical substances to achieve a state of intoxication or a "high." Similarly, behavioral addictions center on compulsively engaging in certain behaviors to get high. In both, abuse or dependence becomes pathological to the point of being harmful to self or others. Tolerance, withdrawal, and craving are similar in both chemical and behavioral addictions.

RESEARCH ON ALCOHOLISM

According to the National Institute on Alcohol Abuse and Alcoholism (NIAAA), about 14 million

TABLE 9-1	DSM-IV Diagnostic Criteria for Substance Dependence

A maladaptive pattern of substance use, leading to clinically significant impairment or distress, as manifested by three (or more) of the following, occurring at any time in the same 12-month period:

(1) tolerance as defined by either of the following:

    (a) a need for markedly increased amount of the substance to achieve intoxication or desired effect

    (b) markedly diminished effect with continued use of the same amount of the substance

(2) withdrawal, as manifested by either of the following:

    (a) the characteristic withdrawal syndrome for the substance (refer to Criteria A and B of the criteria sets for Withdrawal from the specific substances)

    (b) the same (or a closely related) substance is taken to relieve or avoid withdrawal symptoms

(3) the substance is often taken in larger amounts or over a longer period than was intended

(4) there is a persistent desire or unsuccessful efforts to cut down or control substance use

(5) a great deal of time is spent in activities necessary to obtain the substance (e.g., visiting multiple doctors or driving long distances), use the substance (e.g., chain-smoking), or recover from its effects

(6) important social, occupational, or recreational activities are given up or reduced because of substance use

(7) the substance use is continued despite knowledge of having a persistent or recurrent physical or psychological problem that is likely to have been caused or exacerbated by the substance (e.g., current cocaine use despite recognition of cocaine-induced depression, or continued drinking despite recognition that an ulcer was made worse by alcohol consumption)

From American Psychiatric Association. *Diagnostic and Statistical Manual of Mental Disorders: DSM-IV 4th Ed.* Washington, DC, American Psychiatric Association. 1994:181.

adult Americans have an alcohol-use disorder, such as alcohol dependence or abuse. Second only to tobacco, alcohol is the most abused drug in the United States.[3] Its annual economic burden is estimated at $185 billion, calculated from the consequences of alcohol related disorders which include damage to the liver, brain, and other organs, cancer, fetal alcohol syndrome and the life-long deficits it imposes, accidental injury to self and others, property damage, impaired productivity, crime, and broken families.[4]

Much of our knowledge on addictions comes from research on alcoholism. NIAAA, created by Congress in 1970, defined its purpose as coordinating and sponsoring research on "causes, develop prevention measures and treatments for alcohol related problems."[5] Its funding has been consistently increasing to where the appropriation for FY 2002 was $393 million, most of which was scheduled for research grant pro-

jects.[6] Recent research findings in molecular genetics and brain neurochemistry point to common markers for predisposition to substance and behavioral addictions.[7,8] For example, the enzyme, monoamine oxidase (MAO) has been found to have a crucial function in degrading the neurotransmitters dopamine, norepinephrine, and serotonin.[9] All three neurotransmitters are related to satisfying the brain's reward system[10] and to providing the "energy" for the attentional axis from the brain stem to the anterior cingulate cortex (ACC) — a neural region associated with "executive function" or the self regulation of behavior.[11]

Behavioral symptoms of impulsiveness, risk taking, and problems with self-regulation — such as violent or anti-social behavior[12] — are highly associated with early onset of addictive behaviors in both adults and adolescents.[13,14] Research on persons with such behaviors shows an association between genetic variations (mutations or polymorphism) on the dopamine receptor (DRD4).[15,16] Another piece of the genetic puzzle comes from the finding by Blum et al, that the D2 (DRD2) dopamine receptor location may be the "reward gene," which when deficient in dopamine, may lead the person into compulsive efforts to "self medicate" via substance or behavioral addictions.[17,18] The abuse of and dependence on alcohol connected with this condition has been categorized as **Type II alcoholism**[19,20] (as contrasted with **Type I or "milieu limited" alcoholism**, which will be discussed below).

These behavioral symptoms are also the key characteristics of Attention Deficit Disorder (ADD or ADHD).[21] Indeed much of the research on the genetics and biochemistry of ADD indicates that the same genetic neurotransmitter deficits are common to both ADD and Type 2 alcoholism.[22,23,24] Thus, one cause of addictions appears to arise from the genetic neurotransmitter deficiencies in the brain which interfere with executive functions of the frontal lobe, thus leading to poor self regulation, impulsive decisions, and high risk behaviors.[25] At the same time, the "under powered" pleasure center of the brain may lead to efforts to satisfy the pleasure "need" with either substances or behaviors that create temporary "highs." This seems to be the reason why there is a strong correlation between substance abuse patterns and untreated ADD/ADHD.[26,27]

Psychosocial Factors Leading to Addictions

Genetic predisposition or susceptibility does not automatically lead to substance abuse or behavioral addictions. Psychosocial factors can also create the climate or milieu in which such behaviors occur. A common risk factor for "milieu limited" addiction (such as Type I alcoholism) is a severely disturbed childhood.[28] Thus, we see elevated patterns of substance abuse or addictive behaviors among adolescents and adults who were children of alcoholics or abusers of other drugs, as well as among those who were abused and neglected in childhood, and those who came from severely distressed households and families. Psychological factors include depression, poor interpersonal relations, inadequate socialization, oppositionally defiant or antisocial behavior, and learning disabilities. Depression — either endogenous or related to situational factors such as loss, lack of close relationships, or gender identity issues — also is a risk factor for using and abusing drugs or turning to addictive behaviors. In many instances, substances are initially used to get "relief" from "stress." Such stress can consist of feelings of personal, social, or sexual inadequacy (low self-esteem), intrusive traumatic memories from childhood, physical or sexual abuse, or other unpleasant feelings. If the person experiences relief with the use of chemical substances, the onset of such feelings of stress or emotional distress may condition the person to trigger craving for relief.[29]

One link between genetic and environmental factors is the **habituation response** of the neuronal system to pleasurable stimuli in the form or substances or behaviors. The habituation response is the interaction between the pleasurable high of the substance (or behavior) and the subsequent drive (craving)[30] to repeat the experience or to avoid withdrawal symptoms. The habituation response appears to occur more quickly in those genetically affected by neurotransmitter deficiencies.[31]

However, craving does not arise out of a vacuum. Rather, environmental factors usually lead to first use. For example, children and adolescents are powerfully influenced by the behaviors of reference groups such as parents, peers, or other role models. Use and abuse patterns of role models may lead to imitation. If the early experimentation with typical substances, like tobacco or alcohol leads to pleasant outcomes, and/or positive feedback (or lack of negative feedback), the use of that substance or behavior is likely to be reinforced.[32] Research has also shown that the earlier the experimentation with tobacco or alcohol, the greater the risk for subsequent dependence.[33]

IMPLICATIONS FOR TREATMENT

The implications of the aforementioned findings for diagnosis and treatment are enormous. The strong correlation between ADD/ADHD and substance abuse and other risky behaviors should prompt you to use the psychosocial history as a preliminary screening tool for Type 2 chemical addictions as well as for behavioral addiction patterns. (See Chapter 12 for more information on the assessment of ADD.) The strong link between ADD and subsequent substance abuse patterns should also alert you to taking preventive measures, i.e., identifying and treating ADD/ADHD in children before it could lead to experimentation and abuse of substances. Longitudinal research seems to say that treating ADD early, creates an "inoculation effect" against later substance or behavioral addictions.[34] The explanation seems to be that the medication compensates for the deficiency in neurotransmitter flow all along the attentional axis from the limbic system, through the pleasure center to the "executive decision-making center" in the ACC. The implication is that children or adults who are effectively treated for ADD/ADHD are less likely to engage in impulsive risk taking behaviors, tend to engage less in addictive behaviors, and in general will self regulate their behaviors more effectively.

● ●

PATIENT PROFILE 9-1

TOM — WHO ARE YOU?

SETTING: Tom, a 38-year-old man with ADHD, is being treated for fibromyalgia by Moss, the nurse practitioner in a mid-size office in a midwest city. He was taking Adderall for the ADHD but has quit because he said he could handle it by himself without medication. Currently he is taking Prozac, 20 mg. every morning for depression related to the fibromyalgia. His symptoms include: weakness, chronic achy pain and stiffness in neck, shoulders, and back, headaches, weight loss, and exhaustion. His presenting problem today is that sometimes he has "good days and bad days" and wants to feel better and get back to work.

Moss takes a few moments before the appointment and reviews Tom's chart. He notices that within an appointment or sometimes from appointment to appointment, Tom presents as very ill, or feeling great, or with a variety of quickly changing behaviors ranging from depressed, anxious, OK, elated, hyper, to a taking care of business-matter-of-fact demeanor. Moss reads that Tom reports great spiritual strides, traveling to expensive retreats in exotic countries. Moss also notes that Tom tends to seek out high risk activities with high performance stress (sky diving) but then be totally "wiped out" afterwards. Tom reports having great sex with his girlfriend and then not getting along well at all. Sometimes he goes out with a lot of friends and other times he says he has no one to talk with and that he feels very lonely and bored. Moss is puzzled by these ups and downs and the contrast in his demeanor. Moss isn't sure what is going on with Tom.

Moss: How are you today, Tom?

Tom: Not well at all. You know I have my bad days when I just can't do anything. I want to get back to work but I am so exhausted all the time. I feel like I am not my self any more. I used to get out more and now I can barely keep awake during the day.

Moss: *(It sounds like he's having an identity crisis again. His life has changed so much and it is hard for him to adjust to the changes.)* Yes, I know — fibromyalgia can cause severe fatigue. What is your current living situation?

Tom: Sometimes I live with my girlfriend, although recently we broke up. Now I am mostly in my own condo. Dad really wanted to retire but he had to return to the business because I can't work a whole day. We all miss Mom. She 's been dead two years now. She had been the driving force in our investment management business. But I guess I am getting off the subject. When is my energy going to return?

Moss: Over time, you will adapt, but it is important to remember, it's the stress and unrelenting work hours you've worked in the past that in part have caused this disorder. *(That whole family is workaholic. I sense that their busi-*

ness has been deteriorating since the mother died. I know that the brothers are trying to hold it together although they disagree about how to do it. Tom was the peacekeeper for awhile putting out one fire after another. I wonder how he worked those long hours?) Maybe it is time for you to do some relaxing instead of thinking so much about how you need to get back to work. Didn't you used to play tennis regularly?

Tom: That's out now. My legs just won't run around like they used to. I ache too much the next day. I pay for it! I also have some outstanding debts both business and personal. *(He sets aside his laptop and sighs.)*

Moss: *(I think I'll bring up the changes in his status that he experiences now.)* Tom, you seem to have a lot of ups and downs and I wonder if there is anything else going on with you that could be affecting you and causing these changes. Is there anything else going on that you need to tell me about?

Tom: No, just my lowered energy levels.

Moss: OK, I want to double your Prozac prescription and see if that can help. However, remember you need to adapt to this disorder. You are not the person you used to be.

Tom: OK, see ya later. *(Tom grabs his laptop and breezes out of the room.)*

Moss is left with lots of questions about Tom. Then one day his questions were answered. He receives a call from the hospital ER where Tom had been treated for multiple injuries — none serious — after wrapping his Mercedes 280 around a light pole. Blood tests showed both high levels of alcohol and cocaine. Tom was suicidal so he signed himself into a substance abuse treatment unit for detoxification. Ten days later Tom is in Moss's office. He is chagrined.

Moss: So, Tom, it looks like there was something more going on with you. Tell me about it.

Tom: Alright, I should have been more honest with you. I have been abusing cocaine for about a year now and it caught up with me. I also started drinking heavily after breaking up with my girlfriend. Then cocaine helped me feel

better. It all spiraled out of control.

Moss: I am going to refer you to a certified addictions counselor.

Tom: I'd rather just see you. Why can't we just continue like we are?

Moss: Sure you can continue to see me for the fibromyalgia and any new onset of problems. But since I am not trained to treat patients with addictions, it is best that you see a specialist.

POINTS TO CONSIDER:

- Moss has reviewed Tom's chart before the appointment noting once more his questions about Tom's personality changes.

- Moss asks about Tom's living situation because it has changed in the past and with every change, Tom's mood has shifted dramatically.

- Moss treats Tom's exhaustion by doubling his prescription. However, he reminds Tom about his need to adapt to the situation.

- When Tom asks Moss to conduct follow-up addiction treatment, Moss recognizes that this is beyond his area of expertise and refers Tom to a specialist. He does not drop Tom nor treat him judgmentally. He clarifies that he will continue to treat him for fibromyalgia.

• •

Substances

TOBACCO

As stated above, the two most common legal substances abused are **tobacco** and **alcohol**. In terms of their combined impact on public health, they are by far the most damaging.[35] According to NIAAA, tobacco is responsible for more than 400,000 deaths and alcohol for more than 100,000 deaths annually. Nearly 1 in every 5 dollars spent by Medicare, Medicaid, Veterans Administration Medical Centers, and other Federal health entitlement programs is used for health problems related to tobacco and alcohol. Tobacco is known as a **gateway drug.** In other words, nicotine's highly addictive quality conditions the brain to be receptive to other addictions.[36,37] High correlations between first tobacco use and subsequent drug abuse leading to addiction have been amply demonstrated in the research literature.[38,39]

ALCOHOL

As with tobacco, alcohol is easily available. Over the past generation, children have begun to drink alcohol earlier and earlier. Surveys conducted in the year 2000 indicate that 2.5% of 12 year olds report using alcohol, with the percentages going up to 11% by junior high school graduation and to 42% by high school graduation.[40] The use of alcohol among adolescents is associated with a number of public health problems ranging from premature deaths from accidents and other causes, increases in sexually transmitted infections, and carrying weapons.[41] Also at the other end of the age spectrum, recent surveys indicate that "6 to 11% of elderly patients admitted to hospitals exhibit symptoms of alcoholism, as do 20% of elderly patients in psychiatric wards and 14% of elderly patients in emergency rooms."[42] Since women are more susceptible to intoxication than men due to hormonal and metabolic differences, they can develop abuse or dependency with lesser amounts of alcohol than men.[43,44]

CANNABIS[45]

Despite being labeled a "prohibited substance," marijuana is the most widely used illegal drug. In the year 2000, of the 14 million users of illicit drugs, from age 12 on up, 76% reported smoking marijuana in the previous month.[46] The main active chemical in marijuana is THC (delta-9-tetrahydrocannabinol). THC changes the way in which sensory information enters and is processed by the hippocampus. It is used as a "recreational" drug for most users because it produces relaxation or feelings of tranquillity, sometimes followed by drowsiness. However, whether a person derives pleasure or unpleasant feelings is influenced by the mood prior to use, the

expectations, and the setting. This is why enjoying marijuana is a learned response. Medical uses of marijuana, such as an anti nausea agent during chemotherapy, as an appetite stimulant in the treatment of AIDS, or for use in glaucoma have been vigorously opposed by the federal government. Though marijuana itself is not deemed to be physically addictive, it is often an indicator of other substance abuse. Research findings indicate that long-term use of marijuana produces changes in the brain similar to those seen after long-term use of other major drugs of abuse. Alteration in brain chemistry has been shown to produce impairment of critical skills related to attention, memory, and learning. Longitudinal research on marijuana use among young people below college age indicates that those who used marijuana have lower achievement scores than the non-users, more acceptance of deviant behavior, more delinquent behavior and aggression, greater rebelliousness, poorer relationships with parents, and more associations with delinquent and drug-using friends. Research also shows more anger and more regressive behavior (thumb sucking, temper tantrums) in toddlers whose parents use marijuana than among the toddlers of non-using parents.[47] Damage to the lungs is probably the most serious of the several adverse physical effects of marijuana smoking. Due the practice of inhaling deeply and holding the smoke in the lungs, smokers of marijuana absorb much higher levels of tar and carbon monoxide. Heavy users (like heavy tobacco smokers) are likely to have daily cough and phlegm, symptoms of chronic bronchitis, and more frequent chest colds. Use of marijuana during pregnancy has been shown to produce lower birth weight in babies.

HEROIN[48]

Heroin is an opioid that in its pure refined form comes in white or brown powder. Soon after injection or inhalation, heroin crosses the blood-brain barrier where it converts to morphine and binds to opioid receptors. The short-term effects of heroin abuse appear soon after a single dose and disappear in a few hours. The user reports feeling a surge of euphoria ("rush") accompanied by a warm flushing of the skin, dry mouth, and sensation of heaviness in the extremities. Following this initial euphoria, the user goes "on the nod," an alternately wakeful and drowsy state. Mental functioning becomes clouded due to the depression of the central nervous system. A flood of inexpensive and relatively pure heroin from Southeast Asia in recent years has lured younger persons to sniff and snort rather than to inject the drug. Street names for heroin include "smack", "H", "skag," and "junk." Other names may refer to types of heroin produced in a specific geographical area, such as "Mexican black tar." Long-term effects of heroin appear after repeated use for some period of time. Heroin abuse is associated with serious health conditions including fatal overdose, spontaneous abortion, collapsed veins, abscesses, cellulitis, liver disease, and infection of the heart lining and valves. Because many heroin abusers share needles when injecting the drug, they have high rates of HIV/AIDS and hepatitis. Pulmonary complications, including various types of pneumonia may result from the poor health condition of the abuser, as well as from heroin's depressing effects on respiration. In addition to the effects of the drug itself, street heroin may be "cut" or diluted with sugar, starch, powdered milk, quinine, or even poisons like strychnine. The additives do not readily dissolve and can obstruct blood vessels leading to the lungs, liver, kidneys, or brain causing infection or even death of small patches of cells in vital organs. According to the National Institute on Drug Abuse (NIDA), heroin ranks second as the most frequently mentioned drug in overall drug-related deaths.

Opioid analogs include various fentanyl-based designer drugs.[49] The lure of opiates is that they produce a rush of pleasure and a relaxed dreamy state during which all worries seem to disappear. Since opiates are also used for various legitimate analgesic purposes, you may encounter efforts by some patients to obtain prescriptions for various opiate containing medications. The epidemic of OxyContin abuse in 2000 and 2001 is a case in point. (See the discussion of drug seeking patients in Chapter 13.)

STIMULANTS

Stimulants are a class of drugs that enhance brain activity. This class of drugs includes amphetamines and methamphetamines, methcathinone and cocaine. Stimulants are attractive because they produce a sense of energy, euphoria, talkativeness, and alertness. Historically, stimulants were used to treat asthma and other respiratory problems, obesity, and neurological disorders. Because they are highly addictive and dangerous, stimulants are now prescribed for treating only a few health conditions, including narcolepsy, attention-deficit hyperactivity disorder (ADHD), and depression that has not responded to other treatments.[50] Among the many dangers of stimulant abuse are brain damage, psychosis, and death caused by ventricular fibrillation.[51] When used for non-pleasure seeking purposes such as appetite control or for the treatment of ADD/ADHD, dosages have to be carefully titrated to avoid such dangers.

Cocaine, in its various forms — powder, freebase, or "crack" — is the most widely used illicit stimulant. It is highly addictive. Its principal routes of administration are oral, intranasal, intravenous, and inhalation. The slang terms for these routes are respectively, "chewing," "snorting," "mainlining," "injecting," and "smoking" (including freebase and crack cocaine). Snorting is the process of inhaling cocaine powder through the nostrils where it is absorbed into the bloodstream through the nasal tissues. Injecting releases the drug directly into the bloodstream, and heightens the intensity of its effects. Smoking crack involves the inhalation of cocaine vapor or smoke into the lungs where absorption into the bloodstream is as rapid as by injection. The drug can also be rubbed onto mucous tissues. Some users combine cocaine powder or crack with heroin in a "speedball."[52] Some of the most frequent complications are cardiovascular effects, including disturbances in heart rhythm and heart attacks; such respiratory effects as chest pain and respiratory failure; neurological effects including strokes, seizure, and headaches; and gastrointestinal complications, including abdominal pain and nausea.[53]

CLUB DRUGS[54]

Chemically related to stimulants are the so-called **club drugs**, sometimes also known as **designer drugs**.[55] These are synthetic drugs used most commonly by adolescents and young adults who are part of a nightclub, bar, rave, or trance scene. Prominent among the club drugs are MDMA, Rohypnol, GHB, and ketamine.

MDMA is a synthetic, psychoactive drug with both stimulant (amphetamine-like) and hallucinogenic (LSD-like) properties. MDMA's chemical structure (3-4 methylenedioxymeth-amphetamine) is similar to methamphetamine, methylenedioxyamphetamine (MDA), and mescaline.[56] MDMA usually is taken in pill form but some users also snort it, inject it, or use it in suppository form. Street names for MDMA include "Ecstasy," "Adam," "XTC," "hug," "beans," and "love drug." Many problems which MDMA users encounter are similar to those found with the use of amphetamines and cocaine. Psychological difficulties can include confusion, depression, sleep problems, severe anxiety, and paranoia. Physical problems can include muscle tension, involuntary teeth clenching, nausea, blurred vision, dizziness, and chills or sweating. Use of MDMA has also been associated with increases in heart rate and blood pressure. During "raves" in closely confined and crowded conditions persons can develop dehydration and severe hyperthermia which can lead to brain damage or heart fibrillation and death. Research also links MDMA use to long-term damage to those parts of the brain critical to thought, memory, and pleasure.[57]

Rohypnol is the trade name for fluni-trazepam, a benzodiazepine.[58] It has been of particular concern since the 1990s because of its abuse in date rape. When mixed as a colorless liquid with alcohol, Rohypnol can incapacitate victims and prevent them from resisting sexual assault. It can also produce anterograde amnesia, which means individuals may not remember events they experienced while under the effects of the drugs. Street names for Rohypnol are "rophies," "roofies," "roach," and "rope." It may be lethal when mixed with alcohol and/or other depressants.

GHB (gamma hydroxybutyrate) has been abused in the United States for euphoric, seda-tive, and anabolic (body building) effects.[59] It is a central nervous system depressant that was widely available over-the-counter in health food stores to aid fat reduction and muscle building until 1992 . Although now illegal, GHB and two of its precursors, GBL (gamma butyrolactone) and BD (1,4 butanediol), are still obtainable over the Internet, in some gyms, at raves, in night-clubs, at male homosexual parties, on college campuses, and on the street. Street names include "Liquid Ecstasy," "Soap," "Easy Lay," and "Georgia Home Boy." When used for getting high or to perpetrate violence (as in date rape), GHB or its analogs are commonly mixed with alcohol. Onset of action is rapid and an overdose can cause unconsciousness in 15 minutes and deep coma within 30 to 40 minutes. When combined with methamphetamine, there appears to be an increased risk of seizure. GHB may also produce withdrawal effects, including insomnia, anxiety, tremors, and sweating. GHB is not easily detectable on routine hospital toxicology screens.

DISSOCIATIVE DRUGS

Drugs that distort perceptions of sight and sound and produce feelings of detachment — dissocia-tion — from the environment and self rather than hallucinations are called **dissociative drugs**. The most prominent among these are PCP, ketamine and dextromethorphan. They are categorized as "dissociative anesthetics." The dissociative drugs act by altering distribution of the neurotransmitter glutamate throughout the brain. Glutamate is involved in perception of pain, responses to the environment, and memory.

PCP (phencyclidine) was initially developed as a general anesthetic for surgery.[60] It is a white crystalline powder that is readily soluble in water or alcohol. It has a distinctive bitter chemical taste. PCP can be mixed easily with dyes and turns up on the illicit drug market in a variety of tablets, capsules, and colored powders. It is normally used in one of three ways: snorted, smoked, or eaten. When smoked, PCP is often applied to a leafy material such as mint, parsley, oregano, or marijuana. PCP is illegally manufactured in laboratories and is sold on the street by such names as "angel dust," "ozone," "wack," and "rocket fuel." "Killer joints" and "crystal supergrass" are names that refer to PCP combined with marijuana. The variety of street names for PCP reflects its bizarre and volatile effects. At low or moderate doses, PCP produces a rush or increase of energy, feelings of strength, power, invulnerability and a numbing effect on the mind.

In high doses, PCP can make the user aggressive and dangerous to themselves and others. Psychological effects at high doses include delusions and hallucinations. PCP can cause effects that mimic the full range of symptoms of schizophrenia, such as delusions, paranoia, disordered thinking, sparse and garbled speech, a sensation of distance from one's environment, and catatonia (motoric immobility). The physiological effects of high dosages can produce a sudden drop in blood pressure, pulse rate, and respiration. This may be accompanied by nausea, vomiting, blurred vision, flicking up and down of the eyes, drooling, loss of balance, and dizziness. In extreme cases, a PCP overdose can also cause seizures, coma, and death (though death more often results from accidental injury or suicide during PCP intoxication).

Ketamine is an anesthetic that has been approved for both human and animal use in medical settings since 1970; about 90 percent of the ketamine legally sold is intended for veterinary use.[61] Certain doses of ketamine can cause dreamlike states and hallucinations. It has become common in club and rave scenes and has also been used as a date rape drug. It can be injected or snorted or mixed into drinks as a tasteless powder or liquid. Ketamine is also known as "Special K" or "vitamin K." It has a fast onset and lasts about

30-50 minutes. At high doses, ketamine can cause delirium, amnesia, impaired motor function, high blood pressure, depression, and potentially fatal respiratory problems.

Dextromethorphan, when taken in high doses can produce effects similar to those of PCP and ketamine. It is usually found in widely available cough suppressants (like Robitussin). Generally referred to as "Robo" or "DXM", dextromethorphan is often abused by adolescents who drink 4 ounces or more of the cough syrup. Since most OTC cough syrups that have dextromethorphan often contain antihistamine and decongestant ingredients, high doses of these mixtures can seriously increase risks of dextromethorphan abuse. Adverse health effects similar to those of ketamine may be observed.

HALLUCINOGENS[62]

Hallucinogens are drugs that cause hallucinations — profound distortions in a person's perceptions of reality. The molecular structure of hallucinogens is very similar to that of the neurotransmitter serotonin, and their effects come from disrupting the interaction of nerve cells with serotonin. Under the influence of hallucinogens, people see images, hear sounds, and feel sensations that seem real but do not exist. Some hallucinogens also produce rapid, intense emotional swings. Rates of onset, duration of action, and intensity vary from drug to drug. What attracts users to hallucinogens is the subjective perceptual effects, which range from visual distortions and illusory phenomena, prolonged retinal after images, heightened sense of touch and sensuality to marked distortions of time. **LSD** (lysergic acid diethylamide) is considered the typical hallucinogen, and the characteristics of its action and effects also apply to the other hallucinogens, including **mescaline**, **psilocybin**, and **ibogaine**. Users refer to LSD and other hallucinogenic experiences as "trips" and to the acute adverse experiences as "bad trips."

LSD is the most widely used in this class of drugs. LSD is the most potent mood and perception altering drug known. Oral doses as small as 30 micrograms can produce effects that last from 6 to 12 hours. LSD is widely available in the underground drug culture and on college campuses. Since it is so potent, tiny amounts are marketed variously as "microdots," "window panes," or "blotter acid."

LSD's effects are unpredictable and may vary with the amount ingested and the user's personality, mood, expectations, and surroundings. Somatic effects include dizziness, paresthesia, weakness, tremors, pupillary dilation, hyper reflexia, elevated blood pressure and body temperatures, and tachycardia. But the most dramatic effects are emotional and sensory. Psychological and behavioral effects often include extreme lability in emotions and affect in which the user can move from being flooded with feelings of love to being extremely paranoid, with transitions so rapid that the user may seem to experience several emotions simultaneously. LSD also has dramatic effects on the senses. Colors, smells, sounds, and other sensations seem highly intensified. In some cases, sensory perceptions may blend in a phenomenon known as synesthesia, in which a person seems to hear or feel colors and see sounds. On "good" trips, users experience sensations that are enjoyable, mentally stimulating, and that produce a sense of heightened understanding. "Bad" trips, however, may produce terrifying images and nightmarish feelings of anxiety and despair that can include fears of insanity, death, or of losing control. Hallucinogens do not have physiological withdrawal symptoms. Instead some LSD users experience devastating psychological effects that persist after the trip has ended, producing a long-lasting psychotic-like state. **LSD-induced Persistent Psychosis** may include dramatic mood swings from mania to profound depression, vivid visual disturbances, and hallucinations. These effects may last for years and can affect people who have no history or other symptoms of psychological disorder. Some former LSD users report "flashbacks," scientifically known as **Hallucinogen Persisting Perception Disorder** or HPPD.[63] Because HPPD symptoms may be mistaken for those of other neurological disorders such as

stroke or brain tumors, sufferers may consult a variety of clinicians before the disorder is accurately diagnosed. There is no established treatment for HPPD, although some antidepressant drugs may reduce the symptoms. Psychotherapy may help patients adjust to the confusion associated with visual distraction and to minimize the fear, expressed by some, that they are suffering brain damage or a psychiatric disorder.[64]

SEDATIVES AND BARBITURATES

Most sedatives as well as the benzodiazepine tranquilizers, and tricyclics are in this category. Many use these prescription drugs to cope with depression, anxiety, or the pressures of life. Typically they produce a sense of relaxation and a reduction in anxiety. Sedatives or hypnotics are abused because in higher dosages they produce "a state in which mood is elevated, self criticism, anxiety and guilt are reduced, and energy and self confidence are increased."[65] It is important to pay attention to this class of drugs because you may inadvertently be adding to your patients' drug problems. For example Xanax (abrazolam) is frequently prescribed in relatively high doses for extended periods of time for panic attacks and feelings of anxiety. Xanax may result in physical dependence especially if patients self-administer higher doses than are prescribed. (See also Chapter 12.) Two club drugs in the sedative/barbiturate category are the "date rape" drugs Rohypnol and GHB.

Inhalants cover a wide range of gases and volatile substances including amyl and butyl nitrites, anesthesia agents (nitrous oxide, halothane or ether), solvents, paints, sprays, and fuels.[66] Inhalant abuse has been called the poor man's high because it seems to flourish in poverty stricken environments. Adolescents are the most frequent users of inhalants. The attraction of these substances is a quick sensation of warmth, relaxation (of smooth muscles), and mild euphoria to giddiness, sometimes accompanied by visual distortions. Although the nitrites and anesthesia agents are approved for human use, other agents, such as paints, solvents, fuels, and sprays, never were meant to be inhaled and are highly neurotoxic.[67] Brain damage leading to sharp declines in cognitive and social functioning are common after effects of inhalant abuse. Inhalant abusers tend to be very resistant to treatment possibly because of the neurological damage to key brain centers. Damage to air passages and lungs are also common among abusers of solvents, fuels, and some sprays.

STEROIDS

Anabolic-androgenic steroids and other performance enhancing substances like human growth hormone are used widely by adolescents and professional athletes.[68] Cultural pressures for men to be tall and muscular has created pathological dissatisfaction with body image among some adolescents and young men which some have called anorexia nervosa. Generally these are persons with pre-existing personality problems such as narcissistic or antisocial personalities.[69] To compensate for a body that they perceive as too small or insufficiently muscular, such persons (mostly males) may use steroids to achieve a more acceptable physique. To speed up the formation of muscle mass some may raise steroid intake to dangerous levels, causing adverse physical, cognitive, psychological, and behavioral side effects. The adverse physical effects can include fluid retention, cardiac and vascular problems, liver problems (including acute elevations of transaminases, hepatomegaly, peliosis, hepatitis, and cancer), changes in secondary sex characteristics in both males and females, and changes in sexual functioning. When users try to counteract fluid retention with aggressive use of diuretics, severe electrolyte imbalances may produce cardiac failure. Psychologically, users commonly report temporary depression, feelings or acts of aggression (spousal abuse), and manic episodes. Cognitive impairment and distractibility may also increase during episodes of high usage. Since the etiology and use/abuse patterns of steroids differ markedly from most other addictions, dependence is more likely to be con-

ditioned by the underlying psychological condition (i.e., body image distortions leading to excessive exercising or weight lifting) rather than the neurological reward or reinforcement mechanisms underlying most other addictions. Fortunately, users of steroids often are obsessive about keeping meticulous records of dosages and effects. These records can be useful when some of these powerful hormone-like substances produce adverse systemic effects. The high rate of acne among male steroid users can also be a tip-off to possible steroid use/abuse.

Behavioral Addictions

The brain does not seem to differentiate whether messages traveling along the reinforcing pathways are from drugs or behaviors.[70] As in drug addictions, behavioral addictions produce endorphin "highs" that feed the brain reinforcing mechanism. In many instances the body develops tolerance, meaning that the activity has to be increased or intensified to continue to get the "high." Psychological and sometimes physical withdrawal symptoms can be observed, and treatment must address teaching the person to pay attention to the craving for the addictive behavior(s) in order to prevent relapse. In many instances, similar predisposing conditions (genetic, family history, psychosocial, and environmental) will play crucial roles in triggering behavioral addictions. Regardless of the triggering mechanism, once a behavioral addiction is established, it is maintained by similar neurochemical brain reward and reinforcement mechanisms as in substance addictions. Indeed in the final stages of the addictive process — whether substance or behavioral — the pathological reward pathways override the "normal survival behaviors" as the person becomes preoccupied with repeating the addictive behavior.[71] You may also note the same range and frequency of comorbid disorders as in substance addictions.

Some activities such as eating, sexual intercourse, and exercise are a vital part of normal living. A behavior becomes pathological when excessive or compulsive repetition interferes with normal functioning. The DSM-IV uses the term **Impulse-Control Disorders** to describe "the failure to resist an impulse, drive or temptation to perform an act that is harmful, to the person or to others."[72] The DSM-IV applies this description to a number of psychiatric behavioral disorders, including substance abuse, eating disorders, pathological gambling, intermittent explosive disorder (as in domestic violence), trichotillomania (pulling out one's hair), kleptomania (stealing), pyromania (fire setting), and various compulsive sexual behaviors (covered in Chapter 7). Other behaviors which when done compulsively and excessively to the point of being harmful to self others are religiosity,[73] battering (fighting), workaholism, shopping or collecting things,[74] cybermania (excessive computer use),[75] and exercise addiction.[76] Engaging in the behavior appears to release the endorphins that produce the highs. When the high wears off, the person may experience tension, depression, and a craving to repeat the behavior.[77] Below are sketches of two common behavioral addictions: excessive exercising and eating disorders.

EXERCISE[78]

An example, of a benign activity, which can turn into an addictive behavior, is exercise. Many people exercise regularly and derive positive benefits from it. Exercise releases endorphins, which produce a sense of well-being. As such, exercise helps to alleviate stress. The line between a healthy lifestyle and compulsive and excessive exercising is blurred especially for those with a psychological predisposition towards perfectionism and obsessive-compulsive disorders.[79] For such persons, exercise can be used to create an increased sense of control over a specific activity in their lives. It can also be used as means of escape from one's worries and problems. For others, exercise may stem the genetic predisposition for impulsive or risk taking behaviors which take such forms as extreme sports (sky diving, ice cliff or mountain climbing, and the arduous physical exercise routines

to "get in shape" for such sports). If for some reason — like injury — exercise addicts have to halt their exercise regimens, they may experience pronounced psychological withdrawal symptoms. For example, marathon runners, who have to stop running can lapse into deep depression or develop anxiety attacks. The health risks of exercise done to excess are wear and tear on joints that can often require knee or hip repair or replacement surgery. Also problematic are dangerous imbalances in blood chemistry as well as in hormone levels, which in females can lead to amenorrhea.[80]

● ●

PATIENT PROFILE 9.2

FOURTH KNEE SURGERY?

SETTING: Shannell is a 28-year-old single woman and is a certified nursing assistant at a nearby nursing home. She has a history of bulimia as an adolescent and is recovering from her fourth knee surgery. She is being treated at a rehabilitation clinic by her physical therapist, Hillary.

Hillary: So, Shannell, you're here to get some rehabilitation from the fourth knee surgery. You know, that's a lot of knee surgeries. Your orthopedic surgeon says this was the last one. How come four? Are you reinjuring your knee?

Shannell: Well, no. He just can't seem to fix them right. It's both knees. They've never been real strong, so I do knee strengthening exercises.

Hillary: What kind of exercises?

Shannell shows Hillary the standard extension and flexion exercises.

Hillary: That shouldn't be reinjuring them. What else do you do?

Shannell: Oh, sometimes I put weights on my ankles and do the exercises.

Hillary: How many pounds?

Shannell: Two, well, sometimes more.

Hillary: How much more?

Shannell: Not much more.

Hillary: *(Is she dodging my questions? Perhaps I should be more firm with her.)* Three? Four?

Shannell: More, like, more, you know.

Hillary: Exactly how much more, Shannell.

Shannell: Ten or twelve pounds on each ankle.

Hillary: How many repetitions?

Shannell: Well only about 100, sometimes more and I don't do it every day.

Hillary: That seems like too much to me especially with the recurrent knee surgeries. You want to go a little easier on yourself. Tell me more about the exercises you do.

Shannell: *(Big sigh and drops her gaze.)* Well I run, like every day, sometimes twice a day if I've eaten lunch. I feel so good after running. You just can't believe how it makes me feel.

Hillary: What distance do you run?

Shannell: Not much. It depends on what I eat for lunch. Maybe 20-30 miles a day.

Hillary: *(Sure exercise is exhilarating, but this is beyond a healthy exercise regimen. And she was bulimic during her adolescence... Has it returned?)* I see from your medical history that you were bulimic as an adolescent. Is that still a factor here?

Shannell: No, I learned my lesson then. They put me on a strict behavior management program so that now I keep close tabs on my calories and exercise output. That's why I run so much. When I can't run, I feel real anxious and need to spend a couple of hours a day on my Stair Master. I just can't seem to stop. It's like I have to run and if I can't then it's bad, believe me, bad. I feel real anxious.

Hillary: *(Bulimia is pressuring her to exercise excessively thereby continuing to reinjure her knees. Compulsive exercising. Behavioral addiction.)* I understand now. You may be reinjuring yourself with what might be compulsive exercising. I'd like you to see a mental health counselor who is a specialist in this area. You need help in managing your exercise patterns. Would you be willing to see one?

Shannell: Yeah, I guess so. The surgeon said he would not operate on me anymore, so I guess I gotta do so something. My right hip is really hurting now too. Running and exercising is so much a part of me. I just can't seem to control it. I don't think I can stop.

POINTS TO CONSIDER:

- Hillary inquires about Shannell's need for four knee surgeries.
- Hillary asks specific questions of Shannell because she wants to get to the bottom of why Shannell is reinjuring herself.
- Hillary refers Shannell to a specialist because Hillary understands that Shannell needs an expert on addictions.

• •

EATING DISORDERS

Eating is another routine activity of normal living, which can be distorted into pathological, and obsessive-compulsive patterns. In eating disorders the focus on weight and defective body image may be viewed as obsessional in nature, whereas the ritualistic concern about eating habits is analogous to compulsive symptoms.[81] In normal eating, there is a "dynamic process of hunger, feeding, satiation, and satiety," where the state of satiety signals a halt to desire for food.[82] Abnormal patterns of eating include "not eating" or anorexia nervosa and "overeating" or bulimia nervosa. In persons with eating disorders, levels of dopamine, serotonin (5HT), endogenous opioids, or antagonist neuropeptides are quite different from persons without eating disorders. Undereating is characterized by elevated levels of the key neurotransmitter serotonin 5HT. On the other hand, persons who overeat or binge eat have highly elevated levels of the antagonist neuropeptide Y (NPY). Both neurobiological aberrations disrupt the hunger, feeding, satiation, and the satiety cycle.[83]

Both anorexia and bulimia nervosa have many features in common. They both show strong inheritance patterns that often appear in the same individual or in the same families, and share a cluster of psychological traits. These traits include negative affect, behavioral inhibition, tendencies toward perfectionism, high harm avoidance, and an obsessive concern with symmetry. As previously mentioned on the use of steroids, psychological disorders related to

Gender Related Differences in Prevalence of Eating Disorders

Disorder	Females	Males
Anorexia Nervosa	1%	1:6 (males:females) (higher incidence among gay men)
Bulimia Nervosa/ Binge Eating	3-4%	1:20 (males:females) bulimia nervosa 1:2 (males:females) for binge eating

body image,[84] and cultural pressures may be other causative factors.[85] In addition, some sources seem to point to a history of parental psychiatric illness and divorce, or other disturbing life events, (childhood sexual abuse) as precipitating factors.[86,87] Eating disorders usually surface in early adolescence when adolescents are subject to peer pressures. As the psychosocial factors interact with brain mechanisms, two seemingly opposite types of eating disorders not eating or anorexia nervosa, and binge eating and purging or bulimia nervosa can occur. Although psychosocial causes may play an important role in triggering eating disorders, once established as a compulsive pathological routine, neurobiological factors dominate in maintaining them.[88,89] In practical terms, this means that simple exhortations for anorexics to eat more, or for overeaters to not to eat as much, or for bulimics to stop binge eating and purging may in fact produce an intensification of the behavior. One of the dangers for both anorexics and overeaters is their susceptibility to abusing various drugs (like diet pills) to cope with their disorders. Although there is significant gender divergence in eating disorders, the overall occurrence of eating disorders appears to be increasing in both genders.[90] Psychological signs of eating disorders appear to be an obsession with body weight or shape in women, and primarily with body shape in men.[91] In anorexia nervosa, physiological symptoms include amenorrhea in women and loss in bone density in both men and women. Because eating disorders are generally accompanied by other psychiatric disorders, treatment options may need to include a multidisciplinary approach.[92]

Stages of Addiction

Both substance and behavioral addictions have many similarities in the brain neurochemistry as well as in the progression to a dependence that interferes with normal functioning.[93,94] It is easier to determine what kind of intervention or treatment your patient needs when you can identify where a person is along the stage progression. Jonathan Shaffer presents a stage model of addiction and recovery which appears to be common to both chemical and behavioral addictions (See Table 9-2).[95]

STAGE ONE: INITIATION AND EMERGENCE OF ADDICTION

Initial experimentation or occasional use of potentially addictive substances or behaviors does not automatically lead to abuse or dependence. Longitudinal research on young adults shows that even when they have crossed over into abuse or dependence they tend to have high rates of spontaneous remission.[96] However for a number of interactive reasons (e.g., genetic susceptibility, neurobiology of habituation, other underlying psychiatric disorders, and psychosocial circumstances), the initial exposure may provide the entry point into the addictive process.

STAGE TWO: THE LURE OF POSITIVE EXPERIENCES

In Stage Two, the person is deluded by the perception that there are only positive and pleasurable effects derived from using a substance or

TABLE 9-2. Matching Stages with Treatment	
Stage of Addictive Behavior	Possible Treatment Modalities
1. Initiation	Primary Prevention: education, peer resistance training.
2. Positive Consequences	Secondary Prevention: education, counseling, social resistance training.
3. Adverse consequences	Tertiary Prevention: referral to outpatient services. DWI program with mandatory attendance at 12 Step meetings. Possible inpatient for acute situations.
4. Turning Point(s)	Acute Inpatient hospitalization: detoxification followed by outpatient partial care, 12 Step attendance.
5. Active Quitting	Residential Program for chronic abusers followed by partial care, or half way houses (for persons with weak social support), chemical substitute maintenance, counseling, 12 Step attendance, family therapy.
6. Relapse Prevention	Outpatient supervision of medication, 12 Step meetings, family therapy

Adapted from Shaffer, HJ Psychology of Stage Change, In Lowinson JH et al, (Eds) Substance Abuse: A comprehensive textbook. (3rd Edition), Baltimore: Williams & Wilkins: 105.

engaging in a behavior. The neurochemical stimulation in the brain regions connected to the pleasure-reward system elevate mood and allow the person to feel less inhibited, socially or sexually. Positive effects can also be indirect, i.e., through psychological or social reinforcement. As a result of using a substance or engaging in certain behaviors, the person's self esteem and social identity may be enhanced through positive feedback from their peers. The positive experience stage, which reinforces continuation of the behavior, explains the ambivalence or denial of the next stage.

STAGE THREE: ADVERSE CONSEQUENCES EMERGE

According to Shaffer, when negative consequences of their behaviors emerge, persons "in the throes of addiction" tend to be unable to moderate the activity or abstain from it entirely. Instead they tend to dismiss, and to deny negative consequences, or to blame them on others or on circumstances. The use of such defense mechanisms allows them to focus on the perceived benefits or rewards of the substance use

or behavior. In severe cases of denial, the addictive behaviors take precedence over normal regulatory biological survival activities. When this stage of dependence is reached, "the addiction becomes the sole focal point — more important than anything else, including life itself." (p. 101)

STAGE FOUR: TURNING POINTS AND THE EVOLUTION OF QUITTING

The turning point into awareness that the adverse consequences were of their own making, is also considered the end of denial. Often this is precipitated by a major life crisis. In Alcoholics Anonymous (AA), and the various 12 Step support group programs based on it, this is known as **hitting bottom** or **bottoming out.** In the language of the first of the Twelve Steps, addicts have to "admit we are powerless over our [dependency] and that our lives have become unmanageable."[97] However, this awareness in many instances will not produce a rush into treatment or into abstinence. Instead the dependent person may enter into a period of painful ambivalence: knowing that the abuse is directly responsible for their negative life circumstances but still unwilling to completely swear off the addictive activity. Thus, at this stage you may observe sincere efforts by the addict to quit or cut back to "reasonable" levels. Generally such experiments are doomed by the neurobiological tolerance, habituation, and craving mechanism. Failure of such efforts often results in depression and severe self-loathing for not being "strong enough" to either kick the habit or to moderate it.

STAGE FIVE: ACTIVE QUITTING

After the addict recognizes that such efforts are futile they can begin the tasks involved in **active quitting**. Two approaches to quitting are "cold turkey" or "tapering off." Sometimes several attempts are necessary before the quitter is successful. As Shaffer points out (p. 102), active quitting involves conscious changes in life style, including "energetic attempts to avoid the drug [or excessive behavior patterns], gaining social support for personal change, and engaging in some forms of self development that also help to manage stress."

STAGE SIX: RELAPSE PREVENTION

The final stage of quitting involves maintenance of the new positive life style patterns. In substance abuse, total abstinence is the preferred condition. However, for behavioral addictions — such as eating disorders, workaholism, and exercise — moderation must be learned and maintained. Learning moderation seldom happens smoothly. Relapses in response to stressors are common. Sometimes well-meaning efforts to substitute "less dangerous" substances (nicotine, caffeine) or behaviors (physical exercise, work) may maintain addictive patterns from the characterological tendency towards compulsiveness. For many, a combination of inpatient treatment with subsequent regular and long-term attendance in a 12 Step support group are essential for remaining abstinent. In general, successful quitters tend to have multiple, flexible strategies and tactics for maintaining abstinence.[98]

Screening

The survey, which produced the startling statistics at the beginning of the chapter of why primary care health care providers are missing or misdiagnosing patient substance abuse, also revealed the reasons. These are given in Box 9-1. As you can see from the responses, it is not likely to be either easy or even pleasant. Due to the pattern of denial, very few patients are going to volunteer that they have a substance or behavioral abuse or addiction problem. However, the same survey also noted that over 87% of patients who were identified and referred for treatment by their health care provider, seemed glad and satisfied that their health care provider did so.[99] Thus, unless you ask specific questions, you will not find out.

Two simple screening instruments exist. Both were designed originally to screen for alcohol use, but can be adapted to other substances and to behavioral addictions. The first is the venerable four question **CAGE**.[100] It is generally used to inquire further about any evidence coming from a routine medical history questionnaire that there is use or possible abuse of any substance or behavior. If the person gives two or more positive

---

Box 9-1 Barriers to Diagnosing Addictions

1. Lack of adequate training in school, residency programs, or continuing education courses.

2. Skepticism about treatment effectiveness.

3. Patient resistance. (57.7 % of those surveyed say they don't discuss substance abuse because they believe that their patients lie about it. 84.9 % of patients surveyed admitted to lying to their health care provider.)

4. Discomfort discussing substance abuse.

5. Time constraints.

6. Fear of losing patients.

7. Lack of insurance coverage, and fear of not getting reimbursed.

responses to these questions, there is a good chance that the patient has a dependency or abuse problem.

1. Cut down: Have you ever felt that you ought to cut down on your drinking (use of cocaine, marijuana, etc.)?

2. Annoyed: Have people annoyed you by asking you to cut down on your drinking (doing lines, or snorting coke, smoking marijuana, etc.)?

3. Guilty: Have you ever felt badly or guilty about your drinking (using cocaine, smoking marijuana, etc.)?

4. Eye Opener: Have you ever had a drink (snorted coke, smoked marijuana, etc.) first thing in the morning as an eye opener?

A second simple instrument, **TWEAK** was developed specifically for screening pregnant women with a drinking problem.[101] A recent survey noted that women often either do not recognize or cite time constraints and family duties for not admitting to substance abuse addiction.[102] Therefore, the TWEAK, should be used for pregnant women if there is a hint of *any* substance abuse. The first question in this instrument takes into account the difference in effect of alcohol and other substances between men and women. On the TWEAK three "yes" answers are considered to be evidence of a dependency problem.

1. Tolerance: How many drinks (hits) does it take to make you high?

2. Worried: Have close friends and relatives worried or complained about your drinking (use of drugs, smoking marijuana, cigarettes)?

3. Eye Opener: Do you sometimes take a drink (use drugs, smoke marijuana or cigarettes) first thing in the morning to get going or to steady your nerves?

4. Amnesia: Has a friend of family member ever told you things you said or did while you were drinking (or high) that you could not remember?

5. (K) Cut: Do you sometimes feel the need to cut down on your drinking (using drugs, or smoking)?

Both of these screening instruments are really only first pass indicators of possible problems. They rely on the patient's truthful responses. Since denial and secrecy are hallmarks of addiction problems, you need to be especially alert to nonverbal signals, hesitations, or evasive responses. When you perceive that signals of denial are present, it is best to persist with your questioning. You could point out that you noticed a hesitation, or wondered about a nonverbal signal, or the "less-than-straight" answer. Whether a patient will entrust you with information that might put them in a bad light depends in large part on *how* you communicate with the patient. Coming from a position of caring concern will do much to lower or eliminate the patient's fear of disapproval or negative judgment. In the same vein of caring concern, you could point out the negative medical consequences of continued use or abuse on themselves — or for a pregnant woman on the growing fetus. Once the wall of denial has been breached, most persons with addiction problems seem relieved and grateful that the burden of secrecy has been lifted. You can then motivate the person to move to the stage of Active Quitting. You can facilitate that by making a referral either directly into treatment, or to an addictions specialist for a comprehensive assessment of the seriousness of the dependence, prior to treatment.

• •

PATIENT PROFILE 9.3

TWEAK

SETTING: Kim is a 30-year-old pregnant mother of two very active children. She has been under a great deal of stress coping with being a mother and keeping the books for her husband's con-

struction company. She has sought treatment for anxiety by Janet Morely, a physician assistant, at a small rural physicians clinic.

Janet: Hello Kim, how are you today?

Kim: Not good. I just feel overwhelmed all the time, keeping the household together, doing the books, expecting another baby. I often feel anxious and so... *(Kim starts to say something and then is silent.)*

Janet: *(She was going to say something and stopped herself. I wonder what she was going to say.)* Was there something else you wanted to tell me?

Kim: Oh, nothing much. My mother, she can be a nag, thinks I drink too much.

Janet: *(What was that acronym? TWEAK? Let's see how did it go? The first one is **T**olerance.)* I need to know a little more about your drinking. How many drinks does it take to lower your anxiety? To make you feel better?

Kim: Usually about three glasses of wine.

Janet: *(The second one is **W**orried.)* You mentioned that your mother worries that you drink too much. Have any other close friends and relatives mentioned that you drink too much?

Kim: Well, once my husband got on me. He bitched at me for drinking instead of cleaning the house.

Janet: *(The next one is the **E**ye opener.)* Have you ever taken a drink first thing in the morning to get going or to steady your nerves?

Kim: *(Sheepishly)* Yeah. Once in a while I sneak a shot of vodka in my orange juice. It's just to keep away that anxious feeling.

Janet: *(**A**mnesia)* Has a friend of family member ever told you things you said or did while you were drinking that you could not remember?

Kim: No, never.

Janet: *(**K** for cut down)* Do you think you should cut down on your drinking or quit?

Kim: Yeah, but... I just can't.

Janet: Kim, this is a little more serious than a few drinks to "unwind." You are pregnant, and I am really concerned about the effects of your drinking on the health of your baby and you. I think you might benefit from seeing a certified addictions counselor.

POINTS TO CONSIDER:

- Silence is a good facilitator during communication between the health care provider and the patient. Janet uses the silence as a stepping stone for further inquiry.
- Janet remembers TWEAK and uses the format to elicit details of Kim's drinking.
- By making a referral to a certified addictions counselor, Janet is providing the best possible care for Kim as well as taking preventive measures to protect the fetus.

• •

If you are the one who will refer the patient directly to treatment, a more thorough assessment will be required to determine the appropriate treatment modality. The American Society of Addiction Medicine (ASAM) has suggested six Patient Placement Criteria for determining the type of treatment needed for chemical addictions:[103]

1. the level of acute intoxication and likelihood of withdrawal

2. biomedical condition

3. emotional behavior

4. acceptance of treatment

5. relapse potential

6. recovery environment

This assessment allows for the differentiation of the severity of the addiction, psychological factors, such as dual diagnoses, and the psychosocial environment in which recovery and relapse prevention will occur. In the age of medical cost containment, such a screening will allow for a choice of least intensive care appropriate to the stage of addiction. However, that choice may not be in your hands but rather will be made by the care manager of the HMO. Even patients with "good" health insurance may find that their HMO will not approve the "best fit" treatment that you or an addictions specialist might recommend. Often the patient will be sent to an "approved provider" facility regardless of the fit.

Treatment

Treatment options and availability vary widely.[104] Persons with detoxification needs for chemical addictions usually are referred to medical inpatient facilities, even if only for the duration of the detoxification and subsidence of acute withdrawal symptoms. Similarly, addictive behaviors which have reached the stage of serious interference with patient health and normal living are now also treated in in-patient facilities.[105] Sometimes short inpatient stays are followed by treatment in day hospitals, outpatient settings, or referrals to half way houses, or simply to 12 Step or other self-help groups.

Treatment philosophy in the United States has been heavily influenced by two models: the 12 Step philosophy of Alcoholics Anonymous (AA), and the Minnesota Model, which was developed by the Hazelden Foundation. The Minnesota model incorporates the AA philosophy into treatment.[106] Although these approaches were originally designed to treat alcoholism, they have been widely adapted and copied for treatment of many types of chemical and behavioral addictions.

Alcoholics Anonymous began in 1935 as an abstinence-based group-support system with a strong spiritual but non-denominational emphasis. Today 50,000 AA groups exist in North America alone, and the 12 Step literature has been translated into many languages.[107] Alcoholics Anonymous, and the various programs modeled on it, owe much of their success to the straightforward message that the addicted person is "powerless" and must "surrender" and appeal to the "Higher Power" in order to start the road to recovery. The key ingredients of "success" of the program are the structure of "working" the 12 Steps (Box 9-2), the fellowship of the support group, the honesty that it demands, and regular attendance to prevent relapse. Nonetheless, AA and the numerous other 12 Step self help support group programs modeled on it, by

---

Various 12 Step Support Groups

Alcoholics	Alcoholics Anonymous
Relatives of Alcoholics	ALANON
Gamblers	Gamblers Anonymous
Drug Addicts	Narcotics Anonymous
Relatives of Drug Addicts	NARCANON
Eating Disorders	Overeaters Anonymous
Sexual Abuse and Addiction	Sexaholics Anonymous
	Sex Addicts Anonymous
	Sex and Love Addicts Anonymous
	Sexual Compulsives Anonymous
Tobacco Addicts	Nicotine Anonymous
Junk Food Addicts	Junk Food Anonymous (aka Sucrose Addicts Anonymous)
Compulsive Shoppers or Over Spenders	Debtors Anonymous
Workaholics	Workaholics Anonymous
Marijuana Abusers	Marijuana Anonymous
Cocaine Abusers	Cocaine Anonymous

their own definition, are *not* treatment programs. Generally, they become part of more intensive in- or outpatient treatment. Attendance at 12 Step support group meetings is considered essential aftercare for the prevention of relapse. Courts, employee assistance programs, and disciplinary committees of professional health care associations will often mandate compulsory attendance at a specified number of 12 Step group meetings within a 90-180 day aftercare period as part of probation or a plea agreement.

In large cities there are also a number of alternative support groups, like Women for Sobriety (WFS), Men for Sobriety (MFS), Rational Recovery (RR), Moderation Management (MM), S.M.A.R.T. Recovery (SMART), and Secular Organization for Sobriety/Save our Selves (SOS).[108] Although each has a different orientation, most are similar in their 12 Step approach. One of the principal philosophical differences between some of them and AA is that the alternative groups tend to de-emphasize reliance on a "higher power." Some also have rejected the abstinence model in favor of learning moderate use.[109] These alternative groups tend to be available only in large cities, whereas AA and Narcotics Anonymous (NA) tend to have groups meeting regularly even in small communities. Almost all major support groups now have an Internet contact where you can find the nearest group.[110]

Probably the most widely used model for the treatment of chemical and behavioral addictions is the Minnesota or Hazelden treatment model. This model can be applied either in residential inpatient or outpatient settings.[111] It is a holistic approach that seeks to address the psychological, behavioral, social, and spiritual problems of each patient. It incorporates cognitive behavioral therapies, including desensitization to relapse cues, coping skills training, educational lectures, individual and group psychotherapy, motivational enhancement, exercise, stress management and relaxation exercises. The Hazelden approach also incorporates the 12 Step philosophy, with patients working at least the first four steps during treatment. Spouses and other family members are also included in the recovery

process and are encouraged to attend support groups specifically geared to the patient's addiction. Hazelden also maintains a large publishing house that provides high-quality training materials for health care professionals as well as educational brochures on the various types of chemical and behavioral addictions for patients and their families.

Box 9-2 Generic Twelve Steps

(For use with either chemical or behavioral addictions)

1. We admitted we were powerless over_____ — that our lives had become unmanageable.

2. Came to believe that a power greater than ourselves could restore us to a joyous and peaceful way of thinking and living.

3. Made a decision to turn our will and our lives over to the care of this power of our own understanding.

4. Made a searching and fearless moral inventory of ourselves.

5. Admitted to this power of our own understanding, to ourselves and to another human being the exact nature of our wrongs.

6. Were entirely ready to have all these defects of character removed.

7. Humbly asked God of our own understanding to remove our shortcomings.

8. Made a list of all persons we had harmed, and became willing to make amends to them all.

9. Made direct amends to such people wherever possible, except when to do so would injure them or others.

10. Continued to take personal inventory and when we were wrong promptly admitted it.

11. Sought through prayer and meditation to improve our conscious contact with god, as we understood god, praying only for knowledge of his will for us and the power to carry that out.

12. Having had a spiritual awakening as the result of these steps, we tried to carry this message to others, and to practice these principles in all our affairs.

Adapted from AA *The Big Book* 3rd Edition. New York: AA World Services, p 59-60.

THERAPEUTIC COMMUNITY

A group therapy based model is the **therapeutic community.** According to its proponents, this model is "founded on a social learning model that fosters behavioral and attitudinal change as a result of the client's membership in a community. Through this intensive, peer-based approach, the client learns pro-social values and addresses self-destructive, anti-social behavioral patterns."[112] Whether structured as in patient or day programs, therapeutic communities focus on treating adults, adolescents and pregnant mothers as an alternative to incarceration for drug-related crimes or other antisocial activities committed while under the influence of addiction. Typical examples are Daytop Village and Odyssey in New York, and Abraxis in Pennsylvania. Persons referred to these therapeutic communities often have multiple, challenging problems, such as criminal backgrounds, homelessness, dysfunctional family backgrounds, severe education and employment skill deficiencies, and sometimes multiple health problems resulting from their addiction. Thus, these mostly privately run, but publicly funded programs, generally offer services like literacy and job training and also halfway programs to address "reentry" problems similar to those faced by prisoners. The therapeutic community model has come under fire for the harshness of some of the techniques used for resocializing the residents. These techniques included use of confrontation, highly regimented boot camp methods, operating on hierarchical principles, and having to earn privileges and rank through good behavior. Since most referrals to such treatment communities are made through either social service agencies (i.e., for mentally ill homeless persons, or drug abusing pregnant women), or through the criminal justice system, your role will likely be limited to performing a medical or mental health assessment prior to committal.

INDIVIDUAL PSYCHOTHERAPY

Individual psychotherapy has not been the predominant treatment modality for substance abuse or addictive behavior since the 12 Step-based treatment and group therapy oriented programs gained favor in the 1960s.[113] Even before then, observers reported difficulties with voluntary individual psychotherapy for the treatment of substance abuse. They were: premature termination, inconsistent attendance, coming to sessions while intoxicated, reaction to anxiety arousing interpretation leading to relapse, and failure to pay fees due to money being spent on drugs.[114] Given these problems, individual psychotherapy is suggested for persons with problems of substance abuse or pathological behavior addictions *only* a.) to introduce them into treatment; b.) to treat patients with low levels of dependence; c.) to complement other modalities; or d.) to help patients solidify gains following achievement of stable abstinence.[115] Thus, individual psychotherapy is generally not recommended as a stand-alone treatment for serious dependence problems.

RELAPSE PREVENTION

All addictions have a compulsive element. Alcoholics Anonymous makes the point that one can be an alcoholic "in recovery" but never a recovered alcoholic — the message is that the addiction is a lifelong condition. For alcohol and other chemical substances, total abstinence is the goal. This makes sense from the neurochemical perspective. For most substance abusers, a relapse may return the body to the tolerance levels experienced at the peak of addiction despite efforts to moderate the behavior.[116] For a number of behavioral addictions — like overeating, workaholism, or compulsive sex — total abstinence is not a viable option. Instead the addicted person needs to learn to modify the behavior in order to moderate and control it. This is why some, like eating disorders, are quite difficult to control. For most addictions — chemical and behavioral — cognitive/behavioral therapy seems to an essential component of successful treatment.[117] For example, in Shannell's situation in Patient Profile 9.2, a behavior management plan for her compulsive exercising and its relationship to what she has eaten is indicated. Plans for behavioral change are based on classical conditioning, desensitization to cues, and learning substitute behaviors. Cognitive retraining goals are for recovering persons to be able to recognize "relapse warning signs," such as changes in attitude, thinking, mood, and behavior. Another major goal of cognitive behavioral training is to teach the patient effective coping mechanisms for dealing with cravings, social pressures to use, negative emotional states, and cognitive distortions. As part of relapse prevention, patients are taught to develop and to enhance their social network, to work towards a balanced life style, and if necessary to consider pharmacological intervention as a supplement to avoid relapse.

PHARMACOLOGICAL INTERVENTIONS

Pharmacological interventions for substance or behavioral addictions are generally used both during the treatment phase, as well part of immediate after care, and also as part of long range strategies to prevent relapse. In general, they are only one part of more comprehensive strategies.

Given that many substances produce either acute or chronic withdrawal symptoms, pharmacological interventions are routinely used to alleviate the physiological effects. Pharmacological interventions start during the detoxification procedures and may continue for years afterwards. In the treatment of advanced alcoholism, for example, relief from agitation and tremors can be achieved with a variety of drugs, including anticonvulsants and benzodiazepines. In addition, high dosages of B complex vitamins are considered essential to prevent peripheral neuropathy and Wernicke-Korsakoff syndrome.[118] For relapse prevention, prescription medications disulfiram (Antabuse), naltrexone, and acamprosate are available to recovering alcoholics in office practice settings.[119]

Because depression is the most common dual diagnosis disorder in chemical and behavioral addictions,[120] pharmacological interventions have been targeted on dopamine and serotonin receptors. With cocaine addictions, a dopamine agonist, amantadine, has been combined with a tricyclic antidepressant (desipramine) to produce dramatic reductions in relapse.[121] With heroin users, similarly new drugs are being developed to replace the much stigmatized methadone maintenance programs. From the perspective of the health care provider, the onerous regulations for methadone prescription have almost limited this treatment to public clinics. Although methadone is generally considered an effective replacement therapy to counter opiate dependence, the perception among users that public treatment programs are punitive has made for low (25%) participation rates among opiate addicts.[122] One opioid agonist, l-alpha-acetylmethadol, known as LAAM, when combined with buprenorphine has been shown to be effective in reducing opiate craving and relapse.[123] Similarly, naltrexone-buprenorphine combinations are promising.[124] Using sublingual buprenorphine tablets with opioid dependent pregnant women has been found to be well accepted by the mother and the fetus.[125] With a more complete understanding of the neurobiology of addiction, expectations are high that new medications will be developed in the near future to effectively treat a wide range of chemical and behavioral addictions.[126]

Conclusion

The National *Survey of Primary Care Physicians and Patients on Substance Abuse,* mentioned at the beginning of the chapter, found that many health care providers feel they are inadequately prepared for screening addictions. One of the recommendations of the Survey authors is that health care providers receive more training in the assessment and diagnosis of substance abuse and behavioral addictions. We encourage you to seek out continuing education courses in this field to keep yourself abreast of the ever-changing patterns of chemical and behavioral addictions. As a primary health care provider, you can play a vital role through prevention, timely diagnosis, and referral to treatment. By educating your young patients on the effects of drugs, you can frequently prevent experimentation or use from turning into addiction. For screening and diagnosing, you will also want to know symptomology of new fad drugs and behavioral addictions connected to new technologies. In addition, you will want to develop a referral network of addiction experts in your community to assist you in obtaining the appropriate level of treatment for patients with chemical or behavioral addictions.

REFERENCES

1. Survey Research Laboratory at the University of Chicago. Missed Opportunity: National Survey of Primary Care Physicians and Patients on Substance Abuse. New York: Center on Addiction and Substance Abuse CASA April 2000.

2. American Psychiatric Association (1994) *Diagnostic and Statistical Manual of Psychiatric Disorders*: Fourth Edition (DSM-IV). Washington, DC. APA, p 176.

3. Grant BF et al (1994) Prevalence of DSM-IV alcohol abuse and dependence — United States, 1992. *NIAAA Epidemiological Bulletin* No. 35 18:243-248.

4. Harwood H et al (1999) Update of The economic costs of alcohol and drug abuse in the United States. NIH Publication No. 98-4327 1-9.

5. NIAAA's Purpose. Accessed on the Internet at www.niaaa.nih.gov/about/purpose.htm

6. National Institute on Alcohol Abuse and Alcoholism, FY 2002 Budget. Accessed on the Internet at www.niaaa.nih.gov/about/congressional/FY2002.htm

7. Anthenelli RM, Schuckit MA (1997) Determinants and Perpetuators of Substance Abuse: Genetics. In Lowinson JH et al, (Eds.) *Substance Abuse: A comprehensive textbook*. (3rd Edition), Baltimore: Williams & Wilkins: 44-51.

8. Ilveskoski E et al (2001) Association of neuropeptide y polymorphism with the occurrence of type 1 and type 2 alcoholism. *Alcohol Clin Exper Res*, 25:1420-1422.

9. Anthenelli RM, Tabakoff B (1995) The search for biological markers. *Alcohol Health Res World*; 19:176-181.

10. Gardner EL (1997) Brain Reward Mechanisms. In Lowinson JH et al, (Eds.) *Substance Abuse: A comprehensive textbook*. (3rd Edition), Baltimore: Williams & Wilkins: 51.

11. Barkley RA (1998) A Theory of ADHD: Inhibition, Executive Functions, Self Control and Time. In Barkley RA. *Attention Deficit Hyperactivity Disorder: A Handbook for Diagnosis and Treatment* (2nd Ed). New York: Guilford Press.

12. Virkkunen M, Linnoila M (1990) Serotonin in early onset, male alcoholics with violent behavior. *Ann Med*, 22:327-331.

13. Kaminer Y (1999) Addictive Disorders in Adolescents. *Psychiatr Clin North America*, 22:275-288.

14. Wender PH. (1995) *Attention Deficit Hyperactivity Disorder in Adults*. New York: Oxford Univ Press.

15. Ebstein RP et al. Dopamine D4 receptor (D4DR) rcon II polymorphism associated with the human personality trait of novelty seeking. *Nat. Genetics* 1996; 12.78-80.

16. Benjamin J et al. Population and familial association between the D4 dopamine receptor gene and measures of novelty seeking. *Nat. Genetics* 1996; 12:81-84.

17. Blum K et al. Allelic association of human dopamine D2 receptor gene in alcoholism. *JAMA* 1990; 2055-2060.

18. Noble EP. The D2 dopamine receptor gene: a review of association studies in alcoholism. *Behav Genet* 1993; 23(2):119-229.

19. Cloninger CR et al Inheritance of risk to develop alcoholism. In Braude MC et al, eds. Genetic and biological markers in drug abuse and alcoholism. NIDA Research Monograph Ser 1986; 66:86-96.

20. Bohman M, Cloninger R et al. The genetics of alcoholism and related disorders. *J Psychiatry Res* 1987; 21:4:447-452.

21. Barkley RA. *ADHD and the nature of self control*. New York: Guilford Press, 1997.

22. Jessor R, Jessor SL (1977) *Problem behavior and psychosocial development: A longitudinal study of youth*. New York: Academic Press.

23. Donovan JE, et al. Syndrome of problem behavior in adolescence: A replication. *J Consulting & Clinical Psychology*. 1988 56 (5):762-765.

24. Donovan JE. Young adult drinking-driving: behavioral and psychosocial correlates *J Studies on Alcohol*, 1993, 54(5):600-613.

25. Wilens, TE. ADHD and Risk for Substance Abuse Disorders, *NIH Consensus Development Conference on Diagnosis and Treatment of Attention Deficit*

Hyperactivity Disorder, Nov 16-18, 1998, (Program and Abstracts), 181-185.

26. Schubiner H, et al. Prevalence of attention-deficit/hyperactivity disorder and conduct disorder among substance abusers. *J Clinical Psychiatry*, April 2000, 61(4), 244-251.

27. NIAAA. Youth Drinking: Risk Factors and Consequences, *Alcohol Alert*, No 37, July 1997. National Institute on Alcoholism. http://silk.nih.gov.silk/niaa1/publication/aa37.htm

28. Kumpfer KL (1989) Prevention of alcohol and drug abuse: A critical review of risk factors. In *Prevention of Mental Disorder, Alcohol, and Other Drug Use in Children and Adolescents*. OSAP Prevention Monograph-2 DHHS Pub. Washington DC. US Govt Printing Office.

29. Johnson BD, Muffler J. Sociocultural. In Lowinson JH et al, (Eds.) *Substance Abuse: A comprehensive textbook*. (3rd Edition), Baltimore: Williams & Wilkins, 1997.

30. Halikas, JA. Craving in Lowinson JH et al, (Editors) *Substance Abuse: A comprehensive textbook*. (3rd Edition), Baltimore: Williams & Wilkins, 1997. p. 88.

31. Madrid GA, et al (2001) Stress as a mediating factor in the association between the DRD2 Taq1 polymorphism and alcoholism. *Alcohol*, 23, 2:117-122.

32. Hanna, EZ et al (2001 The relationship of early-onset regular smoking and alcohol use, depression, illicit drug use and other risky behaviors during early adolescence: Results from the Youth supplement of the Third Annual Health and Nutrition Examination Survey. 2 *Substance Abuse*, 13: 265-282.

33. Grant BF (1998) The impact of a family history of alcoholism on the relationship between age at onset of alcohol use and DSM-IV dependence. *Alcohol Health & Research World*, 22 (2):144-148.

34. Loney J (1998) Risk of Treatment vs nontreatment. *NIH Consensus Development Conference on Diagnosis and Treatment of Attention Deficit Hyperactivity Disorder* (Nov 16-18, 1998): Program and Abstracts:175-180.

35. The National Center on Addiction and Substance Abuse at Columbia University (1995) *Substance Abuse and Federal Entitlement Programs*. New York: CASA.

36. Taylor RC et al, (2000) Tobacco craving: intensity-related effects of imagery scripts in drug abusers. *Experimental and Clinical Psychopharmacology* 8(1):75-87.

37. Zickler, P (2000) Nicotine Craving and Heavy Smoking May Contribute to Increased Use of Cocaine and Heroin; *Nicotine Research, NIDA Notes*. 15,5.

38. Hanna EZ, et al (2001) The relationship of early- and regular smoking to alcohol use, depression, illicit drug use, and other risky behaviors during early adolescence: Results of from the youth supplement of the Third Annual Health and Nutrition Examination Survey. *J Substance Abuse*, 13:265-282.

39. Califano JA, Booth A (1998) *CASA National Survey of Teens, Teachers and Principals*. New York: CASA.

40. Substance Abuse and Mental Health Services Administration (2001) *Summary of Findings from the 2000 National Household Survey on Drug Abuse*. Table F.42 Percentages Reporting Past Month Alcohol Use, Past Month "Binge" Alcohol Use, and Past Month Heavy Alcohol Use, by Detailed Age Categories: 1999 and 2000. Washington, DC: SAMSHA, Department of Health and Human Services.

41. Johnston LD; O'Malley PM; Bachman JG. (2000) *The Monitoring of the Future National Results on Adolescent Drug Use: Overview of the Key Findings, 1999*. Bethesda, MD: National Institute on Drug Abuse, US Dept of Health and Human Services.

42. NIAAA. (1998) Alcohol and Aging. *Alcohol Alert* No 40 (April 1998). Washington, DC NIAAA.

43. Blume, SB. Women: Clinical Aspects. In Lowinson JH et al, (Editors) *Substance Abuse: A comprehensive textbook*. (3rd Edition), Baltimore: Williams & Wilkins, 1997.

44. Hallman J, Persson P, Klinteberg BAB (2001) Female alcoholism: Differences between female alcoholics with and without a history of additional substance abuse. *Alcohol & Alcoholism*, 36:564-571.

45. NIDA. (2001) Marijuana. *Infofax 13551*. Bethesda, MD: NIDA

46. Substance Abuse and Mental Health Services Administration (2001) Chapter 2: Illicit Drug Use: *Summary of Findings from the 2000 National Household Survey on Drug Abuse*. Washington, DC: SMSHA, Department of Health and Human Services.

47. Grinspoon L, Bakalar JB. Marijuana. Clinical Aspects. In Lowinson JH et al, (Eds.) *Substance Abuse: A comprehensive textbook*. (3rd Edition), Baltimore: Williams & Wilkins, 1997.

48. National Institute on Drug Abuse Research

Report Series.(2000) *Heroin: Abuse and Addiction*. NIH Publication No. 00-4165. Bethesda, MD: NIH

49. Jaffe JH, Knapp CM, Ciraulo DA. Opiates: Clinical Aspects. In Lowinson JH et al, (Eds.) *Substance Abuse: A comprehensive textbook*. (3rd Edition), Baltimore: Williams & Wilkins, 1997.

50. King GR, Ellinwood EH. Amphetamines and other Stimulants. In Lowinson JH et al, (Editors) *Substance Abuse: A comprehensive textbook*. (3rd Edition), Baltimore: Williams & Wilkins, 1997:207-223.

51. NIDA Research Report (1998) *Methamphetamine Abuse and Addiction*: NIH Publication No. 98-4210. Bethesda MD: NIH.

52. NIDA Research Report (1999) *Cocaine Abuse and Addiction*: NIH Publication No. 99-4342. Bethesda MD: NIH.

53. Gold MS. Cocaine (and Crack); Clinical Aspects. In Lowinson JH et al, (Editors) *Substance Abuse: A comprehensive textbook*. (3rd Edition), Baltimore: Williams & Wilkins, 1997:166-199.

54. National Institute on Drug Abuse. (2001) Club Drugs. INFOFAX # 13674.

55. Morgan JP. Designer Drugs. In Lowinson JH et al, (Editors) *Substance Abuse: A comprehensive textbook*. (3rd Edition), Baltimore: Williams & Wilkins, 1997:264-269.

56. NIDA. (2000) *MDMA (Ecstasy)*. NIDA INFOFAX # 13547.

57. Grob CS, Poland RE. MDMA. In Lowinson JH et al, (Eds) *Substance Abuse: A comprehensive textbook*. (3rd Edition), Baltimore: Williams & Wilkins, 1997:269-276.

58. NIDA. (2001) *Club Drugs*. INFOFAX # 13674.

59. NIDA (2001) *Club Drugs*. INFOFAX # 13674.

60. NIDA (1998) *PCP (Phencyclidine)* INFOFAX # 13554.

61. NIDA (2001) *Club Drugs*. INFOFAX # 13674.

62. NIDA (2001) *Hallucinogens and Dissociative Drugs*. Research Report Series. NIH Publication No. 01-4209. Bethesda MD: NIH.

63. American Psychiatric Association.(1994) *Diagnostic and Statistical Manual of Psychiatric Disorders*: Fourth Edition (DSM-IV). Washington, DC. APA: 233

64. Pechnik RN, Ungerleider JT. Hallucinogens. In Lowinson JH et al, (Eds.) *Substance Abuse: A comprehensive textbook*. (3rd Edition), Baltimore: Williams & Wilkins, 1997. 230-238.

65. Wesson DR, Smith DE et al Sedative-Hypnotics and Tricyclics. In Lowinson JH et al, (Editors) *Substance Abuse: A comprehensive textbook*. (3rd Edition), Baltimore: Williams & Wilkins, 1997.

66. Sharp CW, Rosenberg NL Inhalants. In Lowinson JH et al, (Editors) *Substance Abuse: A comprehensive textbook*. (3rd Edition), Baltimore: Williams & Wilkins, 1997:246-263.

67. Kuhn C, Swartzwelder S, Wilson W. (1998) *Buzzed: The Straight Facts about the Most Used and Abused Drugs from Alcohol to Ecstasy*. New York: WW Norton.

68. Johnson LD, O'Malley PM. Bachman JG. The *Monitoring of the Future, National Results on Adolescent Drug Use: Overview of the Key Findings, 1999*. Bethesda, MD: National Institute on Drug Abuse, US Dept of Health and Human Services, 2000.

69. Galloway GP. Anabolic-Androgenic Steroids. In Lowinson JH et al, (Eds.) *Substance Abuse: A comprehensive textbook*. (3rd Edition), Baltimore: Williams & Wilkins, 1997. 308-318.

70. Goodman A (1995) Addictive Disorders: an integrated approach. Part One. An integrated understanding. *J Min Addict Recovery*, 2:33-76.

71. (2001) News Focus: Behavioral Addictions; Do they exist? *Science*; 294:98-981.

72. American Psychiatric Association. (1994) *Diagnostic and Statistical Manual of Psychiatric Disorders*: Fourth Edition (DSM-IV). Washington, DC. APA, p. 618.

73. Halperin DA Sects and Cults. (1997) In Lowinson JH et al, (Eds.) *Substance Abuse: A comprehensive textbook*. (3rd Edition), Baltimore: Williams & Wilkins:337-339.

74. Glick J, Halperin DA Collection and Accumulation (1997) In Lowinson JH et al, (Eds.) *Substance Abuse: A comprehensive textbook*. (3rd Edition), Baltimore: Williams & Wilkins;355-359.

75. Black DW, Belsare G, Schlosser S (1999) Clinical features, psychiatric comorbidity, and health-related quality of life in persons reporting compulsive computer use behavior. *J Clin Psychiatry*. 60(12):839-44.

76. Asp K(1999) Addicted to Sweat. *American Fitness*. Nov 1999.

77. Ratey JJ, Johnson C (1998) *Shadow Syndromes: The Mild Forms of Mental Disorders that Sabotage Us*. New York: Bantam.

78. Asp K (2001) *Exercise or Obsession? Women Talk About When Too Much Goes Too Far*. Mighty Words: Electronic Publishing.

79. Kaminker L (1998) *Exercise Addiction: When Fitness Becomes an Obsession.* New York: Rosen Pub

80. Johnson M (2000) *Understanding Exercise Addiction.* New York: Rosen Pub

81. Korn M (2001) Eating Disorders: New Features and New Treatments. Paper presented at 154th Annual Meeting of the American Psychiatric Association Day 4 — May 8, 2001. Accessed on the Internet at http://www.medscape.com/medscape/cno/2001/APACME/Story.cfm?story_id=2263

82. Gold MS, Johnson CR, Stennie K. (1997) Eating Disorders. In Lowinson JH et al, (Eds.). *Substance Abuse: A comprehensive textbook.* (3rd Edition), Baltimore: Williams & Wilkins, p. 319-330.

83. Sahu a Kalara SP (1993) Neuropeptide regulation of feeding behavior:neuropeptide Y. *TEM;* 4:217-224.

84. Herzog DB, Keller MB, Lavori PW, et al. (1992) The prevalence of personality disorders in 210 women with eating disorders. *J Clin Psychiatry;* 53:147-152.

85. Vandereycken W, Hoek HW (1992) Are eating disorders culture-bound syndrome? In: Halmi KA, ed. *Psychobiology and Treatment of Anorexia Nervosa and Bulimia Nervosa.* Washington, DC: American Psychiatric Association: 19-38.

86. Boumann CE, Yates WR.(1994) Risk factors for bulimia nervosa: A controlled study of parental psychiatric illness and divorce. *Addict Behav;* 19(6):667-675.

87. Horesh N, Apter A, Lepkifker E, et al.(1995) Life events and severe anorexia nervosa in adolescence. *Acta Psychiatr Scand;* 91:5-9.

88. Kaye WH. (1997) Anorexia nervosa, obsessional behavior, and serotonin. *Psychopharmacol Bull.* 33:335-344.

89. Gold MS (1993) Are eating disorders addictions? *Adv Bioscience;*1993 90:455-463.

90. Anderson AE (1999) Gender-Related Aspects of Eating Disorders: A Guide to Practice. *J Gender-Specific Medicine;* 2[1]:47-54.

91. American Psychiatric Association. (1994) *Diagnostic and Statistical Manual of Psychiatric Disorders:* Fourth Edition (DSM-IV). Washington, DC: APA.

92. No author (2000) No Single Answer to Treating Binge Eating Disorder. *Drug & Ther Perspect* 15(5):7-10.

93. Jonas JM, Gold MS (1986) Cocaine abuse and eating disorders. *Lancet* 1(8477):390

94. Goldstein L et al.(1985) Differential EEG activation and pathological gambling. *Biolog Psychiatry;* 20:1232-1234.

95. Shaffer HJ. Psychology of Stage Change. In Lowinson JH et al, (Eds.). *Substance Abuse: A comprehensive textbook.* (3rd Edition), Baltimore: Williams & Wilkins, 1997. 100-106.

96. Grant BF, Stinson FS, Harford T (2001) The five year course of Alcohol abuse among young adults. *J Substance Abuse,* 13:229-238.

97. Alcoholics Anonymous (1995) *Big Book,* 4th Edition.. New York: AA General Services Conference.

98. Marlatt GA, Gordon Jr. eds.(1985) *Relapse Prevention: maintenance strategies in the treatment of addictive behaviors.* New York: Guilford Press.

99. Survey Research Laboratory at the University of Chicago. *Missed Opportunity: National Survey of Primary Care Physicians and Patients on Substance Abuse.* New York: Center on Addiction and Substance Abuse (CASA) April 2000. p 15.

100. Mayfield, D.; McLeod, G.; and Hall, P. (1974) The CAGE questionnaire: Validation of a new alcoholism instrument. *Am J Psychiatry,* 131:1121-1123

101. Russell M, et al (1994) Screening for pregnancy risk drinking. Alcoholism: *Clin & Experiment Res,* 18:1156-1161.

102. "Women often don't know they are addicted," Survey says. *Medscape News,* January 11, 2002, accessed at http://psychiatry.medscape.com/MedscapeWire/2002/01/medwire.0111.Women.html

103. American Society of Addiction Medicine (1996) *Patient Placement Criteria for the Treatment of Substance Related Disorders* (SAM PCP-2) 2nd Edition. Chevy Chase, MD: ASAM.

104. Geller A. Comprehensive Treatment Programs. In Lowinson JH et al, (Eds.). *Substance Abuse: A comprehensive textbook.* (3rd Edition), Baltimore: Williams & Wilkins, 1997. 426-429.

105. Blume, SB. Pathological Gambling. In Lowinson JH et al, (Editors). *Substance Abuse: A comprehensive textbook.* (3rd Edition), Baltimore: Williams & Wilkins, 1997. 330-337.

106. Cook CH (1988) The Minnesota model in the management of alcohol and drug dependency: miracle, method or myth. Part 1. *Brit J Addiction,* 83:625-634.

107. Nace, EP (1997) Alcoholics Anonymous. In Lowinson JH et al, (Eds.). *Substance Abuse: A comprehensive textbook.* (3rd Edition), Baltimore: Williams & Wilkins:383-389.

108. Heser RK, Miller WR, eds. (1995) *Handbook of alcoholism treatment approaches: effective alternatives.* New York: Allyn & Bacon.

109. Horvath AT Alternate Support groups. In Lowinson JH et al, (Eds.). *Substance Abuse: A comprehensive textbook.* (3rd Edition), Baltimore: Williams & Wilkins, 1997. 390-396.

110. See "The Twelve Step Cybercafe," accessed in the Internet on Jan 12, 2002, at http://www.12steps.org/Brochure/menubord/menu.htm

111. McElrath D (1987) *Hazeldon: A Spiritual Odyssey.* Center City, MN: Hazelden Pub.

112. O'Brien WO, Devlin CJ (1997) The Therapeutic Community. In Lowinson JH et al, (Eds.). *Substance Abuse: A comprehensive textbook.* (3rd Edition), Baltimore: Williams & Wilkins:400-405.

113. Brill L (1977) The treatment of drug abuse: evolution of a perspective. *Am J Psychiatry,* 134:157-160.

114. Nyswander M et al (1958) The treatment of drug addicts as voluntary outpatients: a progress report. *Am J of Orthopsychiatry,* 28: 714-727.

115. Rounsaville BJ, Carroll KM (1997) Individual Psychotherapy. In Lowinson JH et al, (Eds.). *Substance Abuse: A comprehensive textbook.* (3rd Edition), Baltimore: Williams & Wilkins, 1997: 430-439.

116. Daley DC, Marlatt GA (1997) Relapse Prevention. In Lowinson JH et al, (Eds.). *Substance Abuse: A comprehensive textbook.* (3rd Edition), Baltimore: Williams & Wilkins: 458-467.

117. Morgenstern J, Longabaugh R (2000) Cognitive-behavioral treatment for alcohol dependence: A review of evidence for its hypothesized mechanisms of action. *Addiction;* 95:1475-1490.

118. Goodwin DW, Gabrielli WV (1997) Alcohol: Clinical Aspects. In Lowinson JH et al, (Editors). *Substance Abuse: A comprehensive textbook.* (3rd Edition), Baltimore: Williams & Wilkins:142-148.

119. Rawson RA, McCann MJ Hasson AJ, Ling W (2000) Addictions Pharmacotherapy 2000: New options new challenges. *J Psychoactive Drugs;* 32:371-378.

120. Allison M, Hubbard RL, Ginzburg HM (1985) Indicators of suicide and depression among drug abusers. Research monograph 68. DHHS publication no (ADM) 85-1411. Rockville, MD: NIDA.

121. Ziedonis DM, Kosten TR (1991) Pharmacotherapy Improves Treatment Outcomes in Depressed Cocaine Addicts. *J Psychoactive Drugs,* 23:417-425.

122. Kuo II Fisher B, Vlahov D (2000) Consideration of a North American heroin assisted clinical trial for the treatment of opiate dependent individuals. *Internat J Drug Policy;* 11:357-370.

123. Barnett PG, Rodgers JH, Bloch DA (2001) A meta analysis comparing buprenorphine to methadone for treatment of opioid dependence. *Addiction;* 96:683-690.

124. Umbricht A et al (1999) Naltrexone shortened opioid detoxification with buprenorphine. History, recent molecular and neurochemical research and future in mainstream medicine. *Drug Alcohol Depend;* 56:181-190.

125. Fisher G, Johnson RE, Eder H et al (2000) Treatment of opioid dependent pregnant women with buprenorphine. *Addiction;* 95:239-244.

126. Kreek MJ (2000) Methadone-related opioid pharmacotherapy for heroin addiction. *Ann NY Acad Sci;* 909:186-216.

CHAPTER 10

Domestic Violence

Domestic or intimate partner violence is a problem with serious health consequences, and in general, its symptoms are not being recognized by health care providers. This chapter aims to sensitize you to the issue of domestic violence and to help you to understand the dynamics, the barriers to identification, to recognize the physical and behavioral symptoms, to give you guidance on how to inquire about it, and recommendations on how to manage it.

The Silent Epidemic[1]

Domestic violence has been called *silent* because it is both hidden and largely unrecognized in spite of recent media attention and coverage. *Epidemic* because the dimensions of the problem are truly staggering. By some estimates about 4 million American women experience a serious assault by an intimate partner during the average 12 month period.[2] Popular misconception sees domestic violence as a phenomenon only of poor and uneducated women. While it is true that past and current victims of domestic violence are over represented in the welfare population, most are there because of debilitating factors related to the abuse.[3] However, the silent epidemic crosses boundaries of age, gender, ethnicity, socioeconomic status and sexual orientation.[4] Women between 19 and 29 with children under 12 are most likely to be abused.[5] Violence also occurs in dating couples, with 20% of adolescents reporting being physically or sexually abused.[6] It is estimated that 10% of professional and working women are victims of battering mates.[7] Intimate partner violence occurs with similar frequency in lesbian and gay relationships.[8] In addition there is evidence that women or elderly with disabilities are at higher risk for abuse at the hands of intimates or caretakers.[9,10] Approximately 3.3 million children a year are exposed to violence by a family member against their mother.[11] Such children are 1500 times more likely to be abused than those coming from homes without partner violence.[12] The long term consequences on the children living in violent households are:

1. **Witnessing domestic violence is the single best predictor of drug abuse, juvenile delinquency and engaging in multiple health risk behaviors.[13,14]**

2. **Boys learn that males are violent and need not respect women. As adults they are 10 times more likely to use violence on their partners. Girls learn that male violence is normal and tend to accept it in adult relationships.[15]**

3. **Depending on their developmental stage, children witnessing domestic violence may develop serious medical and/or psychological problems.[16]**

The economic costs of treating domestic violence are enormous. Estimates put the annual medical cost attributed to domestic violence at more than $2 billion. Annually there are 243,000, or one fourth of all ER visits, 21,000 hospitalizations, about 40,000 clinic visits, and 175,000 disability days, estimated to be attributable to domestic violence.[17,18] According to the National Coalition Against Domestic Violence, domestic violence accounts for more injury to women than from all other causes combined, and around 2,000 women a year die as a result of it.[19] Homicide is the number one killer of pregnant and post partum (1 year) women.[20,21] Some of the statistics are mere estimates because typically health care providers correctly identify abuse in fewer than 5% of the cases.[22]

The last statistic of 95% of cases presented in health care settings not being identified as such is most alarming to some. Citing these data, a March 2001 JAMA editorial argued that all health care professionals must do a better job in all settings to recognize and provide appropriate treatment to victims of domestic or intimate partner violence.[23]

CULTURAL FACTORS

In general, domestic violence is overwhelmingly perpetrated by men onto women, so our discussion reflects that fact. As a society, we need to examine norms and values that appear to tolerate (perhaps even encourage) violent and coercive behaviors in intimate relationships. Historically, in most patriarchal societies social, religious, and even legal norms have encouraged male control over women.[24] This included either explicit or tacit understanding that a husband could physically "discipline" his wife. One attempt to limit the amount of violence a husband could visit upon his wife came in the form of old English "rule of thumb." It forbade a husband to use a stick thicker than a thumb to beat his wife.[25] The cultural and religious stigma about homosexuality has made violence in same sex domestic relationships even more hidden. It is rarely considered, diagnosed or treated by health care providers.

• •

PATIENT PROFILE 10.1

I'M SO SICK OF YOUR JEALOUSY!

SETTING: *Rikki and Maury are two homosexual men in their late 30's, living in a large cosmopolitan city. They have been coming to see Greg, an osteopathic physician for minor health problems for a little over a year. He knows that they have been in a committed relationship for 3 years. Rikki has come into the clinic with a bloody towel around his head accompanied by Maury.*

Greg: What have we here? Let me take a look at that.

As he takes the towel off, Rikki winces. There is a 3 cm gash on his scalp just above his right ear.

Maury: He is so clumsy. He left a kitchen cabinet door open and ran into it.

Rikki groans and rolls his eyes, but does not say anything.

Greg is aware of the tensions in their relationship. He suspects that this explanation given by the partner and Rikki's nonverbal gestures might indicate that this is not what really happened.

Greg: Oh Yeah? Rikki you must have been going pretty fast to get a gash that deep.

Maury: Well, you know how Rikki is, kind of flighty. He moves kind of erratically.

Rikki keeps his eyes down and does not say anything. By now Greg is convinced that he needs to get the two separated if he is to find out what really happened.

Greg: OK, I am going to take Rikki into the surgery room to stitch this up. Maury you wait here.

Maury: Oh, no. I'll come. I want to be with him. .

Greg: Sorry, that's against the rules. It won't take long.

In the surgery room:

Greg: I know you two have had some tensions and fights in the past. Has it become violent? Is that what this is about?

Rikki: He's been so possessive lately. He doesn't want me to see any of my friends any more.

Greg: I understand. So, how did you get that gash on your head?

Rikki: I was on the phone talking to a friend, and we were laughing. Maury got jealous and told me to get off the phone. When I didn't, he got really mad and threw an ash tray at me as hard as he could from across the room.

Greg: I see. Was this the first time that he became violent?

Rikki: Well, he has broken things of mine before when he got mad. A week ago he tried to prevent me from leaving the house. He got pretty rough.

Greg: What do you mean by rough? Did he hit you?

Rikki: Yeah, kind of.

Greg: Where?

Rikki: Right here.

He pulls up his shirt and points to some yellowish green contusions on his ribcage; two along the right side and two in back.

Greg makes a body map outline in the chart and records the injuries.

Greg: Those must have been painful when they were fresh. Anything else?

Rikki pulls up the shirt sleeve on his right arm to reveal some more discolored places along the distal part of his forearm.

Greg: This looks like pretty serious stuff. No one deserves to be hit like this. This is intimate partner abuse.

He then briefly explains about the tendency for such abuse to get progressively worse unless there is early intervention.

Rikki: I can't believe this is happening. We've been together for 3 years. He's always been somewhat bossy, but I just let him. But he has just gotten so controlling over the past few months. He doesn't want me to see or talk to any of my friends any more. He just stays home all the time. It drives me nuts.

Greg: Do you need to leave to be safe?

Rikki: We have this big mortgage on our house. I don't want to walk away from that.

Greg: Do you think he would be open to counseling? There is a fairly good group program for gays and lesbians at the Jackson Center. They have some very experienced counselors there too that specialize in gay-lesbian relationship problems.

Rikki: I didn't know that was available. We have been talking about counseling. Maybe if he hears about this from you, he might go. He thinks I need counseling, too. And that's OK by me. I probably do need it.

Greg: Do you think he'll get mad at you for telling me about the battering?

Rikki: Actually my guess is he will be relieved. He has been ashamed and embarrassed every time he loses his temper. Once it is out in the open, he may be glad. At least I hope so. If not, I guess I would have to think about leaving.

Greg: OK then let's dress this suture, and then we'll talk to Maury.

POINTS TO CONSIDER:

- When Maury answers for Rikki, and when the explanation does not match the seriouness of the injury, Greg knows that the patient must be separated from the "helpful" partner.

- Greg educates the patient on domestic violence, and focuses on safety issues.

- Because he knows that intimate partner violence between same sex couples generally does not get a helpful response from the legal system, Greg suggests individual and group counseling for both partners at a community center.

- Greg remembers to probe if there is likely to be retribution from the partner for revealing the abuse.

• •

The legal system has been under pressure to catch up with the problem of domestic violence. It has taken vigorous advocacy as well as some prominent civil judgments by victims of domestic violence to convince state and local lawmakers to enact laws that allow police to arrest perpetrators of domestic violence. However, in many jurisdictions, victims still find barriers to accessing the legal system, getting protection orders, having those orders served on the batterer, and having those orders enforced.[26] Fear of stalking or retribution by the batterer and lack of confidence in the willingness or ability of the legal system to protect them is cited as the principal reason why victims only report one-seventh of domestic assaults to police, and only

55% of serious injuries.[27] The general consensus is that prompt arrest and incarceration deters those abusers who have much to lose from the social consequences.[28] However, unemployed batterers or those with few social ties tend to become more violent after an arrest.[29] When you treat a victim of abuse, and consider possible legal remedies for the woman's safety, this distinction in economic and social status of the batterer is a crucial variable.

BATTERER PROFILE

What kind of man is a batterer? Although batterers come from all racial, religious, and socioeconomic backgrounds, there are a number of characteristics that fit the general profile of a batterer.[30] He objectifies women, and may not even see them as people or as worthy of respect. Rather he tends to see women as sexual objects or even as his property. A batterer may be outwardly successful, and may be seen as a charming, pleasant, "nice" guy. On the other hand, he may come from a chaotic, abusive family, and have feelings of powerlessness. During the pursuit or "courting phase," he may rush into intimacy, convincing his object of love that she is "the one" and that he cannot live without her. However, once he has "captured" her, the process of exercising control over her behavior, freedom of movement and even her thinking will begin almost immediately using the various techniques detailed in the Wheel of Power and Control (Figure 10-1). Victims have described the abrupt change from romantic pursuer to possessive abuser as a Jekyll and Hyde phenomenon.

The Battering Cycle

Relationships involving domestic violence progress through cycles. The first is the **tension building phase.** During this period, the batterer will accuse the significant other of various (often imagined) wrong doings, and in repeated criticisms tell her she can do nothing right. He will start controlling her behaviors by restricting her basic rights, (not letting her drive or leave the house without him), or even ordering her into isolation. The **violent phase** often starts when the batterer uses any real or imagined objectionable act or behavior as a "reason" to launch into explosive violence. In the early phase of a domestic violence situation, this violence may take the form of breaking or throwing objects, or harming or killing pets. As time goes on, the violence of this phase escalates and is directed more and more against their partner. Frequently, the abuser will be under the influence of alcohol or drugs. Once the abuser has released his tension, there follows a calmer phase, also known as the **honeymoon phase.** The batterer becomes remorseful, apologizes, and may make various excuses for his behavior. He may insist that the violence was not intended, that he really loves his partner, and cannot do without her. He will blame it on alcohol, stress at work, or some other external factor.[31] He will promise (often with real tears) that he will *never* do it again. The honeymoon phase, during which the batterer may become a doting husband and loving father, lulls the victim into believing that the perpetrator is truly sorry, that the violence will end, and things will improve. However, without intervention, legal action or counseling, the tension building phase will recommence until it culminates in another violent explosive phase. Over time the abuse tends to escalate in severity and frequency. The honeymoon periods become shorter or may disappear altogether. It has been suggested that this progression is similar to the addictive process, both in the neurochemical reinforcement process in the brain as well as in the tolerance building process which may dictate an increasing violence level to get the same "rush" or release.[32]

RISK FACTORS FOR BECOMING A VICTIM

How do women or any intimate partners get drawn into violent relationships and why do they stay in them? All too often we tend to blame the victim. To understand these questions, we need to look at the typical profile of the woman attracted to batterers, as well as the psychophys-

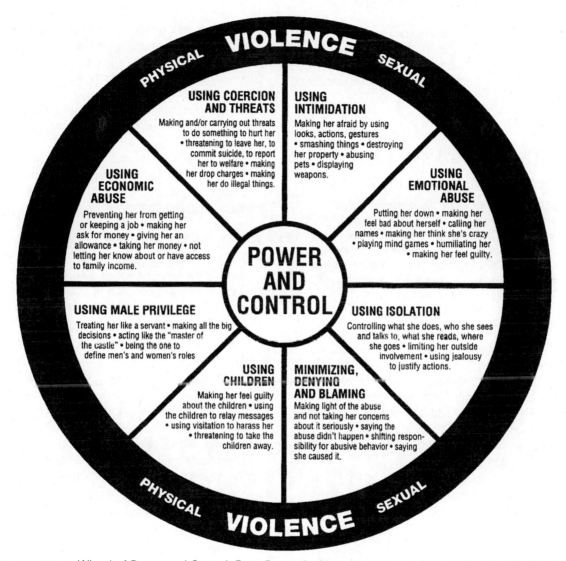

Figure 10-1. Wheel of Power and Control. From Domestic Abuse Intervention Project, Duluth MN, Used by permission.

iological progression of battering that traps the victim.[33] Many women are drawn to men who call forth their vulnerability and protectiveness. Men who had difficult childhoods were mistreated emotionally, sexually or physically, or who have drinking problems, often seduce women into feeling sorry for them. Women who respond to this kind of man often had a pattern in their childhood or adolescence of having taken injured animals or pets and nursing them

back to health. The woman is likely to be even more vulnerable, if in childhood she has been socialized into believing that women are inferior, or that men have the "right" to hit women. This is especially critical if as a child she experienced physical, emotional or sexual abuse, or witnessed domestic violence in her family of origin. Such women as adults are likely to be having feelings of low self worth, and existential guilt. They may be prone to the urge to rescue. They tend to believe that they can compensate for the man's problems by loving him. The man often evokes this response by saying that *only she* can help him, and that he cannot get along without her.[34]

• •

PATIENT PROFILE 10.2

HE SAYS HE'S REALLY SORRY

SETTING: Melody is a 22-year-old college student who has been living with her boyfriend of 1 1/2 years. He is graduating and she is a junior student. Both of them are under a lot of stress because of final exams. They are both Biology majors in a medium-sized mid-Western college. She is a drop in to the student health center and is being seen by Bob, a nurse practitioner.

Bob: Hello, Melody. My name is Bob Jones. I am a nurse practitioner. How can I help you?

Melody: Hi, it's my boyfriend Henry. He was really sweet and very charming when I first moved in with him. Now he's changed into someone else. I am so shocked and unhappy. I can't sleep. I'm so upset and finals are just around the corner.

Bob: One thing at a time. Slowly now tell me how Henry has changed?

Melody: He slapped me. *(Starts crying.)*

Bob: Hmmm. Here's a Kleenex. Is that what caused that red mark on your left cheek?

Melody: Yes.

Bob: Tell me more about this. Has he ever done this before?

Melody: Yes. It started after the first semester that we lived together. Whenever the push is on for exams or projects, he gets really irritable and everything I do seems to upset him. Now the push is on in his classes for graduating with honors. He keeps saying he'll never do it again. I want to believe him and he got me some flowers. He's being really sweet. Do you think he really means it?

Bob: I don't know but this sounds like domestic violence and let me tell you about how this kind of behavior repeats.

He proceeds to tell her about the Batterers Cycle.

Melody: Oh, he's promised he'll never do it again. And he just slaps me, sort of like what Dad used to do to Mom. Not too bad. I'll just be quiet and nice to him and see what happens. Maybe he'll change. We really care about each other.

Bob: Here's a pamphlet on domestic violence. Will you read it and think about what has happened?

Melody: Sure, after finals.

Bob: If anything else happens, will you come back in to see me?

Melody: Yes, and thanks.

POINTS TO CONSIDER:

- Bob continues to question her because he realizes the importance of clarifying the reasons she has come in to the center.

- Bob's non-judgmental and supportive demeanor is essential to facilitate Melody to share more about the relationship and its dynamics.

- Bob realizes that getting out of an abusive relationship sometimes is a long process and continued education is an essential part of helping Melody.

- Bob has available the appropriate educational materials which when given to Melody at this time can reinforce further proactive behavior on her part.

- Bob makes sure Melody knows she can return to the counseling center for help when she needs it.

• •

Once in an abusive relationship, there are many obstacles facing battered women who want to leave. (See Box 10-1.) One obstacle is the intermittent reinforcement of each honeymoon phase. The victim, experiencing the honeymoon phase, convinces herself that the batterer really does love her and needs her. She may truly believe what many victims have said: "I thought if I loved him enough, he would love himself and not hurt me any more." She may also have well founded fears that the batterer will become more violent or even kill her if she attempts to leave. Indeed the greatest danger for homicide is at the point she leaves or shortly after she has left.[35]

Progression of Victimization

The Wheel of Power and Control illustrates the wide variety of techniques used by batterers to intimidate, gain power, and achieve almost total control over the victims. Intermittent violence and physical abuse is used by the batterer to intimidate and control his victim. He will combine direct physical assaults with verbal threats, throwing or breaking objects, harming or killing pets, or simply raising his fists to enforce the other techniques. Relentless psychological abuse, designed to undermine the victim's independence and self-esteem, reinforce the feeling of powerlessness. Whether the abuse is primarily physical, or psychological, or both, most victims tend to go through what has been labeled as a **psychophysiological progression of victimization**.[36] One way to understand this progression is in terms of the batterer's increas-ing need to completely control his victim. There are three stages: the **Injury Stage**, the **Illness Stage** and the **Isolation Stage**. Knowing what goes on in each of these stages can help you identify physical and behavioral symptoms and allow you to plan an effective response.

INJURY STAGE

In the Injury Stage, the batterer is likely to combine verbal abuse and threats or displays of violence, with pushing, shoving, restraining, arm twisting, choking and hitting. The victim may still be employed, and be connected to church, family, and other community ties. However, she is likely to be pressured by him to separate from those outside sources of support, and to rely on him completely for emotional and economic support. Injuries at this stage usually consist of bruises and abrasions, possibly broken ribs. She may have difficulty swallowing or speaking from the attempts to choke or strangle her. The physical symptoms generally will be located on the central part of the body, the outside of the arms, the head, face, and peritoneal area. Often they are not severe, and less than 4% require hospitalization. One clue for you is that the location of the injuries usually is *not* consistent with claims of accidental falls or walking into doors (often provided by the solicitous spouse). Shame and fear of retribution will usually prevent a victim from volunteering the true origin of the injuries, especially if the battering partner is present.

ILLNESS STAGE

During the Illness Stage, the violence and/or the psychological tactics are escalating in severity and frequency. The honeymoon phases may become shorter or disappear altogether. Injuries, like black eyes, dislocated jaw, or broken ribs, or pain from such injuries, may force the victim to miss a lot of work. The batterer may repeatedly "check up" on his partner at the work place to the point of annoyance and disruption. Ultimately, embarrassment and shame over the absences, unexplained injuries, and partner interference may get her to withdraw from work

---

Box 10-1   Obstacles to Leaving an Abusive Relationship

1. Fear and terror of their abuser
2. Low self esteem
3. Lack of money
4. Lack of shelter and housing
5. Batterer's promises to change
6. Isolation
7. Lack of family and social support
8. Lack of access to legal counsel and advocacy
9. History of prior ineffective legal intervention
10. Denial and minimization by victim and outsiders
11. Shame, embarrassment, self blame, and guilt
12. Religious beliefs
13. Wanting to keep family together
14. Protecting the children (by taking the abuse to shield their children)
15. Lack of employment skills
16. Fear of being considered unbelievable or crazy

Adapted from Buel S (1994) Domestic Violence — A Talk by Sarah Buel. Video Produced by Wyeth Ayerst.

and her social network.[37] Physical trauma from the abuse may lead to various complications. Severe head injuries may lead to sinus, hearing or visual problems, or even brain trauma. Rape or "rough sex" may lead to vaginal infections and pelvic inflammations. Pregnant women are especially at high risk from blows or kicks to the abdomen.[38] As the victim succumbs to the stress of constant psychological pressure of repeated battering or threats of battering, she may somatize the stress. In addition to (or instead of) physical injuries, she is likely to complain of atypical physical and emotional ailments, such as myalgia and chronic fatigue, heartburn, irritable bowel syndrome, and sleeping or eating disturbances. Indirectly reaching out to the health care provider, she may refer to the anxiety she is experiencing, or mention that she feels as if she were "walking on eggshells" at home. Unfortunately if domestic violence is not identified as the underlying problem at this stage, the health care provider may simply respond by treating the symptoms — whether they be physical or emotional. Alternatively, a conscientious provider might order more tests to get to the bottom of some mysterious somatic ailment. When such tests show no evidence of a physical cause, the provider may conclude that the patient is either faking it, or is psychologically disturbed. Such labeling could drive the person into the despair of the next stage.

ISOLATION STAGE

This stage begins when the batterer tries to enforce total isolation through all the means shown in the Wheel of Power and Control (Figure 10-1). Verbal abuse at this stage has been compared to brainwashing, and victims have spoken of feeling like prisoners of war. By denying her gainful employment or education, the victim becomes financially totally dependent on the batterer. The batterer will hammer the victim with assertions that she cannot make it on her own. Without resources of her own and without outside support to contradict the abuser's version of "reality," she comes to believe his assertions that she is worthless and that she deserves the abuse. Calling her crazy is one of the psychological battering techniques used by many abusers. Brainwashing has been successful when the victim identifies herself from the perspective of the batterer. Once this perceptual shift has taken place, she internalizes that she is to blame, that she is worthless, that she is crazy, and that no one would believe her if she spoke up about the abuse. If the victim finds that her health care provider also seems to think she is "crazy," this only confirms the batterer's brainwashing. In the despair of hopelessness, she becomes convinced that she cannot make it on her own, that she will never get away, and that ultimately she may die at the hands of her abuser. At that point she lives in a state of almost constant fear and terror for herself and her children.[39]

When a victim has reached this last part of the Isolation Stage, health care providers may have difficulty interpreting certain behaviors. She may show signs of being anxious, hyper vigilant, and jumpy. Her cognitive functioning may become fragmented. She may also be too depressed to be able to concentrate, to organize her thoughts, or to give coherent answers. When faced with these inconsistent behaviors, and when the frightened patient volunteers no infor-

---

POW IMAGE

I feel like I've been a Prisoner of War
and there are all those people
who don't even know me that well,
(and some who know me best)
who are celebrating and hugging me
because I've escaped on my own.
But then there are all these people
who refuse to believe
that there was even a war going on
(just a minor skirmish)
or that I could possibly have been a POW.

*—Anonymous survivor
of domestic violence*

mation about her abuse situation, a health care provider may not relate the symptoms of post-traumatic stress disorder to domestic violence, and instead conclude that the patient needs medication for an anxiety disorder, depression, or possibly delusions. Such an assessment would have the unfortunate effect of perhaps closing the last bridge out of the isolation. If her health care provider misses the domestic violence clues, and appears to confirm the batterer's judgment that she is a mental case, she is likely to be driven deeper into despair. She may cease coming for health care altogether. She is also likely to fall into a pattern of self harming behaviors, including abuse of prescription drugs, alcohol, or other dangerous substances, and believing that there is no way out of the abuse even resort to suicide.

It is important to remember that for many victims in the isolation stage, visits to a health care provider or clinic for treatment of injuries or serious somatic complaints, may be the only contact with the "outside" world. The abuser may change health care providers to avoid arousing suspicion about her injuries. He is also likely to accompany her, and may even insist on being in the examining room with her. If you suspect abuse, it is paramount that you arrange a private and confidential examination with only the victim present. Even when alone with you, the victim out of shame and fear may believe she *cannot* tell you what is going on. However, in most instances sensitive and non-judgmental questions are welcomed, and may produce information you need.

Assessment

There are several keys to correctly assessing domestic violence. One is a willingness to overcome various barriers. Another is paying attention to red flags or inconsistencies between the physical evidence or symptoms and the explanations given either by the patient or the partner. A third is to have protocols for handling domestic violence cases in place in your health care setting.

BARRIERS TO ASSESSMENT

The low identification rates of domestic violence in the medical setting are due to specific barriers.[40] Some barriers to identification are related to the difficulty of getting accurate information from either the victim or the batterer. Some are inherent in the delivery of modern health care. Others relate to personal barriers in the health care provider. First, as mentioned above, a victim paralyzed by fear or shame is unlikely to volunteer a truthful explanatory history about the medical complaints related to abuse. Also, abused victims may be prevented by the batterer from coming to a scheduled follow up visit. In fact, you may not see her for another 3–6 months, usually after another violent episode. Rather than identifying the missed appointment as a red flag for domestic violence, you may see it as lack of interest, or as confirming your suspicion of mental problems. A second barrier on the systemic level may be that cost containment concerns may not reward the time and personal attention needed to elicit information about domestic violence. In such a setting, the temptation may be to just bandage the wounds, treat the somatic symptoms pharmacologically, and go on to the next patient.

Third, many health care providers have personal internal resistance to detecting and providing an appropriate response to a patient who may be a victim of domestic violence. You may fear that you might open a Pandora's Box of troubles for which you might be unprepared, or might not have the time for adequate follow up.[41] You may feel that it is the patient's responsibility to raise the issue, and that it is not your place to probe or intervene. Lack of confidence in identification and management skills may make you overly cautious. There may also be language or cultural barriers.[42] You might fear that by asking a question about possible abuse, you might embarrass or insult a patient who does not have a problem. You may not believe the patient, especially if the alleged assailant is present and seems pleasant, solicitous and concerned. Also some health care providers feel it is an issue between the couple, and that it is not their place to interfere. The fallacy that domestic violence does not happen in higher income families may lead you to ignore even unmistakable symptoms in a patient from a "good" family. This may be a countertransference issue. For example, there is an adage among domestic violence advocates: "The more the batterer looks like you (socially, economically, educationally), the less likely you will be to "see" him as a batterer." This is especially true if you have other social or professional ties to the abuser.

It has also been found that health care providers who have inadequate knowledge about the scope and dynamics of domestic violence may not be aware that domestic violence can occur in same sex or opposite sex relationships, whether married or not. A health care provider may also feel ineffective or helpless when the patient does not take action by seeking counseling or leaving the situation. It is normal to feel frustration when victims seem not to take recommended steps to get out of the violent relationship. When, as frequently happens, the victim goes back to the battering partner, the health care provider might become more judgmental and less supportive the next time. A number of such frustrating experiences might make the provider reluctant to "get involved" when domestic violence is suspected in subsequent patients. Some also fear involvement in legal proceedings. Finally, countertransference may play a part in health care providers who have witnessed or experienced abuse in their own lives. They may feel extremely uncomfortable about investigating something that brings back painful memories or flashbacks. Thus, some former (present) survivors of either childhood or domestic violence abuse might subconsciously not take note of or follow up on even clear evidence of abuse and instead distance themselves from patients in abusive relationships.

CONSTELLATION OF SYMPTOMS

All of these barriers are real, and work against proper identification of symptoms of domestic violence. However, the pervasiveness and tragic consequences of domestic violence place a responsibility on everyone in the health care system to be informed about the constellation of symptoms that point to domestic violence. Here are some red flags for likely abuse situations. One important set of clues is if the patient's intimate partner refuses to leave the examining room, and/or tends to answer all questions for the patient, and when the patient looks at the partner before answering any question. Other clues are if there is an unreasonable delay in seeking treatment, explanations of injury ("ran into door") inconsistent with location of injury, bruises in *various* stages of healing, unexplained stroke in a young woman, and any types of injury related to sexual assault. Indeed, injury to the abdomen and genitals in a pregnant woman should automatically be regarded as a potential abuse symptom. Since most abuse is focused on the abdomen, you will see increased incidence of preterm labor, placental separation, ante partum hemorrhage, uterine rupture, birth defects, and/or fetal fractures.[43]

Box 10-2 presents typical presenting symptoms or characteristics of victims of domestic abuse. These symptoms, presented in the different categories, should be used in combination to see if there is a constellation of signs and symptoms to produce a pattern. For example, the further along in the psychophysiological progression of abuse, the more likely you are to see multiple psychosomatic complaints along with serious injuries and possible signs of psychological disorders, such as anxiety, depression, post traumatic stress disorder, or bizarre behaviors and inconsistent verbal cues. You need to remember that the fear of violence may limit her ability to follow through on a number of health related issues. She may be unable keep medical appointments for herself or her children. She may be constrained from practicing safe sex or using contraceptives. She may not have the money or the transportation to get prescriptions filled. The abuser might prevent her from taking prescribed medicine, and instead take them himself, even samples you might give her. If

---

Box 10-2 Signs and Symptoms of Domestic Violence

PHYSICAL SYMPTOMS
- Acute traumatic injury
- Headaches or hearing difficulty from head trauma
- Joint pains from twisting injuries
- Abdominal or breast pain following blows to the torso
- Dyspareunia or recurrent urogenital infections from sexual assault
- Recurrent sinus infections or dental problems, dislocated jaw or cervical spine
- Bruises or pain in neck or throat from strangulation, also look for bulging eyes
- Bruises or broken bones at various levels of healing
- Chronic abdominal pain, irritable bowel syndrome
- Recurrent sexually transmitted infections and or frequent gynecological problems.

SOMATIC STRESS SYMPTOMS
- Chronic headaches
- Chronic abdominal, pelvic, or chest pains
- Chronic joint and back pain
- Myalgia and chronic fatigue
- Sleeping or eating disturbances
- Heartburn, irritable bowel syndrome
- Exacerbation of chronic diseases like diabetes mellitus, asthma, and coronary artery disease

- Signs of post traumatic stress disorder: anxiety, hyper vigilance, jumpiness, disordered thought process, nightmares
- Depression, difficulty concentrating, feeling numb, suicide attempts or gestures
- Conversion disorders: losing feeling in part of body, temporary blindness

BEHAVIORAL CUES
- Nervous or inappropriate laughter or smiling (possibly tinged with fear)
- Crying, sighing, or hyperventilating
- Anxious, jumpy, furtive looks at the examination room door
- Defensiveness, anger
- Eyes averted or downcast, fearful of eye contact
- Partner: overly attentive or defensive; does not want to leave her alone

VERBAL
- Minimizes seriousness of injuries
- Gives explanations of injuries inconsistent with the actual injury
- Talks about "a friend" who has been abused
- Refers to a partner's "anger" or "temper"
- Refers to partner as being very jealous
- Says she will have to check with partner about any treatment suggestions
- If partner is present, patient will defer to him to answer questions, or look at him before answering questions

---

pregnant, she may be unable to enroll in early prenatal care.

BREAKING THROUGH THE SILENCE

Anne Flitcraft, MD a noted educator on domestic violence, uses the term "bridge out of isolation" to describe the crucial role that health care providers can play for someone trapped in the domestic violence cycle. She writes:

Your response to domestic violence can contribute to

the woman's understanding of the seriousness of abuse and her ability to end the violence. Sharing your concerns about abuse validates the woman's concerns that violence threatens her physical and mental well-being. Listening to her concerns about abuse encourages the exploration of options that contribute to her safety. [44]

The first step is to encourage more information from your patient. Although 90% of identified abused women do not voluntarily confide in their health care provider, they tend to be relieved and willing to discuss it, *if you inquire.*[45] Each health care setting should have established routines for handling domestic violence patients. All office or clinic staff with direct patient contact need to be knowledgeable about domestic violence and how to recognize its symptoms. One way to signal your readiness to explore domestic violence questions is by having materials or even posters on domestic violence along the path that a woman follows in the clinic. Some posters or material could be placed in the ladies' rest room — the one place the abuser is not likely to follow her. All of the above is part of establishing an atmosphere that gives the woman the impression that you and your staff are aware of domestic violence as a health and safety issue — even before she meets you in a confidential examination room.

Experts recommend that you do routine screening of all your female patients for domestic violence. Routine assessment with new patients and periodic reassessment with all patients during regularly scheduled visits provide the best structure to detect those who are in violent, threatening, or highly controlling relationships. Five simple screening questions known by the acronym **PEACE** can be made part of any Intake Questionnaire. (See Box 10-3.) The questions address **P**hysical violence, anxiety and constant fear (**E**ggshells), rape or sexual **A**buse, **C**ontrolling and isolating tactics, and **E**motional or psychological abuse.[46] They can also logically fit into the psychosocial history and/or the review of all systems. The same screening procedures for partner violence can be applied in same sex relationships. If in the written or oral screening, the patient acknowledges even one incident of abuse, you need to make a note in the record to follow up on each subsequent visit. If the intake information or interview reveals a cluster of symptoms listed in Box 10-2, it is appropriate to focus more directly on the role of domestic violence as you evaluate the chief complaint.

Interviewing for Domestic Violence

Health care providers often feel awkward about broaching the subject of domestic violence

---

> **Box10-3 PEACE Questions**
>
> 1. Have you ever been in a relationship in which you have been **P**hysically hurt by a partner or someone you love?
> 2. Have you ever felt you are "walking on **E**ggshells" to avoid conflicts with a partner or someone you love?
> 3. Have you ever been sexually **A**bused, threatened or forced to have sex, or participate in sexual practices when you did not want to?
> 4. Has your partner or someone you love tried to **C**ontrol where you go, what you do, who you talk to or who your friends are?
> 5. Have you ever been **E**motionally abused or threatened by a partner or someone you love?

---

with their patients. Here are a few simple guidelines for sizing up the situation. We have already noted that the "overly" solicitous partner who insists on being present during the physical examination, and who tends to answer all questions you pose to the patient, is a red flag. As long as the abusive partner is present, it is unsafe for the victim to give a truthful account about possible abuse. In fact, asking questions about abuse could put the victim in danger as long as the abuser is present. Thus, a first task in such situations is to separate the patient from the presence of the partner. You may tell him that rules of your office or clinic, require that the partner wait outside during the physical examination. Should he become belligerent in response, you may need to tread lightly, and find a way of getting the patient alone, even for a short time such as having her accompanied by you or an alerted nurse for a urine sample or an X-ray, while the partner waits.

In cases where it is difficult to separate the abuser from the patient, you may have only limited time to deal with this issue. Therefore, you need to be as proficient in determining whether there is or has been abuse, and then addressing immediate safety concerns. In cases where the patient appears frightened or fears for her safety, you may need to assure her of confidentiality, as well as your concern for her safety. Once abuse has been established, there are many questions for follow up. These relate to her medical condition(s), issues of the safety of the woman and her children in the current situation, past history of abuse, and where she is in the psychophysiological progression of violence. The questions in Box 10-4 provide examples for each type of question. They are suggested scripts. Note that all of them are non-judgmental. It is crucial that you not allow your own frustration about her

---

Box 10-4 Domestic Violence Assessment Questions

Preliminary or Indirect
- All couples have disagreements and conflict. What happens when you and your partner disagree? Do conflicts ever turn into physical fights?
- I treat patients in my practice who are being hurt or threatened by someone they love. Is this happening to you?
- Do you ever feel afraid of your partner?

Direct
- Are you in a relationship in which you are treated badly?
- Has your partner ever destroyed things you cared about?
- Has your partner ever threatened or abused your children?
- At any time has your partner hit, kicked, or otherwise hurt or frightened you?

FOLLOW UP QUESTIONS
Current Episode
- What happened? How were you hurt?
- Were alcohol or drugs involved? By whom? Partner? Both you and he?
- Was a weapon involved? (safety issue, especially if firearm was present)
- Are you living with the person who hurt you?
- Do you know where the person who hurt you is now?
- Do you feel you are in danger now?

Abuse History
- Have you been hurt before?
- Do you recall the first time you were hurt?
- Can you tell me about the worst time?
- Can you tell me about the most recent time?
- Have you ever needed medical treatment because of it?

Control and Isolation Issues
- Does your partner threaten to hurt you or others close to you?
- Do you feel your partner isolates you from family and friends?
- Is your partner jealous? Does he explain his controlling behavior by saying that he loves you so much?
- Has your partner ever prevented you from leaving the house, seeing your family/friends, getting a job or getting an education?
- Does your partner watch your every move? Check up on you? Accuse you of having affairs with others?
- Does your partner belittle, insult, or blame you?
- Has your partner forced you to have sex when you did not want to? Forced you to have "rough sex" with him during which you got hurt?

Risk Assessment
- Has your partner become more controlling lately? Increasingly jealous?
- Has the violence become worse?
- Is there a firearm in the house? Does he brandish it or threaten you with it?
- Do you believe your partner is capable of killing you?
- Has your partner threatened to kill you or others close to you?
- Have you ever considered, threatened or attempted suicide? How do you feel about suicide now?
- Have you ever tried to leave? What happened?
- Are you planning on leaving your partner?
- Do you know how to get help if you are hurt or afraid of being hurt?

Questions *not* to ask:
- What keeps you staying with someone like that?
- How long are you going to put up with this?
- What did you do that made him hit you?

staying in such a relationship to come out in your questions.

In many instances, you will not have the time to conduct such an in depth interview yourself. However, if you have a protocol for dealing with domestic violence for your office or clinic, it should specify a follow up procedure. Ideally it should include summoning a domestic violence advocate immediately. Some clinics, ER facilities, or offices now have trained domestic violence advocates on their staff (usually a social worker or nurse). This person can then complete the more time consuming tasks, such as a complete psychosocial history, risk assessment and safety planning. If there is time pressure, i.e., the abuser is waiting outside, such a history may need to be taken while you are conducting the physical examination. If you do not have someone on staff trained as a domestic violence advocate, it is recommended that you establish a good working relationship with the nearest domestic violence program or shelter. Many will agree to dispatch an advocate immediately to work with the patient while she is still in the clinic or office.

Treat, Document, Educate — Don't Rescue!

What do you do after you have established that domestic violence is present in your patient's life? The first task is to treat the patient's medical condition(s) and document your findings. You need to conduct a thorough physical examination to determine the extent of injuries or bruises to parts of the torso normally covered by clothes. You also need to conduct a urogenital examination, looking for evidence of forcible rape, or violent insertion of foreign objects into the vagina or anus. If the patient is pregnant, you need to look for abdominal trauma and rule out possible injury to fetus or uterus. Due to the common practice of the abuser taking the victim to different providers to avoid detection of abuse patterns, you also need to inquire about other medical professionals who have treated her. This means obtaining names of all clinics and health care providers she has visited, or from whom she received medications.

When the extent of abuse becomes apparent, your emotions of outrage, sympathy and caring may be aroused. You may be tempted to rescue the victim. While understandable, this would be a mistake that could leave you frustrated, angry, and possibly disgusted with your patient. *It is **not** your function to get her to leave the batterer. She needs to reach that decision herself.* Your pushing her before she is ready will sabotage the critical work she herself needs to do before she can decide to leave. Remember, due to the barriers listed in Box 10-1, usually it takes multiple attempts at leaving the domestic violence situation before a survivor succeeds in resisting the batterer's pressure to return.

• •

PATIENT PROFILE 10.3

...BECAUSE I LOVE HIM

SETTING: *Rhonda is a 27-year-old married woman with two children, 5 and 3. She is currently being followed because she is pregnant. She has been treated on and off for 3 years for minor bruises and abrasions in a large urban medical office. She is often seen by Sue, a physician assistant, who is aware of the domestic violence and has been talking with her about it for 2 years now. Alerted by the staff that Rhonda had come in with a black eye, Sue tried to summon a domestic violence advocate from the nearby shelter, but was told that both were unavailable.*

Sue: Hi Rhonda, let's take a closer look at that black eye. Did he hit you again?

Rhonda: Yes. Day before yesterday.

Sue: That must have really hurt. Did you get hurt anyplace else?

Rhonda mutely raises her arms to show some bruises on the distal sides of her forearms. Sue marks the locations on the body map she has pulled out.

Sue: Did he choke you?

Rhonda shakes her head.

Sue: Did he kick you or punch you in the abdomen?

Rhonda again shakes her head.

Rhonda: I fell when he hit me, but I don't think I hurt the baby. At least the children didn't see him do it. They were all in bed. He came in late, drunk as usual.

Sue: We are doing an ultrasound anyway, so we'll take a closer look to make sure the baby is OK.

Rhonda: OK.

Sue: I know its hard to think about leaving while you are pregnant, because your whole body wants to make a family. But I am worried about you and the baby. Should we think of taking out a protection order and get him out of the house? Would that be safe?

Rhonda's eyes widen with fear.

Rhonda: Oh no. That would just make him madder. No telling what he would do.

Sue: Do you need a break? Do you want to go to the shelter?

Rhonda: No, I don't think I want to do that right now. He's been really nice since he hit me, and promised he won't do it again. He is under a lot of stress right now. I need to stand by him.

Sue: OK, I understand. I am really concerned for your safety and that of the baby and also your kids. You know, after this little honeymoon, it is probably going to get worse. Let's talk about safety. Could you call the police if he starts his threatening behaviors?

Rhonda: Naw, if he heard me talking to the police, he would really get mad. He might kill me.

Sue: Do you have close neighbors who know?

Rhonda: Yes, the people next door. I think Linda knows. She has asked me several times if she can help — like keep the kids, when he is really drunk.

Sue: If she is willing, maybe you could work out a signal with her, so she could call the police, when he comes in drunk and looks like he is going to get violent. What kind of code word could you use so she would know to call for the law?

Rhonda: Well, as soon as he walks in and starts to threaten me, I could say I had to call Linda because she was expecting me. Then if I can make the call, I could tell her that I could not come, and the signal would be that I left little Stevie's shoes at her house. That would be the signal for her to call the cops.

Sue: Good. Now let's think of some other safety issues. Can you safely pack and store a bag with a change of clothes for you and the kids in case you need to leave quickly? Where will you keep it?

Rhonda: I have to think about that. Maybe Linda can keep it.

Sue: You know you can call the domestic violence program or go to the shelter any time you need to. I am going to write their number down on the back of the card for your next appointment. Remember to not get cornered either in the kitchen, the bathroom, or any room where he keeps guns. In general, when you think he is going to get violent, try to stay in rooms that have another exit so you don't get trapped. Rhonda, nobody deserves to be hit. That includes you and this baby.

Rhonda's eyes fill with tears.

Rhonda: You must think I am crazy. I don't know why I stay with him. I guess it's because I love him, and I keep hoping that if I love him enough, he is going to start loving himself, and wouldn't want to hurt me or the kids any more. I wish he wouldn't drink.

Sue squeezes her hand.

Sue: No, you are not crazy. I know how hard this must be for you. I am just worried about you and the unborn baby. I just want to be sure that you will take steps to keep yourself, the baby and the children safe.

Sue completes her physical examination. The eye exam and the ultrasound reveal no abnormalities.

Sue sends Rhonda on her way with: You know that any time you are ready, I am here for you.

Rhonda: *(again with tears in her eyes)* Thanks. You have no idea how much that means to me. I feel so alone most of the time.

POINTS TO CONSIDER:

- Sue cognizant of the abusive situation, tries to make it a team effort.
- With pregnancy as a risk factor for increased abuse, Sue focuses on safety concerns for the mother and the fetus.
- Sue is not trying to rescue Rhonda but offers her safety alternatives and lets Rhonda make the decision about how to keep herself safe.
- Understanding the tenuous hold on sanity of someone in Rhonda's position, she offers Rhonda the assurances that symbolize the bridge out of isolation.

GIVING ASSURANCES

But there are certain things you, or an expert in domestic violence with whom you consult, can do to assure her physical and emotional needs while she is in your office or clinic. You can create a supportive environment. Assure her of confidentiality and privacy. Let her tell her story. After listening to her, tell her clearly that she is not crazy. This is a crucial reassurance that will help her to counteract the batterer's brainwashing efforts. Point out to her that she is a **survivor.** Commend her for taking the first step toward improving her life and that of her children. Affirm that she did the right thing by telling someone about the crime that is occurring to her. Emphasize that no one has the right to hurt others, and that no one deserves to be beaten or threatened with violence no matter what responsibility she feels she has for the "problems" in the home.

By being supportive, pointing out the danger to herself and her children, and setting in motion other procedures for helping her, you communicate to her that she is not alone. The recognition that you, your staff, and/or a domestic violence advocate understand how difficult her situation is, and that you stand ready to assist her in planning for her safety, offers her hope that she will survive when she leaves the situation. This is the **bridge out of isolation** that will help the survivor counteract the feeling of being trapped in a sea of helplessness and hopelessness. If she feels understood and cared for, she may be able to take the first steps in the sometimes lengthy process of empowerment for her to reach freedom from abuse and move towards regaining control over her life.

You or a domestic violence advocate can also provide her with information about the community resources available for battered women and their children. You might review with her a brochure from the nearest shelter or Coalition on Domestic Violence. However, giving her a brochure to take home might endanger her safety if the batterer later finds it. You might simply write the number of the nearest domestic violence shelter or of the advocate on one of your business or appointment cards. If you have an advocate present, she can identify options, and devise a safety plan. In many locales, the legal advocate will help the abused person make a report to the police, and/or walk her through the legal system to obtain a court order of protection. The advocate can also explain her medical and legal rights to the woman. For example, the batterer can be made legally liable for the cost of treating the injuries and even for counseling she may need. Free legal assistance is usually also available through the nearest office of the state Legal Aid Society. Because the batterer has restricted her education and employment, she may need to

---

Assurances to Give to a Victim Who Says She Cannot Leave Now

- "You are not crazy."
- "You deserve better than this."
- "I am afraid for your safety (and the safety of your children)."
- "It will only get worse."
- "I am here for you when you are ready to leave."

apply for welfare and work training programs after she leaves him.

DOCUMENTATION

It is imperative that you clearly document your findings from the physical examination and the history. Using a simple front and back body map, clearly indicate locations of injuries or wounds, and label them. Always reference any injuries drawn on the body map in the medical record and link them to the "suspected violence." If a woman comes in with somatic symptoms only, and you have indications from her that they are connected to the stress of being in a domestic violence relationship, your documentation should use the phrase "related to suspected domestic violence." If a distraught victim spontaneously narrates the circumstances of the abuse, it is recommended that you quote the victim's own words and relate them to the injuries or somatic complaints. Such direct quotes are called **excited utterances** in legal terminology,

---

Box 10-5 Sample Documentation

Pt states she was "punched" in the left shoulder two times, beaten on her arms while covering her head and face, and stabbed with a screwdriver in her back.

Pt states husband screamed at her "I am going to kill you" at least three times, while trying to strangle her.

Physical examination of the skin reveals a 3 cm swollen ecchymotic area on left anterior shoulder consistent with a wound from a direct hit. There are three linear ecchymotic areas on each side of the neck consistent with strangulation marks from fingers. There is a closed puncture wound medially near vertebrae of left scapula consistent with stab wound from a blunt instrument. The lateral surfaces of both arms are discolored with blue and red contusions consistent with the blunt trauma as described by patient. See locations marked on body map. X-rays of right and left humerus were without evidence of fractures.

---

and they carry weight in court proceedings. Report all laboratory findings and note that they were ordered in connection with injuries or somatic complaints "attributed to domestic violence" as illustrated in Box 10-5. If possible, incorporate the notes from the interview by a domestic violence advocate directly into the record, or at least reference that such an interview was conducted. It is critical to have as many details as possible, because such a record can become evidence against the batterer in subsequent legal proceedings.

Before she leaves your office or clinic, schedule a follow up visit in the near future. Given the rate of no-shows, you might flag your office staff to call the home before the next appointment — and without saying anything about domestic abuse— remind the patient to come for her follow up appointment. If the batterer is present in the clinic, you should also impress upon him the importance of her receiving follow up treatment for the presenting symptoms.

SAFETY PLANNING

Before the end of the first visit, you need to review her situation with her. Your primary aim here is *not* to get her to take action, but simply to focus on safety for herself and her children. First and foremost is her immediate safety if she returns to the home. You, or the domestic violence advocate could discuss a plan on how to get out of the house during a violent incident. Box 10-6 contains the major elements of a safety plan. She may need important documents if she and the children are forced to flee the house with only their clothes on their back. She will need such documents if she later has to apply for welfare assistance or a medical card for herself and her children. Your office can help by having the person who takes the information on her insurance and means of paying, also ask for the driver's license and social security card and make a copy for the medical file.

You and she need to know, that the immediate period after she leaves, or after the batterer has been forced out of the home by police or a

---

Box 10-6   Safety Plan

SAFETY DURING A VIOLENT INCIDENT:
- Stay out of rooms with no exit.
- Avoid rooms that may have weapons.
- Select a code word that alerts children, friends or neighbors to call the police if in immediate danger.
- Practice how to get out of your home safely.
- Keep purse and car keys readily available.
- Have access to clothes.
- Teach children how to use the telephone to contact the police and the fire department.
- Have the police file a report. Write down the officers' names. This way you can get in touch with them again later if you have questions about what happened.
- Get medical attention if needed.

SAFETY WHEN PREPARING TO LEAVE:
- Leave suitcase and copies of essential documents with neighbor or friend.
- Open a savings account to increase independence.
- Rehearse an escape plan.
- Practice it with your children.

SAFETY WITH AN ORDER OF PROTECTION:
- File an Order of Protection with the court to prevent stalking.
- Keep your protection order on or near you at all times.
- Give your protection order to police departments in communities where you visit family or friends.
- Inform your employer, minister, closest friends and relatives that you have a protection order in effect. Show them pictures of the abuser.
- Ask for help screening telephone calls at work.
- Call police immediately if order is violated.
- Change locks on doors and windows. Have outside lighting with movement sensors installed.
- Have smoke alarms and fire extinguishers installed. Plan an escape route from second floor or apartment in case of fire.
- Change phone numbers, screen calls, have caller ID blocked.
- Carry a noise maker or personal alarm. Vary your route to and from home.
- Inform landlord, neighbors of situation and ask that police be called if abuser shows up.
- Let those who care for children know who is allowed to have contact with them. Take copy of the protective order to the school, and inform teachers, counselors, and principal of the order.
- Keep copies of protection order in case original is lost or destroyed.

ITEMS TO CONSIDER TAKING WHEN LEAVING:
- Identification, birth certificates, social security cards, school and vaccination records, money, checkbook, ATM card, credit cards, bank books, house and car keys, driver's license and registration, medication, welfare identification, work permits, green card, passport(s), divorce papers, medical records, lease or rental agreements, house deed, mortgage payment book and insurance papers.

Adapted from Domestic Violence: There's No Excuse (2001) Brochure produced by Women's Aid in Crisis, Inc. PO. Box 2062, Elkins, WV.

---

court order, is the most dangerous time. Most murder/suicides in abusive relationships happen at this juncture. Hence safety planning is critical.

Conclusion

Treating patients who are in domestic violence situations is a necessary part of health care. Given the high number of medical incidents related to domestic violence that go unrecognized in the health care system, it is imperative that health care providers become part of the solution rather than part of the problem.[47] The first part of a solution is to create increased awareness not only among health care providers, but all support personnel. Your office or clinic staff will need periodic training. Your receptionist/telephone opera-

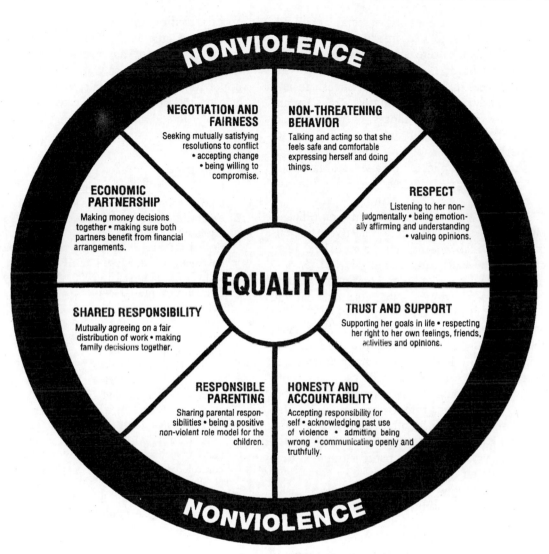

Figure 10-2. Wheel of Non Violence and Equity. From Domestic Abuse Intervention Project, Duluth MN, Used by permission.

tor needs to be alert to the verbal cues of distress of someone who "can't come in," but wants to know what to do for some of the physical or somatic conditions of abuse listed in Box 10-2. Generally, the local shelter or state Coalition on Domestic Violence will be glad to provide training on how to recognize and respond to patients who are potential or actual victims of domestic violence. They will train your staff to be sensitive

to the need for non-judgmental support of the victim. Their trainers will help you set up a protocol for alerting everyone in the office or clinic, especially if the batterer is present. They will give you emergency phone numbers for summoning a domestic violence advocate to the office or clinic as quickly as possible.

Managing patients who have been abused can be quite frustrating and stressful. You and staff members may have strong visceral and emotional reactions to the injuries you see, the descriptions of severe abuse you hear, or the look of terror or hopelessness you see in the patient's face. In fact, such experiences can create **secondary post traumatic stress** symptoms, i.e., sleep disturbances, even flashbacks and anxiety attacks, for staff members who are themselves survivors of violent abuse. Such feelings may be complicated by a sense of failure, if the abuse victim is not ready to leave the batterer.

The stress on you and those in your office or clinic will lessen if you have effective protocols in place which specify what part of the team effort each staff person will play. After any encounter with a particularly horrendous example of domestic violence, it is essential that you pay attention to the emotional stress of yourself and those who worked with you. We suggest that after any such incident you take time at lunch or after office hours to debrief yourself and those members of the staff who came into contact with the abuse survivor and/or the batterer. Unless you do this promptly, you and other staff members are likely to build up resistance and internal barriers to acknowledging symptoms of domestic violence in your patients the next time you encounter them.

No matter how well you perform these tasks, encounters with victims (and perpetrators) of domestic violence are neither easy nor rewarding in the short run. Remember the goal of the office visit, or clinic encounter is *not* to get the woman to leave the abuser. Rather it is to treat and document the injuries, and educate the survivor on the options and community resources available to her. A second task is to do a risk assessment and safety planning. A third major goal is to provide the emotional assurances and support to help her break the stranglehold of isolation, and increase her self confidence so *she* can make choices to move towards gaining control over her life. The survivors of intimate partner violence coming into your office or clinic need your active participation in lifting the veil of shame and secrecy, and in giving them hope that they can gain control, and create lives free from violence. (See Figure 10-2.) This is a team effort in which you, trained advocates, and your staff work with the victims as you treat their injuries, supportively listen to their stories, and educate them on the options available to them. This is how you can collectively build that bridge out of their isolation.

REFERENCES

1. Dirlam ME (2000) Domestic Violence: The Silent Epidemic. *Primary Care Case Reviews,* 3 (1), 12-19.
2. American Psychological Association (1996) *Violence and the Family: Report of the American Psychological Presidential Task Force on Violence and the Family.* Washington, DC: APA, 10.
3. Tolman RM, Raphael J (2000) A review on welfare and domestic violence. *J Social Issues,* 56(4):655.
4. CDC & Nat Institute of Justice (2000) *Extent, Nature, and Consequences of Intimate Partner Violence.* Washington, DC: NIJ.
5. US Dept of Justice (1998) *Violence by Intimates: Analysis of Data on Crimes by Current or Former Spouses, Boyfriends, and Girlfriends.* Washington, DC: Dept of Justice.
6. Silverman JG, Raj A, Mucci LA, Hathaway JE (2001) Dating violence against adolescent girls and associated substance use, unhealthy weight control, sexual risk behavior, pregnancy, and suicidality. *JAMA.* 286:572-579.
7. Eisenstat S, Bancroft L. (1999) Domestic Violence. *New England J Med;* 341:886-892.
8. Burke LK, Follingstad DR (1999) Violence in lesbian and gay relationships: theory, prevalence, and correlation factors. *Clin Psychol Rev,*19(5):487-512.
9. McFarland J et al (2001) Abuse assessment screen reliability (AAS-D): measuring frequency, type, and perpetrator of abuse toward women with physical disabilities. *J Women's Health Gender Based Med,* 10(9):861-866.
10. Werfel PA (2001) When seniors suffer. Elder abuse emerges as new EMS dilemma. *J Emergency Med Serv,* 26(10):48-53.
11. American Psychological Association (1996) *Violence and the Family: Report of the American Psychological Presidential Task Force on Violence and the Family.* Washington, DC: APA. 11.
12. Department of Justice, Bureau of Justice Assis-

tance. (1993) *Family Violence: Interventions for the Justice System.* Washington, DC: Dept of Justice.

13. DuRant RH, Smith JA, Kreiter SR, Krowchuk DP. (1999) The relationship between early age of onset of initial substance use and engaging in multiple health risk behaviors among young adolescents. *Arch Pediatr Adolesc Med,* 153:286-291.

14. US Department of Education (1998) *Violence and Discipline Problems in US. Public Schools: 1996-1997* Washington, DC: US Dept of Education Publication.

15. Pelcovitz D (2000) Psychiatric disorders in adolescents exposed to domestic violence and physical abuse. *Am J Orthopsychiatry;* 70(3):360-369.

16. Reynolds MW et al (2001) The relationship between gender, depression, and self esteem in children who witnessed domestic violence. *Child Abuse Neglect,* 25(9):1201-1206.

17. Bureau of Justice Statistics (1997) *Violence-Related Injuries Treated in Hospital Emergency Departments* (NCJ-156921):5.

18. Burge S (1999) Women's Health — violence against women. *Prim Care,* 21:67-81.

19. National Coalition Against Domestic Violence *1995 Statistical Survey on Domestic Violence in the Health Care System.* Duluth, MN: Domestic Abuse Intervention Project.

20. Murphy SL (2000) Deaths: final data for 1998 *Natl Vital Stat Rep.* 48(11):1-105.

21. Weiss H (2001) Causes of traumatic death during pregnancy. *JAMA,* 285(22):2854-2855.

22. Rodriguez MA, Bauer HM, McLoughlin E et al (1999) Screening and Intervention for intimate partner abuse – practices and attitudes of primary care physicians. *JAMA;* 282:468-474.

23. Frye V. (2001) Examining Homicide's Contribution to Pregnancy Related Deaths. Editorial. *JAMA.* 285:1610-1611.

24. Morgan R (2001) *The Demon Lover: The Roots of Terrorism* New York: Washington Square Press.

25. Goldberg S (1993) *Why Men Rule: A Theory of Male Dominance.* Chicago: Open Court.

26. National Center for the State Courts (1996) *Examining the Work of State Courts, 1995: A National Perspective from the Court Statistics Project.* Washington, DC: National Center for the State Courts.

27. American Bar Association, Commission on Domestic Violence (2002) Domestic Violence Statistics. Accessed on the Internet at www.abanet.org/domviol/stats.html

28. Zorza J (1992) The Criminal Law of Misdemeanor Domestic Violence. *J Crim Law & Criminology.* 83:66.

29. Buzawa E, Buzawa C, Eds (1996) *Do Arrests and Restraining Orders Work?* Thousand Oaks, CA: Sage Publications. 48-49.

30. Dutton D (1995) *The Batterer: A Psychological Profile* New York: Basic Books.

31. Testa M, Leonard KE (2001) The impact of husband physical aggression and alcohol on marital functioning: does alcohol "excuse" the victim? *Violence Victim,* 6(5):507-516.

32. Irons R, Schneider JP (1997) When is domestic violence a hidden face of addiction? *J Psychoactive Drugs,* 29:337-344.

33. National Coalition Against Violence. The Problem. Accessed on the Internet at http://www.ncadv.org/problem/

34. Domestic Abuse Intervention Project (1994) Guidelines for Avoiding an Abusive Relationship. (Handout). Duluth, MN: Domestic Abuse Intervention Project.

35. CDC (2000) *Women's Health. Domestic violence Statistical Survey,* taken from National Coalition Against Domestic Violence. Atlanta, Centers for Disease Control and Prevention.

36. Flitcraft A et al (1992) *Diagnostic and treatment guidelines on domestic violence.* Chicago: Am Med. Assoc.

37. Lloyd S, Taluc N (1999) The effects of male violence on female employment. *Violence Against Women,* 5(4):370-392.

38. Martin SL et al (2001) Physical abuse of women before, during, and after pregnancy. *JAMA.* 285(12):1581-4.

39. Raphael J (2000) *Saving Bernice: Battered Women, Welfare, and Poverty.* Boston: Northeastern Univ.

40. Davis RE, Harsh KE (2001) Confronting barriers to universal screening for domestic violence. *J Prof Nursing,* 17(6):313-320.

41. Sugg NK, Inui T (1992) Primary Care physician's response to domestic violence: Opening Pandora's Box. *JAMA;* 267:381-387.

42. Barcelona de Mendoza VB (2001) Culturally appropriate care for pregnant Latina women who are victims of domestic violence. *J Obstet Gynecol Nursing,* 30(6):579-588.

43. Sheridan, DJ (1996) Forensic documentation of battered pregnant women. *J Nurse Midwifery,* 41(6):467-472.

44. Flitcraft A, Paranteau K (1993) *Project Safe: A physi-*

cian's guide to domestic violence. Domestic Violence Training Project & Connecticut Coalition Against Domestic Violence. New Haven, CN: Project SAFE.

45. Webster J, Stratigos SM, Grimes KM (2001) Women's responses to screening for domestic violence in a health care setting. *Midwifery,* 17(4):289-294.

46. Women's Health Advocacy Project (1997) *Guidelines for Using PEACE questions for domestic abuse.* Lewisburg, WV: Family Refuge Center.

47. Sharps PW et al (2001) Health care providers' missed opportunities for preventing femicide. *Prevent Med,* 33(5)373-380.

CHAPTER 11

Child Maltreatment: Abuse and Neglect

The scale of abuse and neglect of children is of concern to policy makers, the legal system, and health care providers. This chapter first reviews statistics, legal definitions and reporting requirements, how and why it occurs, and the barriers to identifying and treating abuse. It also examines the impact of abuse and neglect on children at various developmental stages, and the resulting somatic, emotional, and behavioral symptoms. This chapter outlines the initial identification process, including interviewing a child victim, the elements of a medical examination, and evidentiary documentation. It provides guidelines for coordinating the team effort, or consulting a specialist. Lastly, it suggests precautions for self care related to the stress of treating abused and neglected children.

The Scope of the Problem

In the previous chapter we examined the challenge presented to the health care provider by patients who are in domestic violence situations. Another serious problem facing the health care profession is children who are abused or neglected. There are strong statistical correlations between substance abuse, domestic violence and child maltreatment. Thus, the presence of one of these conditions ought to alert the health care provider to look for signs for the other two. Since all three are covered by a code of secrecy,[1] recognition by health care providers of any of the three requires special skills.[2]

Under the mandate of the federal Child Abuse and Prevention Act (CAPTA) of 1974,[3] a coalition of federal public institutions, like the National Clearinghouse on Child Abuse and Neglect and the National Child Abuse and Neglect Data System (NCANDS) monitor annual state supplied figures on the type and incidence of maltreatment, the types and ages of victims, and the types of perpetrators of abuse and neglect (Box 11-1). Three National Incident Surveys (NIS) using sampling techniques compiled detailed reporting data from all 50 states in 1979 (NIS-1), 1986 (NIS-2) and 1993 (NIS-3). NIS-3 showed an alarming 2/3 increase of reported cases between 1986 and 1993.[4] After a 1993 high of just over 1 million confirmed maltreatment cases, or a victimization rate of 15.3%, statistics show a steady annual decrease to where in 1999 the victimization rate was 11.8% and actual number of confirmed cases was 826,162.[5] (See Table 11-1.) More children suffer from neglect than from any other single form of abuse,[6] with children under one year old being at greatest risk for fatal outcomes.[7] Around 80% of the victims were abused by their parents, with mothers committing about 44.7% of various types of maltreatment.[8] In children under one year old, about 70% of the abuse was by female providers of child care, with about 64% of that being neglect.[9] Fathers or other male perpetrators were responsible for 22% of all abuse and 62% of sexual abuse.[10] Taking race and ethnicity as variables in the incidence of child maltreatment, the NCANDS statistics show that the victimization rate among African Americans was 25.2%, American Indian 20.1%, Hispanics 12.6%, Whites 10.6%, and Asian Americans 4.4%.[11]

Box 11-1 Child Maltreatment: Victims and Offenders

- Child protective service agencies received reports of maltreatment on more than 3 million children in 1996, resulting in about 1.6 million investigations.
- Reports from professionals were more likely to be substantiated than those from non-professionals (51% vs. 35%).
- 19% were age 2 or younger, 52% were age 7 or younger, 7% were age 16 or older.
- Neglect was the most common form of maltreatment among all age groups (58%).
- Older victims were more likely to have experienced physical abuse (29%) or sexual abuse (15%).
- Females were three times more likely to experience sexual abuse than males. Perpetrators of sexual abuse were predominantly male (around 60% male only vs. less than 15% female only and around 25-30% both male and female).
- 80% of the perpetrators of maltreatment were parents of the victim. Younger children were more likely to be abused by females than males. The disparity between female and male was greatest in neglect cases with children under 2 (70% to 10%.) In many instances both parents were involved.
- 1,077 children died due to abuse and neglect, 76% of them under age 4.
- 16% of victims were removed from their homes.

Source: U.S. Department of Health and Human Services. (2001) Child Maltreatment 1999: Reports from the States to the National Child Abuse and Neglect Data System. Washington, DC: U.S. Government Printing Office.

Definitions

The term **maltreatment** has come into use as being more comprehensive than either the words of abuse and neglect. "Victims of maltreatment are defined as children who are found to have experienced substantiated or indicated maltreatment or are found to be at risk of experiencing maltreatment."[12] Under the federal Child Abuse and Prevention Act (CAPTA),[13] four general categories of maltreatment are recognized 1) physical abuse, 2) sexual abuse, 3) neglect, and 4) emo-

tional maltreatment. The older definition of **child abuse and neglect** is "Any recent act or failure to act on the part of a parent or caretaker, which results in death, serious physical or emotional harm, sexual abuse, or exploitation, or an act or failure to act which presents an imminent risk of serious harm."[14] Box 11-2 sets out the principal elements of each category of maltreatment.

In order to distinguish the difference between actual harm and the risk for harm, two new definitional standards were developed for the collection of data for NIS-2 in 1986. The **Harm Standard** requires that an act or omission result in demonstrable harm in order to be classified as abuse or neglect. Exceptions are made in only a few categories where the nature of the maltreatment itself is so egregious that the standard permits harm to be inferred when direct evidence of it is not available.

The **Endangerment Standard** was developed to supplement the perspective provided by the Harm Standard. The central feature of the Endangerment Standard is that it allows children who were not yet harmed by maltreatment to be counted in the abused and neglected estimates. The Endangerment Standard is slightly more lenient than the Harm Standard in that it includes maltreatment by adult caretakers other than parents in certain categories, as well as sexual abuse perpetrated by teenage caretakers. The Endangerment Standard was used in both the NIS-2 and the NIS-3, and the improvement in the ability of those reporting abuse to recognize the more subtle symptoms accounts in part for the substantial increases in the reported incidence of maltreatment between 1986 and 1993.[15]

Although CAPTA established national standards, there are some definitional variations from state to state. For example, some states have an exemption for poverty as a cause of neglect/abuse, others have a religious exemption for "good faith" failure to treat a child medically. Some cultural religious practices can lead to charges of abuse. For example, the African Muslim practice of female circumcision (also known as female genital mutilation), sometimes practiced by immigrants, is illegal in the United

TABLE 11-1 Victimization Rates by Maltreatment Type (1999)

	Physical Abuse	Neglect	Medical Neglect	Sexual Abuse	Psychological Maltreatment	Other Abuse
Population of children 0-18	67,421,449	67,421,449	48,311,250	67,421,449	65,892,458	49,715,250
No. of victims	166,626	437,540	18,788	88,238	59,846	219,549
Rate	2.5	6.5	0.4	1.3	0.9	4.4
No. of states reporting	49	49	38	49	48	33

*Excerpted from Table 2–5. Child Maltreatment 1999: Reports From the States to the National Child Abuse and Neglect Data System. Washington, DC: US Department of Health and Human Services.

States and can lead to charges of abuse. Similarly, as discussed in Chapter 2, healing techniques regarded as perfectly normal within a specific subculture, are sometimes seen as abuse or neglect in American society. Such practices can confuse the presentation of symptoms. See Patient Profile 11.1.

• •

PATIENT PROFILE 11.1

WHAT IS SHE SAYING?

SETTING: *Sammy and his mother have come to a drop in emergency clinic because he has broken his wrist falling out of a tree. She says he's 10 years old, but he looks more like 8. Since there is a large Vietnamese population in the area, he is most likely Vietnamese. Lynn is a physician assistant who does the initial patient assessment.*

Lynn: So what do we have here? Your son was climbing a tree, fell and broke his arm?

Mother: Nods affirmatively.

Lynn: Well, kids will climb trees. So off with your shirt young man so I can check out your shoulder. It might be hurt too. *(What are those welts on his back? What could have caused those marks? What a strange pattern. They look like repetitive and severe scrapes. Could this be child abuse?)*

As Lynn points to the welts and tries to communicate with the Mother, the Mother becomes more

agitated and keeps saying what sounds like "gaw-sha."

Lynn: *(I am not getting anywhere. I don't know if she understands me and I certainly do not understand her. We'll need to get a translator in here since my Vietnamese is very limited.)*

Box 11-2 Elements of Child Maltreatment

PHYSICAL ABUSE:
Beatings with an object, scalding, burning, severe physical punishment
Munchausen by proxy (inflicting harm to feign or induce illness)

SEXUAL ABUSE:
Incest, rape, statutory rape, sexual assault by relative or stranger, fondling of sexual areas, exposure to indecent acts, sexual rituals, involvement in child pornography or prostitution, insertion of foreign objects into mouth, anus or vagina, forcing child to perform oral sex or other unnatural acts

CHILD NEGLECT:
Intentional or unintentional failure to perform appropriate parenting or caretaker functions: physical, nutritional, emotional, supervisory, medical, educational neglect or abandonment.

EMOTIONAL MALTREATMENT:
Verbal abuse, belittlement, symbolic acts to terrorize a child (e.g., locking up child in dark closet or basement) lack of nurturance, or availability by caregiver.

Later after receiving translation assistance from a local Vietnamese priest, Lynn learns that Sammy had a cold last week, and the treatment in their culture for a cold is to scrape with a spoon on the neck and shoulders to "disperse wind."

Lynn: *(I am so glad that I asked for help and the priest was available to do so. I almost turned them in for child abuse.)*

POINTS TO CONSIDER:

- Lynn realizes that she may need a translator in this interview because the mother does not speak English well enough for her to make an appropriate assessment especially since child abuse needs to be ruled out.

- Lynn keeps an open mind and defers any judgment until she can understand the nature of the "strange pattern" of marks. She knows that it is vital to be familiar with the cluster of essential characteristics of child abuse for proper diagnosis and treatment.

• •

The line between acceptable forms of proper discipline and physical or mental abuse is subject to individual interpretation. According to research by Melvin Kohn the type of discipline used is also influenced by the occupation of the parents (usually the father).[16] In general, parents who have occupations that allow them creativity and individual expression tend to encourage the same in their children. They tend to use withdrawal of privileges or affection to correct misbehavior. On the other hand, parents in occupations that are tightly supervised and which demand strict adherence to the rules, tend to insist on conformity and strict obedience with their children. They are more apt to use physical punishment for disciplining their children.

Either physical or psychological punishment can turn into extreme forms of discipline. Non-physical punishment in the form of isolating or locking up a child for extended periods of time, sometimes without food, is maltreatment. Spanking or whipping a naked or partially naked child, is not only physical abuse, but can become sadistic sexual molestation.

Sexual abuse is defined as: "The employment, use, persuasion, inducement, enticement, or coercion of any child to engage in, or assist any other person to engage in, any sexually explicit conduct or simulation of such conduct for the purpose of producing a visual depiction of such conduct."[17]

The American Academy of Pediatrics adds to this that it is abuse because the child "cannot comprehend, is developmentally unprepared, and cannot give consent" to sexual activities which are forced on it.[18] The inability to give consent is a critical issue because of the enormous power differential between adults and children. When the abusing adult is also a trusted and familiar figure, as is true in 90% of child sexual abuse cases, it is very difficult for a child to distinguish between good touch and bad touch or to resist sexual advances. Coercion may range from co-opting a child's compliance through the promise of extra attention and love from the perpetrator, to brutal force and threats of harm for disclosure. In either case, we have to assume that the child was incapable of giving legal consent to the sexual advances of the adult.

Risk Factors in Child Abuse

Analysts have pinpointed several psychosocial issues in producing the environment in which abuse occurs.[19] Accordingly they categorize the potential of abuse associated with factors related to parents, children, families, and the environment. No single psychological profile appears to be typical of perpetrators of child maltreatment. Since many perpetrators experience behavioral and emotional difficulties which are often the consequences of child abuse, it is not surprising that the most consistent finding in the child abuse literature is that maltreating parents often report having been physically, sexually, or emotionally abused or neglected as children.[20] As Abraham Maslow noted long ago, individuals who have not had their own needs met as children, will have difficulty meeting the needs of their children.[21] This is not to say all who have been abused will abuse their children. Most do not.[22]

The likelihood of general abuse/neglect of children is also directly related to the psychosocial situation of the parent/care giver of a child.[23] Low income families have the highest rates of abuse and neglect. Young single parents have the highest poverty rate. A young mother, with few economic resources and little social support may have few parenting skills. She is more likely to react inappropriately or abusively to the frustration of caring for an infant than a married middle class mother surrounded by loving relatives and friends. (See Chapter 1, Figures 1-1 and 1-2.) However, maltreatment also is more common in low income families with large numbers of children.[24] In poor communities, health facilities are often inadequate, and continuity of care is lacking or inaccessible. For example, if services are geographically dispersed, parents without transportation may find it impossible to obtain prenatal, or regular pediatric care for children. You may see such a child only when something is seriously wrong, thus leading to the charge of medical neglect.

Certain children are physically and emotionally more vulnerable than others to maltreating behavior. Even tempered infants and children are easier to care for than a colicky infant, or a hyperactive child. Children with difficult temperaments, those who are perceived as different, as well as children with handicaps or disabilities are at increased risk for physical and sexual abuse as well as neglect.[25] (See Chapter 3 on Human Development for discussion of children with difficult temperaments.)

Drug abuse by one or both parents is another major risk factor. It is likely to impact the ability to properly care for children, and create chaotic and dysfunctional families. Drug abuse in conjunction with some of the psychological characteristics listed above, may then create the climate for severe abuse. Drug use by a pregnant mother also directly affects the health and temperament of the neonate. For example, crack addicted infants tend to be hyper excitable, and thus, are likely to be very difficult to parent. Similarly as

pointed out in the last chapter, children in domestic violence situations are almost automatically at risk for physical harm as well as severe psychological trauma.[26]

It is important to understand that these risk factors are both cumulative as well as interactive. No *one* factor causes abuse. For example, most children in poverty stricken homes are cared for by loving parents. It is usually only when several adverse psychosocial factors converge in a family situation that the probability of abuse/neglect increases.

Identifying Abuse

Recognition of maltreatment by various professionals has improved considerably since the first National Incidence Survey in 1979. A concerted campaign by a coalition of federal state agencies is credited with distributing good training materials to professionals. The improvement has been especially noticeable in the school environment where large numbers of children are available for observation each day. School personnel now are the largest single source of reports of maltreated children (54%); more than all other sources combined. There is still concern among policy makers that identification of maltreatment in medical settings is limited more to the "battered child syndrome," i.e., serious injuries, rather than psychological or behavioral symptoms of abuse or neglect. Indeed the Institute of Medicine of the National Academy of Science has called for better training of health care providers to sharpen their skills in identifying various types of maltreatment.[27]

BARRIERS

The barriers to identifying child maltreatment in the medical setting are similar to those for domestic violence. Health care providers may lack confidence because they were not adequately trained to handle cases of maltreatment. There may be emotional barriers. For example, even in the face of physical or verbal evidence of maltreatment, it may be hard to acknowledge that an adult — who is supposed to protect a child — would deliberately harm or molest that child. Time pressures in the medical setting might convince some providers to limit their action to treating the abuse injuries, but hesitate about getting into assessing the child for concomitant emotional trauma. They may feel that the social workers should "handle it." In addition, health care providers who themselves are survivors of child maltreatment, may unconsciously block out evidence of abuse. Lastly, managing cases of child physical or sexual abuse is emotionally draining and stressful. Repeated exposure to egregious cases of maltreatment can cause secondary post traumatic stress disorder, possibly leading to aversion to becoming involved in another stressful abuse case.

TEAM APPROACH

For all these reasons, we suggest a team approach for following up on suspected physical or sexual abuse cases similar to the model presented for domestic violence in the last chapter. There should be in place an office or clinic protocol, which specifies who is to be involved and how the requirements for legal notifications will be fulfilled. It is suggested that all clinics and hospital emergency rooms designate pediatric abuse specialists to be trained in interviewing, and examining maltreated children and in recording such information. Most medium sized communities will have specialists who are skilled in interviewing children who have been abused or neglected. Some are pediatricians who have specially equipped examination rooms for collecting forensic evidence from abused children. At the very least, offices or clinics should establish a referral procedure with such an expert in the community. In addition, the local Domestic Violence Coalition or domestic abuse shelter usually will have not only trained interviewers, but also will know what pediatric specialists can perform child abuse medical examinations and collect forensic evidence. Either the domestic violence shelter or Child Protective Services may be able

to send a trained interviewer to your office or clinic while the child is there. Lastly, there is a National Child Abuse hotline number to find the nearest child maltreatment pediatric specialist or a skilled interviewer (1-800-352-6513).

SYMPTOMS

What do you look for in identifying physical or sexual abuse? Many of the symptoms of physical abuse are similar to those seen on the adult victims of domestic violence, i.e., injuries to the head and the outer surfaces of arms, bruises and welts on the torso and the legs, or broken ribs or long bones. Also obvious are round burn marks, where a lit cigarette was pushed into the flesh of the child (sometimes justified by the abuser as punishment for misbehavior). Less obvious is **shaken baby syndrome**. Shaken-slam or shaken-impact baby syndrome may more accurately reflect the combination of internal and external injuries because shaken infant or baby syndrome tends not to occur in isolation, but is associated with other kinds of abuse and neglect. It is usually inflicted on infants and babies under 2 years old by a parent with a low frustration tolerance that violently shakes and hits, or throws the baby to get it to stop crying. Because it is the leading cause of serious head injuries to infants under one year old, the Committee on Child Abuse and Neglect of the American Academy of Pediatrics (AAP) suggests than *any* serious head trauma in children under two be investigated for abuse.[28] Others suggest that retinal hemmorrhages in children under two should automatically raise an alarm for potential abuse.[29] Unfortunately, unless there are obvious external bruises or injuries, a correct diagnosis is missed in up to one third of the cases.[30] Associated behavioral symptoms such as poor feeding, vomiting, lethargy and/or irritability are often attributed to viral illness, feeding dysfunction, or colic. Since many of the symptoms of shaken baby syndrome are subtle (see Sidebar), the AAP Committee suggests the formation of a diagnostic team comprising "specialists in pediatric radiology, pediatric neurology and/or pediatric neu-

---

Clinical Features to Look for in Shaken Baby Syndrome

Immediate subtle

Subdural hemorrhage

  may be prominent in the interhemispheric fissures

  may be visible only as cerebral edema with subarachnoid hemorrhage

Retinal hemorrhage

  most common and reliable indicator, esp. if bilateral

Diffuse axonal injury

  common but difficult to observe

Possible associated abuse symptoms

Bruises

  shoulders

  neck and throat

Fractures

  Skull—multiple, bilateral, diastatic, crossing suture lines

  Spine—long bones, hands, feet, ribs

Late sequelae

Chronic extra-axial fluid collection

Cerebral atrophy

Cystic encephalomalacia

Excerpted from Committee on Child Abuse and Neglect, American Academy of Pediatrics(2001) Shaken Baby Syndrome: Rotational Cranial Injuries- Technical Report (Policy Statement) Pediatrics, 108,1:206-210.

rosurgery, ophthalmology, and a pediatrician who specializes in child abuse" (p. 208). It also recommends the formation of regional networks of such specialists for rural or underserved areas that can be activated as needed. The Committee recommends a combination approach of high technology (MRI, CT scans, pupillary dilation), and investigation of psychosocial stresses any time unusual head trauma or retinal hemorrhages are seen.

SEXUAL ABUSE

Equally difficult to detect at first glance are cases of sexual abuse in children. Because sexual abuse is psychologically more damaging than physical abuse alone,[31] it is crucial that you understand some of the issues. First is the **"secrecy issue."** In almost all cases, the child is either coerced or coopted into keeping the sexual abuse secret. In coercion, the perpetrator will use threats of physical harm to the child, or actual harm to a pet or destruction of a favorite toy to insure the silence of the child. Sometimes a perpetrator will threaten to abuse a younger sibling of the victim to keep an older child from telling anyone. A perpetrator may coopt a child by promising spe-

cial "rewards." These may range from extra attention to being called "daddy's special girl." They come at the price of keeping it secret. Once the abuse has become chronic, the perpetrator reinforces fear with the message: "If you tell, no one will believe you, and no one will love you."

PATIENT PROFILE 11.2

CAN I TELL HER?

SETTING: Carrie, 15-years-old, is seeing her physician, Elizabeth Maloney for headaches. Dr. Maloney has only seen Carrie twice in a small suburban office which specializes in pediatric care. She feels that she has established good rapport with Carrie although she notices Carrie seems hesitant at times to answer her questions and sometimes wonders what Carrie might be withholding.

Dr. Maloney: Hi Carrie, what can I do for you today?

Carrie: Hi, Dr. Maloney. I still have headaches and now my stomach is bothering me. I just don't have an appetite. *(Can I tell her about my step-dad? The bastard jumps on me when Mom goes to her church meetings. Of course, he* *does give me the CDs I want and lots of pocket money. Guilt money. The last time I told him it had to stop, he threatened to go after my little sister. This doctor is nice, but I've only seen her a couple of times. Will she call me a slut — like Mom did? Tom (Carrie's new boyfriend) is really upset and said he'd kill my step-dad if it continues. Something's got to be done. I really want it to stop.)*

Dr. Maloney: *(Boy I can hear the wheels churning in her brain. I wonder what she needs to tell me?)* I need to talk with you more about your headaches and how your stomach feels but first, Carrie, sometimes I feel like there's something you want to tell me and then you don't. Is there anything you'd like to talk with me about?

Carrie: *(Oh no, here we go.)* Yes, as a matter of fact there is . . .

And Carrie proceeds to tell Dr. Maloney about the sexual abuse.

POINTS TO CONSIDER:

- Dr. Maloney has applied her intuition and follows through on it by directly asking Carrie an open-ended question.

- The open-ended question produced results and now Dr. Maloney can proceed according to clinic protocol.

- Aware of the legal reporting requirements of the case, Dr. Maloney calls the local center of the Coalition on Domestic Violence to request that an advocate come to the office and debrief Carrie.

- Knowing that Carrie will need sexual abuse counseling, she also makes a referral to a specialist.

• •

No matter how the abuse occurs, the child does not feel free to tell any one else about it. This goes against the natural inclination of children to share and talk about what is going on in their lives. The burden of keeping such a terrible secret has several short term and long-term psy-chological and behavioral consequences. The secrecy mandate, especially from a close adult tends to bring the realization sooner or later that what they are doing is "wrong." They will internalize the message "I am bad." or "it's my fault." The longer the secret sexual abuse goes on, the greater the feelings of guilt and shame. The child is likely to feel soiled and dirty after each encounter. The child may feel trapped because they feel that if they reveal the abuse, "Everyone will think I am damaged goods." This in turn has devastating consequences on self-esteem.

The severity of sexual abuse is directly related to the factors listed in the Sidebar below. The general rule is that the frequency, closeness of the perpetrator, and depth of penetration are the key factors. Frequency may range from a one-time molestation to repeated rapes over many years. Generally, the closer the perpetrator is as a biological relative, the deeper the psychological impact. Sexual abuse is also rated on the basis of the depth of penetration. However, sexual abuse may range from inappropriate touch-

---

Severity of Sexual Abuse As a Function of:

1. Frequency

2. Depth of penetration (penile penetration or penetration with foreign objects of the vagina, mouth and/or anus)

3. Closeness of the perpetrator as a biological relative

4. Geographical proximity, availability of victim, lack of supervision

5. Frequency of threats to rape or harm the victim or others

6. Perpetrator's mental status (if perpetrator is developmentally disabled, schizophrenic, or an alcoholic/drug addict, victim can rationalize, "He didn't know what he was doing.")

7. Reaction of significant others when child confides about the abuse.

ing or fingering the genitals to penile penetration of vagina, anus or mouth, or the insertion of foreign objects into either the vagina, anus or mouth.

What happens when a child tries to communicate about the abuse to another significant person is also a major determinant for severity of long-range psychological damage. For example, a child trying to tell the non-abusing parent or another adult may encounter disbelief, indifference, or angry accusations that she is fabricating this for attention, or other manipulative motive. Even worse, she may be blamed for "seducing" the perpetrator. An unsuccessful attempt to confide the awful secret to someone else leads the victim to questioning her own reality, to not trusting adults, to feeling trapped, and to depression and possible suicidal ideation or actions. The psychological impact of sexual abuse tends to stay with survivors into adulthood, resulting in much higher incidence of various psychological and behavioral problems from mood disorders to dissociative identity disorders.[32]

DEVELOPMENTAL ISSUES

The meaning of sexual abuse varies for victims according to their stage of life development. For children under six years there is little sexual meaning. The major reaction to painful abuse at that age is feelings of betrayal and hurt. On the other hand, a child that young who is coopted into non-painful abuse may also feel special for being singled out for attention. Children between ages six and preadolescence tend to be aware of the sexual implications of the abuse and will generally recognize that it is wrong. Fear and hurt are intertwined with a sense of violation of their bodies and their private space. Preadolescents and adolescents normally experience several inherent developmental conflicts between their emerging sexuality, their gender identity and their relationships with their parents. Sexual abuse severely interrupts the development of a healthy sexuality, leading in some cases to inappropriate or pathological sexual behaviors. Girls who have suffered abuse may become alienated from their own femaleness, and may come to hate all men. Boys molested by pedophiles (usually male) may feel sexually flawed. If forced over time to participate in oral or anal sex, they may wonder if they are homosexual. [33]

The hidden incidence of date rape among adolescents and young adults also has lasting impact. [34] In addition to feeling sexually violated, victims also tend to have feelings of helplessness and loss of control. In most cases of rape, the perpetrator is known to the victim. Often fearing that they will be blamed, the victim is likely to not report the incident(s). Shame and guilt may also keep them from seeking either medical or mental health care for the results of the rape. The results may range from pregnancy, STIs, pelvic inflammation, to persistent psychological trauma and depression.

Indicators of Sexual Abuse

Sexual abuse presents in many ways, and some symptoms may be so general that they could indicate non-abuse stressors, or physical or psychological abuse. It may be the result of examining a child (or adult) who presents with some of the physical symptoms listed in Box 11-3. Or the psychosocial history may reveal some of the behavioral indicators listed. Sometimes during a physical examination the patient may hint at abuse by talking about a friend who is being sexually abused. Occasionally a child may actually confide to you that she has been sexually abused. Without such an admission, you need to remember that you need to consider the weight of a *cluster* of physical and behavioral symptoms. Nonetheless, the American Academy of Pediatrics suggests that because of the secrecy issue "a high level of suspicion may be required to recognize the problem."[35] Once you suspect that sexual abuse has occurred, we suggest that you activate the protocol for interviewing the victim, collecting medical evidence, documenting your findings, and fulfilling the legal requirements for reporting.

Box 11-3 Indicators of Sexual Abuse

1. PHYSICAL (RECENT OR ONGOING)
- irritation, itching, scratching or bruising in the genital area
- pain or bruises in the inside upper thigh or pelvic area
- vaginal, penile or anal discharge
- difficulty urinating
- chronic urinary tract infections or pain in the bladder or kidneys
- stomach or chest pain
- semen around genitals or blood and semen on clothes
- STIs, pelvic inflammatory disease
- headaches
- very tense in upper thighs, refusing to relax or abduct legs for vaginal examination
- tense buttocks muscles refusing to relax for anal examination

Adolescent and adult survivors of sexual abuse (evidence of older chronic abuse)
- vaginitis, vaginismus
- endometriosis
- pelvic inflammatory disease
- spastic colon, irritable bowel syndrome, megacolon (in males who were sodomized)
- physical abnormalities

2. BEHAVIORAL
Young children
- regressive behaviors: thumb sucking, temper tantrums
- enuresis
- encopresis
- excessive crying
- fear of being left alone
- excessive clinging to a parent

- sudden fear of a specific person and avoidance behaviors (hiding in closets)
- head banging
- talks of a "friend" who was sexually abused
- withdrawal, running away
- unusual and developmentally inappropriate interest in sexual play (humping, wriggling on male person's lap, spreading legs in provocative manner, public masturbation)
- overly aggressive to adults
- trying to excessively please adults (Daddy's little "love girl")

Adolescent or adult survivors of sexual abuse
- appetite and/or sleep disturbance (nightmares, sleep walking)
- school or work problems
- alludes to trouble at home but then clams up (the family secret)
- depression
- hypervigilant, anxious, jumpy
- suicidal threats or attempts
- sexually provocative or overly promiscuous
- becoming a "shut in"
- substance abuse
- promiscuity, prostitution
- complete rejection of sex, frigid, or other sexual dysfunction
- major depression, phobic anxiety regarding intimacy
- post traumatic stress disorder
- dissociative symptoms (esp. if rape and violence involved)
- seeking out abusive relationships
- low self-esteem

Child Interview

Interviewing and examining children who have been sexually abused and collecting and recording evidence is a specialized procedure.[36] Pediatric offices and large public clinics are increasingly aware that they need to have a "child friendly" examination room, or be able to create one on demand. Such a room or area should be equipped with the specialized instruments and equipment listed in Box 11-4. If pediatric abuse specialist(s) are available within the facility, they should be brought in on the case as soon as sexual abuse is suspected or indicated. This is espe-

---

Box 11-4   Materials and Equipment Needed for Examination and Evidence Collection

1. Routine examination equipment
2. Appropriate laboratory slips and cultures
3. Blood collection equipment
4. Small speculum suitable for use with child or adolescent females
5. Wood's Lamp (ultraviolet illuminator)
6. Evidence collection kit
7. Paperwork for all medical and evidence collection
8. Anatomically correct dolls
9. Hidden or unobtrusive video camera (optional)

---

cially important in cases of rape or other sexual trauma where forensic evidence needs to be collected in a timely manner.

If for various reasons, such as the time of night, or lack of availability of a pediatric abuse specialist, you cannot refer, your office, or clinic will need to perform such examinations and forensic evidence collection. Thus, you and other staff members need to be familiar with the protocol for interviewing and examining a sexually abused child, as well as for collecting and preserving the evidence. Ideally, the protocol will specify the roles of other "team" members, such as assembling the specialized instruments listed in Box 11-4 in a private examination room, and making legal notification phone calls. Such a team effort will also reduce the stress on you.

INTERVIEWING PRECAUTIONS

Cases of sexual abuse are fraught with a number of potential interviewing hazards. In cases where the child or adolescent was violently raped or otherwise physically traumatized, the physical examination, and the collection of forensic evidence may retraumatize the victim. This means that the whole team needs to be especially sensi-

tive to the child's trauma, confusion, shame and fears. The victim needs to know that they can confide in you and your team, and that you will believe, protect and not blame them. Child abuse experts agree that before the formal medical examination procedure begins, the interviewer/examiner should take a few moments to attend to the emotional welfare of the victim and make the following five **assurances**. It is important that you **reassure** the victim that

1. You believe what they have told you.
2. You know it is not their fault.
3. You are glad that they told you about it.
4. You are sorry it happened.
5. You will do your best to protect and support them.

These assurances are especially important to a child whose previous efforts to communicate about the abuse, had not been believed, or they have been blamed, or threatened. Since you as the listener may find the child's condition and revelations upsetting, giving these assurances may also calm your own emotional turmoil. If the child expresses a preference for someone to be in the room to lend support during the examination, the wish should be accommodated, if feasible. However, care must be taken that it is not a family member who might inhibit the child from speaking. The child's posture, facial expression, and how the child cues on the parent/guardian before speaking are key clues. The adult's nonverbal cues to the child (supportive vs anxious or threatening) are the other determinant for inclusion.

In interviewing traumatized children, it is important not to create **false memories**. These are imaginary scenarios that can be created by children in response to suggestive or leading questions.[37] Great care should be used interviewing making sure to use short open-ended questions such as

1. Do you want to tell me about it?
2. Is there anything else you want to tell me about it? (for follow up)
3. Have you told any one else about it?

Listen and let the child tell what happened. In situations of sexual abuse, it is helpful to have anatomically correct dolls available. Sometimes children will spontaneously talk about the abuse and reveal the identity of the abuser. For young children, it is often easier for the child to tell you what happened by using anatomically correct dolls to show you what the perpetrator did. When the child answers, avoid showing strong emotions, such as shock, anger, or disbelief. In fact, you should reassure the child periodically that she can confide in you and that you will believe, protect and not blame her. In an extended interview, you also need to provide at regular intervals short rest periods, and give the child opportunity to go to the bathroom or have some refreshment. During such breaks the child may want to play with toys or dolls. The younger the child, the more frequent such breaks should be. Again, the aim here is to calm the child and prevent retraumatization.

In general, in interviewing children, you should be aware that you may be the first person to interview the child about the abuse event(s). The child may have difficulty in revealing these events to you for several reasons. If they have been coerced or coopted into secrecy, they may fear retaliation or may think they are being disloyal if they talk about it. The child may feel embarrassed, guilty or be too shy to talk to outsiders. You also need to be aware that young children may be unable to understand the questions, or lack the vocabulary to explain what happened. The Academy of Pediatrics guidelines suggest that children under three not be interviewed.

Medical Examination

Years of research have produced general consensus about the medical procedures in child sexual abuse cases.[38] The examination procedure for all child abuse — whether physical or sexual — should consist of a thorough physical examination, with special attention to genital, perineal, and anal areas. In some cases a thorough exami-

nation will reveal that what was initially suspected to be physical abuse, was actually a combination of physical and sexual abuse. As you proceed with the examination, it is essential that you gently explain each step of the process and the reason for it. This will minimize additional trauma. Be especially careful with the words you choose, because young children tend to interpret statements literally. The child should never be restrained, however, in cases of extreme agitation, you might consider sedating the child.

When examining the genital and anal areas you should explain to the child why you are looking at or touching these private areas. If the outer area indicates trauma, you may want to check if the hymen has been penetrated. When checking for internal damage in a small child it is best to use a small speculum that has been warmed. Careful attention should be given to any discharge, odors, evidence of foreign objects, tears, or skin tags, and tenderness. In case of sexual abuse of a male child, the glans and scrotal area should be examined for erythema, bruises, suction marks, excoriations, burns and lacerations of the glans and frenulum. In both girls and boys the area around the mouth or even head hair should be carefully examined for evidence of recent oral sex. Similarly the anal and perineal areas should be carefully checked for both trauma and possible fluid evidence. In cases of chronic abuse, you may also see signs of STIs, which may present as discharges, lesions, reports of painful urination, or even fever in the case of pelvic inflammation.

In cases of date rape frequently there is alcohol or drugs involved. However, single or clusters of symptoms like vertigo, temporary amnesia, bradycardia, respiratory depression, orthostatic hypotension, hypothermia, acute respiratory acidosis, or possibly seizures and coma should alert the examining provider to the possibility that so-called date rape drugs were involved (see discussion in Chapter 9). In that case, toxicology tests for any one of the three most common club drugs GHB (gamma-hydroxybutyrate), Rohypnol (flunitrazepam), or K (ketamine hydrochloride) should be ordered.[39,40]

Evidence collection is crucial if the last sexual abuse encounter took place *less* than 72 hours prior to the examination. Passing a Wood's Lamp over the child may determine the presence of external body fluids or semen that may need to be collected as physical evidence. If evidence collection is indicated, caution is again indicated for small children to prevent trauma. It is suggested that for collecting rectal evidence that only one rectal swab be used. If the child or adolescent female is too traumatized for a full pelvic examination, you can obtain evidence specimen by gently swabbing the exterior vaginal areas using a moist swab or a pipette. Frequently overlooked are sources of DNA evidence left by the perpetrator in clothing, like torn underwear, a robe or blanket the child may have been wrapped in when she was brought in, or any material the victim may have used to stop the bleeding or seepage of fluids. Any evidence should be carefully labeled and preserved for lab analysis.

Documentation

Carefully recording your findings in all child abuse cases is essential to protecting the child against accusations of having fabricated the charges of abuse. Clear and detailed recorded findings are also needed by CPS and legal authorities for taking action against the perpetrator(s). A simple body map lends itself well to documenting the location of injuries. Reference any drawings, using the child's own utterances to explain injuries, where possible. This is true even if you are video recording the procedure. You also need to estimate and record the age of injuries, by noting the color of a hematoma and the degree of healing in an abrasion, or burn. In cases of sexual abuse, any injury in the genital areas, such as damage to the hymen or internal tears should be illustrated with separate drawings. As evidence is collected, odors or discharges should be noted together with an informed judgment as to their nature and origin. The results of any findings from use of the Wood's Lamp, other diagnostic techniques, as well as the procedure for the collection of specimens needs to be recorded. Usually the examination rooms of pediatric abuse specialists are outfitted with built in video cameras and microphones so that the whole procedure can be made into a visual record. If such a pre-installed system is not available, you may still consider placing a video camera on a tripod in the corner of the interviewing/examination room and let the tape run unattended. However, you still need to produce a detailed written record even if you use recording devices.

Legal Reporting Requirements

As stated above, all states mandate reporting child maltreatment from any professional who has reasonable cause to believe that a child is being neglected or abused; or believes upon examination that a child has been seriously physically injured, sexually abused or sexually assaulted; observes a child being subjected to conditions that are likely to result in abuse or neglect; or knows of or suspects institutional abuse and neglect.

In a health care setting, you are most likely to find out about abuse during an interview and examination. In that case *you* will be responsible to assure that proper notification is made.

Persons Required to Report Child Maltreatment

All members of the various health care professions

Mental health professionals

Dentists

Alternative healers

School teachers or personnel

Social service workers

Child care workers

Clergy

Law Enforcement personnel

Depending on how the child was brought in and by whom, you will need to determine if legal reporting was already done. It is best *not* to rely on hearsay ("She heard her say that it was reported.") or speculation ("I think it was reported.") It is prudent to call in a second or third report, rather than to miss reporting at all.

In most cases the most efficient way to report a case of child abuse and neglect is to call the Child Protective Services (CPS) of the nearest office of the Department of Human Services in your state. Generally, they will take the next step to investigate, and when warranted, notify the police. If you call in an expert on child abuse, they will generally tell you the person to be notified or will do it for you. In some locations where you have effective cooperation between the Coalition on Child Abuse, CPS, and law enforcement authorities, notification of one agency will automatically trigger notification of other appropriate agencies.

• •

PATIENT PROFILE 11.3

OUT OF THE BLUE . . .

SETTING: Dorrie is a 4-year-old being treated for a second ear infection at a pediatric clinic in a large urban hospital. John, the physician assistant, has treated Dorrie since she was born. The child clings to her mother, Ann, as they both talk about Dorrie's symptoms.

John: So, Ann, I think she is recovering well from the cold and ear infection, however, do be sure to keep her on plenty of liquids so she doesn't dehydrate.

Ann: OK, John. Is there anything else I should be watching for?

John: No, that's about it . . .

Out of the blue Dorrie interrupts John and says:

Dorrie: He tried to put his pee pee in my, you know, down there.

Both John and Ann are stunned and look at Dorrie then at each other. Ann has a look of horror on her face.

John: *(This must be examined very carefully now. Whatever steps I take now, can have many repercussions. I need to call Dr. Wilson in on this now to assure the following examination occurs correctly according to the clinic protocols. How is Ann reacting to this disclosure? She looks stunned too. This must be quite a shock for her. After Dr. Wilson examines Dorrie, I will talk with Ann.)*

POINTS TO CONSIDER:

• John has the normal reaction of being stunned, however he also realizes great sensitivity is needed in this situation.

• John is aware that certain steps need to take place now and is remembering the names of specialists in the area of sexual abuse.

• John is correct in reminding himself that he needs to follow clinic protocol in this matter.

• John realizes that Ann needs some assistance as well as Dorrie.

• •

Conclusion

Abuse, especially sexual abuse of children, is likely to be *the* most emotionally stressful issue you will encounter as a health care provider. And it will happen to you more often than you think possible.

Therefore, you and other members of the health care team involved need to be especially supportive of each other when you deal with child abuse cases. We suggest that you debrief each other as soon as possible, but no later than the next day. Because there may be delayed and/or hidden reactions, it would be useful to agree to monitor your own and each other's emotional state of well being. You may need to do follow up debriefings. Such mutual support after an emotionally upsetting case of abuse can create a strong sense of closeness between team members. The creation of this feeling of solidarity is essential to your continued willingness to deal with the next case of child abuse.

REFERENCES

1. Stacey W, Shupe A (1983) *The Family Secret: Domestic Violence in America.* Boston, MA: Beacon Press.

2. Panel on Research on Child Abuse and Neglect (1993) *Understanding Child Abuse and Neglect.* (Commission on Behavioral and Social Sciences, National Research Council) Washington, DC: National Academy of Science Press.

3. Public Law 93-247.

4. Sledlak AJ, Broadhurst DD (1996) *Executive Summary Of The Third National Incidence Study Of Child Abuse And Neglect.* (National Center on Child Abuse and Neglect, Administration on Children, Youth and Families) Washington, DC: US Department of Health and Human Services.

5. Table 2-3 Victimization Rates, 1990-1999. In *Child Maltreatment 1999: Reports From the States to theNational Child Abuse and Neglect Data System.* Washington, DC: US Department of Health and Human Services.

6. Table 2-4: Maltreatment Types, 1999. In *Child Maltreatment 1999: Reports From the States to the National Child Abuse and Neglect Data System.* Washington, DC: US Department of Health and Human Services.

7. Table 4-3: Maltreatment Fatalities by Age and Sex, 1999. In *Child Maltreatment 1999: Reports From the States to the National Child Abuse and Neglect Data System.* Washington, DC: US Department of Health and Human Services.

8. Table 3-2: Perpetrator Relationship to Victim. In *Child Maltreatment 1999: Reports From the States to the National Child Abuse and Neglect Data System.* Washington, DC: US Department of Health and Human Services.

9. Office of Juvenile Justice and Delinquency Prevention (1999) As primary caretakers, females were the primary perpetrators of maltreatment (Figure). In Child protective service agencies received reports on more than 3 million maltreated children in 1996. *1999 National Report Series, Juvenile Justice Bulletin.* Accessed at www.ncjrs.org/html/ojjdp/2000_5_2/child_09.html

10. Table 3-4: Perpetrator Relationship to Victims by Maltreatment Type, 1999. In *Child Maltreatment 1999: Reports From the States to the National Child Abuse and Neglect Data System.* Washington, DC: US Department of Health and Human Services.

11. Table 2-10: Victimization Rates by Race and Ethnicity, 1999. In *Child Maltreatment 1999: Reports From the States to the National Child Abuse and Neglect Data System.* Washington, DC: US Department of Health and Human Services.

12. National Clearinghouse on Child Abuse and Neglect Information provides State by State summaries at www.calib.com/nccanch/services/statutes.htm# More detailed information on state statutes is available at www.calib.com/nccanch/pubs/stats00/define.pdf

13. 42 USC 5101 et seq; 42 USC 5116 et seq. (West Supp. 1998).

14. 42 USC Par 5106g(2) (West Supp. 1998).

15. Childrens' Bureau (1999) *10 Years of Reporting Child Maltreatment.* (Administration of Children Youth and Families) Washington, DC: Dept of Health and Human Services.

16. Kohn ML (1977) *Class and Conformity: A Study in Values,* 2nd ed. Homewood, IL: Dorsey Press.

17. 42 USCA Par 5106g(4) (West Supp 1998).

18. Committee on Child Abuse and Neglect, American Academy of Pediatrics (1999) Guidelines for the evaluation of sexual abuse of children: Subject Review. *Pediatrics,* 103,1:186-191.

19. Office of Juvenile Justice and Delinquency Prevention (1999) Children as Victims *Juvenile Justice Bulletin.* Accessed on the Internet at www.ncjrs.org/html/ojjdp/2000_5_2/child_09.html

20. Goldstein AP, Keller H, Erne D (1985) *Changing the Abusive Parent.* Champaign, IL: Research Press, 14.

21. Maslow AH (1970) *Motivation and Personality.* New York: Harper and Row.

22. National Clearinghouse on Child Abuse and Neglect Information *Understanding Child Abuse And Neglect.* Accessed on the Internet at www.calib.com/nccanch/pubs/usermanuals/basic/section3.cfm

23. Bethea L (1999) Primary Prevention of Child Abuse, *Family Physician,* 62:1591-1602.

24. Sledlak AJ, Broadhurst DD (1996) Distribution of Child Abuse and Neglect by Family Characteristics. In *Executive Summary Of The Third National Incidence Study Of Child Abuse And Neglect.* (National Center on Child Abuse and Neglect, Administration on Children, Youth and Families) Washington, DC: US. Department of Health and Human Services.

25. Childrens' Bureau (1999) *10 Years of Reporting Child Maltreatment*. (Administration of Children Youth and Families) Washington, DC: Dept of Health and Human Services.

26. Kerker BD, Horwitz SM et al (2000) Identification of Violence in the Home: Pediatric and Parental Reports. *Arch Pediatric, Adolescent Med.* 154,5:457-462.

27. Cohn F, Salmon ME, Stobo J, Editors (2001) *Confronting Neglect: The Education of Health Professionals on Family Violence*. (Committee on the Training Needs of Health Professionals to Respond to Family Violence, Board on Children, Youth, and Families, Institute of Medicine), Washington, DC: National Academy Press.

28. Jenny C et al (1999) Analysis of missed cases of abusive head trauma. *JAMA*, 28:621-626.

29. Committee on Child Abuse and Neglect, American Academy of Pediatrics (2001) Shaken Baby Syndrome: Rotational Cranial Injuries - Technical Report (Policy Statement) *Pediatrics*, 108,1:206-210.

30. Kivlin JD (2001) Manifestations of Shaken Baby Syndrome. *Curr Opin Opthamology*, 12,3:158-163.

31. Briere, J (1996) The lasting effects of sexual abuse. In *Therapy for Adults Molested as Children*. New York: Springer Publishing.

32. Frothingham TE, Hobbs CJ et al (2000) Follow up study eight years after diagnosis of sexual abuse, *Arch. Diseases of. Childhood.*, 83: 132-134.

33. Moody CW (1999) Male Child Sexual Abuse. *J Pediatric Health Care*, 13,3:112-119.

34. Rickert VI, Wiemann CM (1998) Date Rape among adolescents and young adults. *J Pediatric Adolesc Gynecology*, 11,4:167-175.

35. Committee on Child Abuse and Neglect, American Academy of Pediatrics (1999) Guidelines for the evaluation of sexual abuse of children: Subject Review. *Pediatrics*, 103,1:187.

36. Bernet W et al Practice parameters for the forensic evaluation of children and adolescents who may have been physically or sexually abused. *J Am Acad Child Adolesc Psychiatry* 1997 Mar;36(3):423-442.

37. Yapko MD (1994) *Suggestions of Abuse: True and False Memories of Childhood Sexual Trauma*. New York: Simon & Schuster.

38. Atabaki S, Paradise JE (1999) The medical evaluation of the sexually abused child: lessons from a decade of research. *Pediatrics*,104,1:178-186.

39. O'Connell, Kaye L, Plosay JJ (2000) Gamma-Hydroxybutyrate (GHB): A Newer Drug of Abuse. Americ Fam Physician.62:2478-2482.

40. Hoffman RJ et al (2001) Common methods of illicit preparation of Ketamine: Gas chromatography/mass spectrometry analysis of products. *J Toxicology, Clin Toxicology*, 39,3:267.

CHAPTER 12

Mental Disorders

This chapter examines the barriers of fear, stigma, and denial about mental illness that inhibit discussion between provider and patient and provides guidance for overcoming the barriers. It briefly explains the organization and use of the *Diagnostic and Statistical Manual of Mental Disorders* (DSM-IV) and reviews various diagnostic screening instruments developed to facilitate assessment of mental disorders. The chapter addresses the two most commonly presented mental problems in primary care: depressive and anxiety disorders, calling attention to the wide range of organic and psychosocial factors that can cause and exacerbate these disorders. It also spells out the need for a collaborative effort for treatment and continuity of care, especially for those with chronic mental disorders.

Societal Beliefs About Mental Illness

The primary care provider is usually the first contact for mental health services. The two most commonly presented mental health disorders are depression and anxiety.[1] However, the rate of recognition and treatment of these disorders in primary settings is low.[2] Several factors contribute to the latter: the stigma attached to the label of mental disorder; health care providers' perception of psychiatric disorders; and the health care providers' lack of familiarity with the use of the DSM-IV.[3]

STIGMA

Fear of being labeled crazy often delays or even prevents patients from revealing any symptoms that might suggest psychiatric problems. Indeed, until modern times, mental illness was seen either as demonic possession or as a sign of serious moral failing. The 1999 *Surgeon General's Report on Mental Health* traces American negative attitudes on mental illness to three major sources.[4] The first, the acceptance in the 19th century of Descartes' split between body and mind, led to separating medical disorders from mental health disorders. This split and the subsequent discoveries in microbiology and organic causes of disease led to neglect of psychosocial factors. It may also have led to a heightened perception that mental illness is somehow under voluntary control, hence a weakness or character defect. The second is the historical or innate fear of someone engaged in aberrant behaviors, which produces avoidance or denial. For example, people who talk to themselves out loud in public or say they are hearing voices or start yelling for no apparent reason make us uncomfortable, and we may want to avoid them. In our mind, we may label such persons as mad, crazy, or insane. Both the labeling and the social isolation create a powerful stigma around mental disorders. Denial by the person with the difficulty, by their family, and sometimes even by the health care provider is the common reaction to labeling someone as mentally ill. The third reason, primary care providers' lack of familiarity with the system of assessment in DSM-IV leads them to overlook mental disorders.

FEAR OF DISCLOSURE

Many cultures do not encourage emotional self-disclosure. Certainly the American cultural imperative to be strong, especially for men, does not encourage it. Instead, a person in an emotional crisis may be told to "get over it," "pull yourself together," "you can handle it." The message is don't be weak or don't show weakness. Revealing "unacceptable" feelings such as fear, anxiety, panic, depression, confusion, helplessness, or hopelessness is frowned upon, in part because it makes others uncomfortable. The cultural norm is for a person to pretend that everything is fine. However, denial or minimizing by the person in response to the fear of being stigmatized may be counterproductive. Well-meaning messages on self-reliance often prevent persons from seeking the emotional support that would help them get through a difficult situation. For example, a job loss can induce painful feelings of anger, confusion, depression, and loss of self-esteem, which when shared, normally resolve after a short adjustment period. However, persons who routinely suppress such feelings may develop maladaptive behavior patterns. Some argue that the high rates of depression and anxiety in the United States[5] (perhaps worldwide)[6] are the result of this tendency not to reveal inner turmoil.

Family members, friends, and coworkers also tend to deny or minimize the mental problems they see in others. Those who first observe that a person is not functioning "normally" may initially pretend not to notice. If it is an adult and the behaviors are somewhat outside the norms without being bothersome to others, the person may be labeled eccentric. When the behavior or thought processes become too obvious or disruptive to be ignored, the family may shift to minimizing or using colloquial euphemisms to label such behavior. For example, a child with developmental disabilities may be called a "slow learner." Someone with hallucinations may be described as "having a spell." This tendency to minimize also applies to self-labeling when persons come to their health care providers. A person with anxiety or panic attacks may report a "bad case of nerves." Depression is often identified as a problem of low or no energy. The fear of stigma also applies to psychiatric medications that may be associated with being crazy or having something "wrong in the head." Especially in

rural areas, but also in some urban subcultures, patients may refer to "nerve pills," anything from antidepressants to anxiolytics to antipsychotics. Patients usually use such euphemisms because they are embarrassed or fear being stigmatized. Use of vague or indirect descriptors often indicates ignorance of their problem and possible treatment options. When a patient uses such euphemisms, the health care provider should regard them as important clues to how to proceed. Any such indirect hints should prompt you to ask follow-up questions to obtain an explanation or further information. For example, after hearing a patient refer to a bad case of nerves, you might ask in a neutral tone of voice, "What happens when you have a bad case of nerves?" When you ask in an empathic manner and use terms that are neither judgmental nor stigmatizing, the patient is more likely to provide accurate information.[7]

FEAR OF DISCRIMINATION

Another barrier to revealing an emotional or mental problem is the often justified fear of prejudice and discrimination in the workplace (see Chapter 5). For years the insurance industry and business associations have lobbied to prevent parity in reimbursement for treatment of mental disorders. The message is that mental health disorders somehow are not as valid as medical problems. While the federal Americans with Disabilities Act has created improved access for persons with physical disabilities, the battle is still being fought by activists to extend that protection to persons with mental disabilities. Most small businesses have no programs or policies to accommodate persons with mental disorders or disabilities. Many health plans have no coverage for treatment of outpatient psychiatric disorders. On the other hand, many large corporations recognize that their employees' mental health is a crucial factor in work productivity and the reduction of absenteeism. They have set up **employee assistance programs** (EAPs), and many include mental health counseling in the benefit package for their employees. These offer nondiscriminatory and confidential referral services for substance abuse and sometimes for other mental health needs. In effective programs there is a boundary to protect confidentiality that prevents details about an employee's referral, diagnosis, or treatment from getting back to the supervisor, fellow coworkers, or the company. A court decision in 2001 confirmed that EAP records are protected by client–therapist privilege, thus alleviating fears of misuse of EAP information either by the company or insurance carriers.[8] However, in general, unless there is a supportive atmosphere or understanding at work about mental problems, employees are afraid to admit to such problems, even when they are justified by a life crisis.

• •

PATIENT PROFILE 12.1

I CAN'T CATCH MY BREATH

SETTING: *Barbara, a 28-year-old single mother of a 1-year-old, works as a laboratory technician in a large medical clinic. Her ex-boyfriend, who is the father of her child, also works at the clinic. She seeks help at the obstetrics and gynecology clinic in her suburban neighborhood rather than her workplace so as to avoid embarrassment and fear of losing her job. She is seen by Patti, a physician assistant, who provides all her routine gynecological care. Barbara begins by saying she believes she is having panic attacks.*

Patti: So you believe you are having panic attacks. I know they can be very frightening. Tell me what you feel during one of these attacks.

Barbara: Well, my heart starts beating really fast and I start sweating. I feel like my heart is going to explode in my chest. Sometimes I feel sick to my stomach and I can't catch my breath. I feel like I'm going to die. *(I sure hope she doesn't think I am crazy.)*

Patti: That must be very upsetting to you. How often do these attacks occur?

Barbara: They vary a lot but usually about once a week. What worries me the most is not know-

ing when the next one is going to happen. I've had some at work and sometimes I can derail them. Other times I just have to ride them out. I had a bad one last week and decided it was time to get help.

Patti: I am glad you decided to come in and get help. How do you derail these panic attacks?

Barbara: You'll laugh at me, I know. I use one of the breathing techniques I learned in the birthing class. That seems to help. *(She does seem interested in what I think is happening. What a relief!)*

Patti: Show me these breathing technique.

(Barbara demonstrates the breathing technique.)

Patti: When did the panic attacks start?

Barbara: I was pregnant and had just broken up with my boyfriend. He is also the father of my child. Then I started to get scared and worried about the future. You know, being all alone, having this baby on my own, with no support.

Patti: Indeed, that is a lot of responsibility for anyone. A normal response is to feel anxious about a situation like that. Have the attacks gotten worse or more frequent since then?

Barbara: They seem to come in clusters. I'll have a bunch of them and then for a week or two none.

Patti: Do you find that certain situations trigger them?

Barbara: Stress at work triggers them. Also worrying that I might run into my ex-boyfriend sure sets them off. But lately they just come out of the blue.

Patti: Do these panic attacks stop you from going out or going to work?

Barbara: Not at all.

Patti: You may indeed have a panic disorder. I would like you to get some laboratory blood work done to rule out any thyroid problems. Do you want to get that done here or at your workplace?

Barbara: I'd prefer here because I don't want them to know about this.

Patti: Now there are a number of ways we can manage these attacks. One technique that many people have found helpful is to reduce other stressors or their impact as much as possible. Have you done anything to reduce your stressors?

Barbara: I talked with my supervisor about taking one day off a week twice a month and she agreed.

Patti: How about other stressors?

Barbara: I have been able to do a trade with another mother for baby-sitting, and we started a young mothers club for support. We set aside a time for an hour of play time with our children and we rotate who watches them while the rest of us take walks, watch videos on parenting and sometimes just have lunch and exchange stories.

Patti: That's great! I am sure getting some support will help. What else?

Barbara: I am doing a trade with another lab technician for housecleaning. She cleans my house and I baby-sit her baby so she can do errands or whatever.

Patti: It sounds like you have already taken some very important steps towards reducing stressors. Add to your breathing techniques an emphasis on the exhale. Anxious people often do not exhale sufficiently. If you continue to have panic attacks, I may refer you for more in-depth counseling. Would you be willing to try counseling?

Barbara: I guess if the other stuff doesn't help.

Points to Consider

- Patti elicits a focused history and details on the symptoms.
- Patti uses effective communication techniques with Barbara: open-ended questions, empathy, and reassurance.
- Patti makes additional suggestions for stress reduction while offering other management suggestions.
- Engaging Barbara in thinking about other stress management techniques increases the likelihood that she will change her own behavior and thus reduce the stressors in her life.

• •

PROVIDER BARRIERS

When patients or families do seek help from their primary health care provider, they may do so cautiously and indirectly to gauge the response. Previous adverse or unsympathetic reception by a health care provider may make patients hesitant about what information on their mental health they reveal and how they reveal it. Indeed some health care providers have some internal resistance to discussing mental illness. Discomfort stemming from the social stigma of mental illness may make them reluctant to identify a possible mental problem in a patient. Others feel they lack the training or interviewing skills to conduct an effective mental health assessment. Still others worry that if they explore a person's mental condition, the patient may start rambling and the provider may lose control of the interview. Some health care providers feel that they need to focus on physical problems and that psychiatric problems are not part of their practice. This particular bias may be unconscious and related to the relatively low emphasis given to the psychiatric and psychosocial components in medical training. It may seem simpler to search for an organic cause of a patient's illness rather than to venture into the confusing area of psychological or environmental causes.

Patients fearful of consequences of being labeled mentally ill may deliberately encourage their health care providers to focus on physical causes rather than mental anguish or pain. Thus, patients may display a fake cheeriness to hide depression or other mental problems. If you do get fooled by the patient's performance, you may miss crucial information (see Patient Profile 12.2). When a patient's answers portray a situation that seems just a little too perfect, you may have to rely on your intuition to alert you to a discrepancy between the words and cheery facade and the other clues. For example, when patients habitually suppress their mental distress, the body may manifest the struggles within the mind and produce real physical symptoms. This process by which the body produces somatic symptoms that cannot be explained adequately on the basis of physical and laboratory examinations is called **somatization**.[9] (See Chapter 13.) When somatization is suspected, you should pause in your search for organic causes of physical illness to explore possible psychosocial stressors. With time, most health care providers can develop the sensitivity—some call it a sixth sense—to follow up on indirect nonverbal clues.[10] Chapter 4 discusses the importance of letting patients tell their story. Health care providers, strongly oriented toward the orderly and logical search for symptoms, may fear this will encourage the patient to wander off into irrelevant detail, producing little if any usable information about symptoms. When you get an indication of mental problems, you may wish to use one of the assessment tools discussed later in the chapter. Of course, ruling out organic causes is necessary and appropriate, but it comes after establishing whether a mental disorder is present.

The balance is between the desire for efficiency and the need to have the patient participate fully in finding the relevant facts. If the health care provider is too directive, the patient may feel resentful about not being allowed to talk. If the practitioner is too casual, the patient's communication may ramble. Thus, the challenge, especially regarding mental disorders, is to have the patient narrate a focused symptom history. Of course, if despite your best efforts the patient keeps going off on tangents, that in itself may be a sign of a mental disorder.[11]

DSM-IV

This section addresses the third factor cited for the low rate of identification by health care providers who are not practitioners of psychiatry: lack of familiarity with the system of assessing and classifying mental disorders used in the standard reference, DSM-IV. At this writing (August 2002) the manual is in its fourth revised edition, known as **DSM-IV-TR** (text revised).

MULTIAXIAL SYSTEM

The classification approach of DSM-IV is based on the assumption that mental disorders have biological, medical, psychosocial, and gender-related aspects along with their psychological and behavioral manifestations. Indeed, DSM-IV comments on the body–mind split by recognizing that "there is much physical in mental disorders and much mental in physical disorders."[12] This central assumption is the basis for the **multiaxial system**, which assesses the patient across five dimensions, or axes (Box 12-1). According to DSM-IV, the "multiaxial system provides a convenient format for organizing and communicating clinical information, for capturing the complexity of clinical situations, and for describing the heterogeneity of individuals presenting with the same diagnosis."[13] In general, medical disorders tend to be defined through symptom presentation, structural pathology, and deviance from the physiological norm. DSM-IV defines a **mental disorder** as "a clinically significant behavioral or psychological syndrome or pattern that occurs in an individual and that is associated with present distress (e.g., a painful symptoms) or disability (i.e., impairment in one or more areas of functioning), or with a significantly increased risk of suffering death, pain, disability, or an important loss of freedom."[14]

DSM-IV goes on to point out that no matter what the original cause, "it must currently be considered a manifestation of a behavioral, psychological or biological dysfunction in the individual,"[15] rather than a reflection of cultural, religious, or political conflicts between the individual and society.[16] In many instances expected and unexpected stressful events cause a temporary loss of equilibrium from which the person recovers, generally within 6 months. When the disruption in functioning is transient, it is called an **adjustment disorder**. DSM-IV also classifies mental disorders by identifying etiology, severity, and especially duration.

Axis I includes the mental disorders and adjustment orders and "other conditions that may be a focus of clinical attention."[17] Since

---

Box 12-1   The Five Axes of the DSM-IV Multiaxial System

Axis I   Clinical Disorders
          Other conditions that may be a focus
          of clinical attention
Axis II   Personality Disorders
          Mental retardation
Axis III General medical conditions
Axis IV   Psychosocial and environmental
          problems
Axis V   Global assessment of functioning

---

many disorders have considerable overlap in symptoms, etiology, behavior, or mental functioning, DSM-IV addresses the problem of **differential diagnosis**. Disorders are divided into the broad categories shown in Box 12-2. The text describes the diagnostic features; subtypes and/or specifiers; recording procedures; additional descriptive features; associated laboratory findings; associated physical examination findings; general medical conditions; culture, age, and gender features; prevalence date; course disorders; and familial patterns. DSM-IV highlights key factors for making a differential diagnosis. Each diagnosis is generally recorded as a three-digit code followed by two decimals. The number after the first decimal specifies the subtype within a category, and the second records the severity. For example, under the category mood disorders, a major depressive disorder can occur as a single episode or recurrently. That element is coded in the first decimal after the diagnostic code. The severity of the disorder, in the second decimal, ranges from mild to severe. Thus, a major depressive disorder (296) with recurrent episodes (.3) that are moderate (2) would be coded 296.32.

Axis II is reserved primarily for **personality disorders** and **mental retardation**. In complex cases, there may be multiple conditions to report. Axis II is also used for noting "prominent maladaptive personality features and defense mechanisms,"[18] such as "histrionic personality features" or "frequent use of denial." However, frequently there are no diagnoses to report on Axis II, and this is coded with V71.09. If the diagnoses are deferred, 799.9 is coded until additional information can be obtained.

Axis III reports current medical conditions that are relevant to the understanding and management of the patient's mental disorders. Generally, the names of the medical conditions are written in with the ICD-9 codes added in parentheses. This Axis provides an opportunity to record the medical factors, which may be comorbid with the mental disorder. For example, in the elderly, coexisting dementia and depression may complicate an accurate diagnosis. It is the task of the health care provider to identify and record on this Axis medical conditions as distinct from psychosocial factors.

Axis IV provides an opportunity to list the **psychosocial and environmental problems** that appear to play a role in the etiology or main-

---

Box 12-2   DSM-IV Major Diagnostic Categories

Disorders usually first diagnosed in infancy,
    childhood, or adolescence
Delirium, dementia, and amnestic and other
    cognitive disorders
Mental disorders due to a general medical condition
    not elsewhere classified
Substance-related disorders
Schizophrenia and other psychotic disorders
Mood disorders
Anxiety disorders
Somatoform disorders
Factitious disorders
Dissociative disorders
Sexual and gender identity disorders
Eating disorders
Sleep disorders
Impulse control disorders not elsewhere classified
Adjustment disorders
Personality disorders
Other conditions that may be a focus of clinical
    attention (V-codes)

tenance of the condition. If there are multiple problems such as extreme poverty, limited access to health care, and family conflict, they would all be listed on Axis IV. DSM-IV groups such problems into the following categories:[19]

Primary support group: relationship problems or events in the family, such as death, divorce, marital conflict, health problems, inadequate discipline, parent–child conflict, child maltreatment, sibling rivalry.

Social environment: inadequate social support, living alone, difficulty with acculturation, discrimination, adjustment to life cycle changes (e.g., retirement).

Educational problems: illiteracy, academic problems, discord with teachers or classmates, inadequate or dangerous school environment.

Occupational problems: unemployment, threat of job loss, stressful work schedule, difficult work conditions, job dissatisfaction, job change, discord with boss or coworkers.

Housing problems: homelessness, inadequate housing, unsafe neighborhood, discord with neighbors or landlord.

Economic problems: extreme poverty, inadequate finances, insufficient welfare support, inability to get affordable child care.

Access to health care: inadequate health care services, no or inadequate health insurance, no transportation to health care services.

Legal system problems: arrest, incarceration, litigation, victim of crime, problems with parole officer.

Psychosocial and environmental factors: exposure to disasters, war, other hostilities; discord with nonfamily caregivers, such as counselors, social workers, physicians; unavailability of social service agencies.

Axis V is also known as the **global assessment of functioning** (GAF) (Box 12-3). This instrument for measuring the severity of dysfunction quantifies the patient's ability to function in the psychological, social, and occupational realms along a continuum from 1 to 100, with lower numbers indicating lesser ability to function. The GAF is also used as a comparative measure, that is, as an overview of the progress or regression from a year ago to the present. Health care providers can use periodic measurements to track declines in functioning and progress from an acute crisis back to normal functioning.

Assessment

Assessment of mental disorders can be frustrating and complex. One reason for the difficulty in identifying mental disorders is the wide range of psychoemotional and behavioral signs or symptoms of impairment of normal functioning. **Signs** are the provider's "observations and objective findings, such as a patient's constricted affect or psychomotor retardation." **Symptoms** are the "subjective experiences described by patients, such as depressed mood or lack of energy." A **syndrome** is a "group of signs and symptoms that together make up a recognizable condition."[20] To catalog the signs, clinicians use various versions of the **Mental Status Examination**. The long version is used primarily for a comprehensive psychiatric evaluation in cases of serious mental disorders, such as dissociative disorders or psychosis. Periodic administration of the instrument provides reference measurements of improvements or deterioration over time in a person's identified condition. Generally divided into the nine categories shown in Box 12-4, it describes the patient's appearance, speech, actions, and thought processes.[21]

Shorter versions often called **mini mental state examinations** are used to assess the patient's cognitive functioning and relationship to reality (Box 12-5).[22] They are used to measure impairment in cases of delirium, dementias, and/or amnestic disorders, due either to medical conditions or substance abuse.[23] For a person who seems disoriented or confused, a provider might first ask just a few questions to check a patient's orientation to person, time, and place, such as these:

Box 12-3   DSM-IV Global Assessment of Functioning (abbreviated)

100–90	Superior functioning in wide range of activities		ment in reality testing or communication (speech is illogical, obscure, or irrelevant)
90–81	Good functioning; absent or minimal symptoms	30–21	Inability to function in almost all areas (stays in bed, no job, no friends); behavior influenced by delusions or hallucinations or inappropriate communication or judgment
80–71	Slight impairment; symptoms transient, expectable reactions to psychosocial stressors		
70–61	Some difficulty in social, occupational, or school functioning; mild symptoms (depressed mood, insomnia or anxiety)	20–11	Some danger of hurting self or others (suicide attempts without clear expectation of death; being aggressive and violent or manic) or intermittently failing to maintain adequate personal hygiene; or gross impairment in communication (incoherent or mute)
60–51	Moderate difficulty in social, occupational, school functioning; moderate symptoms (flat affect, circumstantial speech, panic attacks)		
50–41	Serious impairment in social, occupational, school functioning; serious symptoms (suicidal ideation, obsessional rituals)	10–1	Persistent danger of hurting self or others or persistent inability to maintain minimal personal hygiene, or serious suicidal act with clear expectation of death
40–31	Major impairment in several areas: work, school, family relations, judgment, thinking, or mood; some impair-	0	Inadequate information

Adapted with permission from APA (1994) Diagnostic and Statistical Manual of Mental Disorders, Washington, DC: American Psychiatric Association.

- What is your name?
- What is my name?
- What building are you in?
- What city are you in?
- What day of the week, month, year is it?

Inability to provide correct answers to such simple questions is a signal to conduct more detailed assessment.

Assessment Shortcuts

Insurance companies require DSM-IV multiaxial assessment and diagnosis codes for reimbursement of treatment of mental disorders. However, most primary care providers find DSM's multiaxial system too strongly oriented toward psychiatry and too cumbersome.[24] The first effort to make DSM more user friendly for primary care physicians produced a condensed version for primary care providers, the **DSM-IV-PC**.[25] It focuses on the eight most common psychiatric disorders seen in primary care. It presents diagnostic **algorithms** for evaluating depression, anxiety, cognitive abnormalities (dementias), substance abuse, somatization, sleep and sexual disorders, body dysmorphic and eating disorders, and psychosis. The algorithms are designed to facilitate the process of making a differential diagnosis.[26] Regarded as still too difficult to use, it was found languishing in most primary care offices.[27] Recognizing time constraints and the lack of experience of most primary care providers with psychiatric assessments, researchers have endeavored to develop more user-friendly instruments for assessing mental disorders in the primary care setting. The **PRIME-MD**, a psychiatric screening instrument based on the DSM-IV-PC, was specifically designed for primary care settings. On the

---

Box12-4 Mental Status Examination

I. General description
   A. Appearance
   B. Overt behavior and psychomotor activity
   C. Attitude
II. Mood and affect
   A. Mood
   B. Affect
   C. Appropriateness of affectl
III. Speech characteristics
IV. Perception
V. Thought content and mental trends
   A. Thought process
   B. Thought content
VI. Sensorium and Cognition
   A. Consciousness
   B. Orientation and memory
   C. Concentration and attention
   D. Reading and writing
   E. Visuospatial ability
   F. Abstract thought
   G. Information and intelligence
VII. Impulsivity
VIII. Judgment and insight
IX. Reliability

Adapted from Kaplan HI, Sadock BJ (1998) *Synopsis of Psychiatry*, 8th ed. Philadelphia: Lippincott, Williams & Wilkins, 1998;250–254.

average it would take a physician about 8.5 minutes to administer the 26 yes–no questions about symptoms the patient had in the past month.[28] This assessment process was still considered too long for the PRIME-MD to be used routinely. To reduce the time further, a self-report instrument modeled on the PRIME-MD was developed. The **Patient Health Questionnaire** (PHQ) is a three-page questionnaire covering the five most common groups of psychiatric disorders encountered in primary care: depression, anxiety, substance abuse, somatoform disorder, and eating disorders. Its five subsections can be used together or separately to target specific disorders. It requires only about 3 minutes of provider time to score and assess after the patient has completed it.[29]

More recently an electronic hand-held self-report device for screening mental disorders has come into use; it requires no provider time to administer or score. The **Quick PsychoDiagnostics Panel** (QPD) screens for nine mental disorders: major depression, dysthymic disorder, bipolar disorder, generalized anxiety disorder, panic disorder, obsessive compulsive disorder, bulimia nervosa, alcohol and substance abuse, and somatization disorders.[30] The QPD panel also assesses suicide risk. The hand-held device is about the size of a textbook. The 59 core questions of the QPD panel are displayed one at a time on a large LCD screen, and patients record their answers by pressing either a True or a False button. When responses suggest a possible disorder, the test branches into modules that probe for more information. Questions are short and geared to sixth grade reading level, so that most patients can complete the test in the waiting room in about 6 minutes. The patients' responses are analyzed and printed immediately as a diagnostic report that the physician can review before seeing the patient. The report resembles a familiar blood chemistries report and can be used by any physician without any special training. The report includes scores and reference ranges for each diagnostic category and the specific symptoms marked by the patient. Any scores out of range are called to the provider's attention.[31]

These self-administered instruments have had their validity tested in extensive studies and are considered reliable but not foolproof. Thus, each instrument still needs some personal follow-up. However, they are time-saving devices for providers whose primary specialization is not in psychiatry. Instead of a lengthy and possibly awkward screening interview, primary care providers or specialists like obstetrician–gynecologists or surgeons can use one of these structured instruments to screen for a variety of disorders. In addition to the broad screening instruments listed, a number of scales measure specific conditions, such as depression, anxiety, or substance abuse. They are discussed later in this chapter and in Chapter 9.

Box 12-5 Mini-Mental State Examination Questionnaire

Orientation (score 1 if correct)

Name this hospital or building. _____

What city are you in now? _____

What year is it? _____

What month is it? _____

What is the date today? _____

What state are you in? _____

What county is this? _____

What floor of the building are you on? _____

What day of the week is it? _____

What season of the year is it? _____

Registration (Score 1 for each object correctly repeated)

Name three objects and have the patient repeat them. Score number repeated by the patient. Name the three objects several more times if needed for the patient to repeat correctly (record trials _____). _____

Attention and calculation

Subtract 7 from 100 in serial fashion to 65.

Maximum score = 5 _____

Recall (score 1 for each object recalled)

Do you recall the three objects named before? _____

Language tests

Confrontation naming: watch, pen = 2 _____

Repetition: "No ifs, ands, or buts" = 1 _____

Comprehension: Pick up the paper in your right hand, fold it in half, and set it on the floor = 3 _____

Read and perform the command "close your eyes" = 1 _____

Write any sentence (subject, verb, object) = 1 _____

Construction

Copy the design below = 1 _____

Total MMSE questionnaire score (maximum = 30) _____

Reprinted from Kaplan & Sadock (1998), 319 based on adaptation from Folstein MF, Folstein S, McHugh PR. Mini-mental state: A practical method for grading the cognitive state of patients for the clinician. *J Psychiatr Res* 12: 89, 1975.

MOOD AND ANXIETY DISORDERS

Mood disorders and **anxiety disorders** are the two most common disorders in primary care settings. DSM-IV divides mood disorders into depressive disorders, bipolar disorders, and two disorders based on etiology: mood disorder due to a general medical condition and substance-induced mood disorders.[32] Anxiety disorders are divided into generalized anxiety disorder, acute stress disorder, posttraumatic stress disorder (PTSD), obsessive-compulsive disorder, various phobias, and panic disorders. In addition, the DSM-IV also identifies generalized anxiety disorder due to a medical condition or substance abuse.[33]

Mood and anxiety disorders may occur simultaneously or sequentially, or one can be superimposed on and mask the other. Each can have an organic, psychosocial, or mixed etiology. For example, genetic neurochemical imbalances can predispose persons to either mood or anxiety disorders. Similarly, prescription medications, over-the-counter drugs, drug interactions, and herbal supplements can cause symptoms of either depression or anxiety. Medical problems or substance abuse can cause depression, anxiety, or both. Systemic poisoning from neurotoxins is one of the recent additions to environmentally produced medical conditions that can produce acute and chronic symptoms of depressive or anxiety disorders.[34,35] In the psychosocial realm, an adjustment disorder in response to a crisis such as death, loss, failure, disappointment, or breakup of a relationship can include depression and/or anxiety. The initial symptoms of depression or anxiety may be intense, but generally lessen or resolve on a timetable that often depends on the person's coping ability and the amount of available social support. Serious, often chronic psychosocial stressors, such as childhood maltreatment, severely dysfunctional family life, grief overload, poverty, or homelessness, can cause long-lasting or recurrent disorders such as dysthymia, cyclothymia, bipolar disorder, major depressive disorder, anxiety, and phobia disorders, including PTSD. Thus, common psychosocial etiologies may be the link between simultaneous depressive and anxiety disorders in a patient. For example, as pointed out in Chapter 11, persistent sexual abuse in childhood or adolescence can produce a range of recurrent or chronic anxiety disorders in adults, such as panic attack, PTSD, various phobias, obsessive-compulsive disorder, or a chronic generalized anxiety disorder. In addition, such abuse can trigger a range of other psychiatric disorders, dissociative identity disorder, somatic disorders, or sexual dysfunctions, to mention a few. Similarly, as shown in Chapter 10, ongoing domestic violence can trigger concurrent depressive and anxiety disorders.

Depressive Disorders

Sometimes health care providers receive vague or contradictory signals from depressed patients about their mental condition. Part of the difficulty is that frequently patients themselves are unable to identify their internal processes. For example, patients may report a single symptom, such as fatigue, anorexia and weight loss, insomnia, or gastrointestinal symptoms. These nonspecific symptoms may lead the health care provider to pursue a medical workup. Other patients may make vague statements like "I just can't seem to get going." In both cases, the health care provider may disregard the possibility of treatable depression. While not ignoring the possibility of biomedical problems, the health care provider

should also include questions about psychosocial stressors in the patient's clinical history interview. One way to allay a patient's fear of stigma or of revealing secrets is to normalize the situation. A nonthreatening statement like "everybody has stress these days" can be followed by "what is stressful in your life right now?" Subsequent questions can focus on how stress affects work performance and relationships at home. This leads into queries about how a stressor affects the patient's own behavioral patterns and how the patient feels about these effects. For depression, probing for the four **vegetative signs of depression** is an effective way to get a profile of a patient's functioning level (Box 12-6). Answers to these questions will allow the practitioner to gauge the severity of impairment fairly easily. Another way to gauge the severity of depression is to use the 21-item Beck Depression Scale.[36] While no laboratory studies can definitely diagnose major depression, specific testing can rule out other medical conditions that may mimic or exacerbate depression. These tests include complete blood count, chemistry profile, urinalysis, thyroid function, and serum B_{12} and folate levels.[37]

While the four vegetative signs are fairly reliable indicators of depression for adults, you may need to look for other or additional indicators in children, adolescents, and elderly persons. Chapter 11 discussed changes in developmentally appropriate behavior in children in response to maltreatment. Depressed children

---

Box12-6 Vegetative Signs of Depression

1. Change in eating patterns: eating more or constantly; or no interest in eating, no appetite; or craving sweets or chocolates
2. Change in sleeping patterns: disturbed sleep patterns, waking up, not being able to go to sleep, early morning awakening, oversleeping
3. Low energy: unable to get out of bed or get going, unwilling to go to work or school
4. Anhedonia: inability to enjoy, especially food, sex, life, the company of others

may suddenly become very shy or quiet or more introverted. Some also regress in development, exhibiting such behaviors as bed wetting, clinging behavior, or fear of the dark. Such changes in behavior should prompt questions about recent losses or possible maltreatment.

Depression in many adolescents can often be gauged fairly well by the four vegetative signs, that is, changes in eating and sleeping, anhedonia, and lowered energy levels. However, some adolescents react paradoxically to depression. Instead of becoming more quiet and withdrawn, they may act out aggressively, fighting with parents, siblings, and fellow-students. Instead of **anhedonia**, they may engage in hedonistic or risk-taking activities, becoming sexually promiscuous and abusing substances or engaging in self-injurious behaviors, such as cutting themselves. Emotional volatility of adolescence can exaggerate mood disturbance to the point of suicide risk over the breakup of a relationship or the death of a friend. Hence, a necessary question when you have identified depression in an adolescent has to be "are you thinking of hurting yourself?" If the answer is yes, it is essential to follow up to assess the seriousness of the threat with questions about whether the person has any concrete plans and to develop a safety plan or a **no-suicide contract**, sometimes also known as **contract for life**. If the patient refuses a safety plan and a no-suicide contract, immediate hospitalization is indicated.

Although adolescents are especially at risk for suicidal ideation and attempts, health care providers should assess for suicide whenever they note a cluster of the factors listed in Box 12-7. Ask these questions: Have you ever thought of hurting yourself? Have you ever been suicidal? Any positive responses should prompt the following:

- A thorough examination of a patient's mental state
- An inquiry about depressive symptoms, suicidal thoughts, intents, plans, and attempts
- Taken together, a lack of future plans, giving away personal property, making a will, and having recently experienced a loss generally indicate increased risk of suicide[38]

Box12-7 Factors Associated with Suicide Risk	
RANK ORDER	FACTOR
1	Age (45 and older)
2	Alcohol dependence
3	Irritation, rage, violence
4	Prior suicidal behavior
5	Male
6	Unwilling to accept help
7	Longer than usual duration of current episode of depression
8	Prior inpatient psychiatric treatment
9	Recent loss or separation
10	Depression
11	Loss of physical health
12	Unemployed or retired
13	Single, widowed, or divorced

Reprinted with permission from Kaplan HI, Sadock BJ (1998) *Synopsis of Psychiatry* (8th Ed) Baltimore, MD: Lippincott, Williams, & Wilkins, 870.

If clear indications exist that the patient is suicidal, the next step is to discuss hospitalization. Other options include intensive outpatient treatment depending on the amount of social support available for the patient. Creating a safety plan related to the no-suicide contract is an essential part of treatment for a person who exhibits suicidal ideation.

DEPRESSION IN THE ELDERLY

Depressive disorders are fairly common in elderly persons but are often misattributed to aging by both the patient and the health care provider.[39] (They are present in about 15% of older persons in adult community settings and in nursing homes.)[40] Somatic symptoms may be due to coexisting chronic medical conditions and age-related changes. When major depression coexists with dementia, it can make an accurate differential diagnosis difficult, because dementia in its early stages mimics depression.[41] Many commonly prescribed drugs, including antihypertensives, hormones, anticonvulsants, steroids, digitalis, antiparkinsonian agents (levodopa), antineoplastic agents, and reserpine for therapeutic use with hypertension and psychotic states, can bring on depression. Similarly, stimulants, when withdrawn, produce a depressive syndrome. Causes of depression are listed in Box 12-8.

Selected medical disorders that may cause depression in the elderly include neurologic disorders like Parkinson's disease, multi-infarct dementia, stroke, and Alzheimer's disease. Also, mood disorders can accompany debilitating disorders and diseases such as cancer, leukemia, cardiovascular disorders, endocrine disorders of hypothyroidism and hyperthyroidism, Cushing's disease, Addison's disease, malnutrition, metabolic disorders, and viral infections, such as hepatitis and herpes zoster. Chronic pain from arthritis or cancer can lead to alcohol or drug abuse and depression.

In the psychosocial arena, multiple losses, ranging from deaths of spouses and cohort friends to loss of health and independence, are common causes of vegetative signs of depression in the elderly (see Chapter 8). Loss of appetite can lead to nutritional deficits and contribute to feelings of low energy. Anhedonia can lead to withdrawal from social interaction. Nutritional deficits, lack of social interaction, and certain drug interactions can produce pseudo-dementia. When someone responds to questions with "I don't know" or "I don't care" in a flat and unemotional voice, it may be an indication of both pseudo-dementia and depression.

An elderly person with symptoms of major depression is also likely to have a history of episodes of depression or even lifelong dysthymia. Since the usual age of onset of depression is before age 40, an apparent first episode of depression in an older patient should prompt a thorough evaluation to exclude other underlying

---

Box 12-8   Causes of Depression
MEDICAL AND NEUROLOGICAL

Neurological	Alzheimer's disease, dementia, epilepsy, migraines
Systemic	Viral and bacterial infections
Endocrine	Menses related, postpartum, hypothyroidism
Inflammatory	Systemic lupus erythematosus, rheumatoid arthritis
Vitamin deficiencies	Folate, vitamin B_{12}
Other	Cancer, renal disease, AIDS

PHARMACOLOGICAL

Cardiac and antihypertensive medications	Clonidine, digitalis
Sedatives and hypnotics	Barbiturates, benzodiazepines
Steroids and hormones	Corticosteroids, oral contraceptives
Stimulants and appetite suppressants	Amphetamine
Psychotropic drugs	Butyrophenones
Neurological agents	Levodopa, baclofen
Analgesics and anti-inflammatory drugs	Ibuprofen, opioids
Antibacterial and antifungal drugs	Ampicillin, tetracycline, streptomycin
Antineoplastic drugs	C-Asparaginase, vincristine
Miscellaneous drugs	Choline, anticholinesterases

This box is representative rather than exhaustive. Adapted from detailed tables of causes of depression in Kaplan HI, Sadock BJ. *Synopsis of Psychiatry* 8th Ed. Philadelphia, PA: Lippincott Williams & Wilkins. 1998, 530-531.

disease and medication effects.[42] Careful attention must be given to the medical history and medications to see if the onset of depressive symptoms coincided with the initiation of new medication or changes in the current regimen.[43]

● ●

PATIENT PROFILE 12.2

EVERYTHING'S JUST FINE

SETTING: Amelia is an 87-year-old widow who came to the United States from Austria at age 36. She has lived alone for many years in a small house in the suburbs of a large city. For the past 30 years, she has received all of her health care needs from the same physician. Her annual check-ups have become special occasions. She has her hair done the day before and spends the morning of her appointment carefully choosing her outfit and getting her makeup just right.

Dr. Branch: Hello, Amelia. It is good to see you. You look so well and so young! How do you do it?

Amelia: (Radiating cheerfulness.) This is a new dress. It was such a good deal I couldn't pass it up. *(I must remember to tell my children that the doctor had marveled at how well I am doing and how young I look.)*

(Small talk ensues, during which she tells him with a warm and cheerful smile that everything is just fine.)

Dr. Branch: *(I know she just loves to visit and this is a social event for her, but I must get on with the physical examination.)* Let's get started with your examination, Amelia.

After completion of the physical examination, Dr. Branch records his findings while Amelia is helped by the nurse to dress. Dr. Branch notes that Amelia has had a weight loss of 30 pounds over the past 3 years, which has accelerated since her last annual visit. In reviewing her medical history, he pays attention to the number and frequency of falls she has had; the most recent fall resulted in a fracture of the left hip. He continues to read on and reviews the discharge summary from that hospitalization, which reports "advanced osteoporosis, depres-

sion, and nutritional deficits." He recalls that all of her children live out of state and she has few surviving friends for social contact. He will take extra time with Amelia today and carefully discuss his concerns, including a discussion of depression and weight loss; talk with her about the laboratory procedures she needs; and how social and community resources can help her.

Points to Consider

- Dr. Branch realizes how important it is for him to establish rapport with Amelia, and he recognizes the significance of the visit to her.

- He reviews previous notes from routine office visits as well as discharge summaries from recent hospitalizations.

- Depression is one of the most common reversible causes of weight loss in the elderly, so Dr. Branch will address the depression and her weight loss.

- Dr. Branch will communicate to his office staff to initiate contact with the appropriate community resources.

● ●

Anxiety Disorders

Anxiety is the other commonly seen disorder in primary care. Anxiety disorders cause great distress and can severely impair functioning. In general, the various anxiety disorders and conditions are distinguished by the symptoms, the objects or events feared, and the stressors (Box 12-9). The psychosocial causes of anxiety disorders generally include a precipitating event or stimulus to which an appropriate response is fear. It becomes an anxiety disorder when the specific fear becomes generalized, free floating, and persistent.

Physical symptoms of anxiety can manifest as tachycardia, chest pain, dyspnea, dizziness, muscle tension, headache, tingling or numbness in extremities, nausea, epigastric pain, frequent urination, and excessive sweating. Substance

Box 12-9 Symptoms of Anxiety

These are usually rated none, mild, moderate, or severe for the past week, including today.

1. Difficulty breathing, fast breathing, or choking
2. Trembling inside or outside
3. Heart racing or pounding
4. Numbness or tingling in extremities
5. Feeling hot (sweating)
6. Agitated, irritable
7. Shaky or wobbly on feet
8. Fears of impending doom or future calamity
9. Unable to relax
10. Feeling terrified, scared
11. Nauseous or nervous stomach, knot in the gut area
12. Cold sweats
13. Dizzy, light-headed, feeling faint
14. Fears of dying, losing control, passing out
15. Face flushed

intoxication, over-the-counter cold preparations, caffeine, and prescribed medications can precipitate anxiety symptoms. As discussed in Chapter 9, abuse of and/or withdrawal from after heavy chronic use of any of these substances can also produce anxiety attacks. Similarly, too much caffeine can produce caffeine intoxication, with jumpiness, irritability, tachycardia, fast breathing, and jumbled thoughts.[44] Certain drugs, either singly or in interaction, can cause some of the symptoms of anxiety. Also a number of medical disorders can mimic anxiety symptoms: endocrine disorders, such as hypothyroidism, hyperthyroidism, and hypoglycemia; cardiovascular problems and arrhythmias; pulmonary embolism; and some neurologic disorders. The challenge of assessing anxiety symptoms lies in deciding how much diagnostic testing and how many procedures may be appropriate to rule out medical problems. Knowledge of the medical diseases that can produce or mimic anxiety disorders can help you make an accurate diagnosis and avoid unnecessary testing. Early recognition

of an anxiety disorder can reduce the patient's discomfort, medical expenses, iatrogenic complications, and anxiety-related complications. Prompt diagnosis can also reduce substance abuse, as many patients self-medicate with alcohol and benzodiazepines to reduce their anxiety symptoms.[45] A short standardized screening questionnaire, the Beck Anxiety Inventory (BAI) can be used for the assessment of anxiety.[46]

After organic or drug-induced causes of the patient's anxiety (Box 12-10) have been ruled out, look for causes in the psychosocial history of the patient. From the psychosocial perspective, anxiety disorders can be more difficult to identify than depression. One reason is that the range of symptoms for anxiety disorders is more extensive and less coherent than those for depression. Fear of being stigmatized is another reason many patients, especially men, are reluctant to disclose an anxiety or panic disorder. Thus, you must listen closely for descriptive statements of feelings or body sensations when you elicit the symptoms and the psychosocial factors from the patient. Statements like these are red flags: "My heart feels like it is racing sometimes." "I feel smothered." "I can't catch my breath." "I worry all the time." "My nerves are so bad." Such remarks should prompt you to follow up: "What has been going on just before you felt this way?" "Is it hard for you to breathe sometimes?" "What do you worry about?" "Do you feel nervous?" Sometimes men refer to a knot in their gut or throat. Women often say they feel fearful and shaky. Women who are in abusive situations may exhibit signs of anxiety and depression simultaneously.

Anxiety can have its roots in the remote past and be cognitively inaccessible. This may make it necessary to probe the patient's early childhood. For example, as pointed out in Chapter 3, disruption in the parent–infant attachment through abandonment, neglect, or abuse can produce anxious ambivalent attachment patterns. Similarly, early childhood diseases, such as asthma, epilepsy, cancer, and heart disorders, or long hospitalizations at an early age can produce an adult burdened with anxiety and various phobias.

Box 12-10 Disorders Associated with Anxiety

NEUROLOGICAL DISORDERS
Cerebral neoplasms
Cerebral trauma, postconcussive
syndromes
Cerebrovascular disease
Subarachnoid hemorrhage
Migraine
Encephalitis
Cerebral syphilis
Multiple sclerosis
Wilson's disease
Huntington's disease
Epilepsy

SYSTEMIC CONDITIONS
Hypoxia
Cardiovascular disease
Cardiac arrhythmias
Pulmonary insufficiency
Anemia
Endocrine disturbances
Pituitary dysfunction
Thyroid dysfunction
Parathyroid dysfunction
Adrenal dysfunction
Pheochromocytoma

Virilization disorders of females
Inflammatory disorders
Lupus erythematosus
Rheumatoid arthritis
Polyarteritis nodosa
Temporal arteritis

DEFICIENCY STATES
Vitamin B deficiency
Pellagra

MISCELLANEOUS DISORDERS
Hypoglycemia
Carcinoid syndrome
Systemic malignancies
Premenstrual syndrome

**FEBRILE ILLNESSES AND
CHRONIC INFECTIONS**
Porphyria
Infectious mononucleosis
Posthepatitis syndrome
Uremia

TOXIC CONDITIONS
Alcohol and drug withdrawal
Amphetamines

Sympathomimetic agents
Vasopressor agents
Caffeine and caffeine withdrawal
Penicillin
Sulfonamides
Cannabis
Mercury
Arsenic
Phosphorus
Organophosphates
Carbon disulfide
Benzene
Aspirin intolerance
Neurotoxic poisoning

**IDIOPATHIC PSYCHIATRIC
DISORDERS**
Depression
Mania
Schizophrenia
Anxiety disorders
Generalized anxiety
Panic attacks
Phobic disorders
Posttraumatic stress disorder

Adapted from Cumming JL (1985) *Clinical Neuropsychiatry.* Orlando FL: Grune & Stratton, 214.

*ANXIETY DISORDERS IN CHILDREN AND
ADOLESCENTS*

According to some observers, anxiety disorders may be more common in children and adolescents now than 50 years ago.[47] The principal causes for this increase seem to be mostly psychosocial. Higher divorce rates causing family disruptions and frequent relocations may be factors. But the perception that the world is a more dangerous place as a result of terrorist activities, school shootings, and television violence may also contribute to the higher rates of anxiety among children and adolescents.[48] Anxiety in children and adolescents may not cause the same signs and symptoms as in adults. In children, anxiety may produce signs of behavioral inhibition, so that the child may appear extremely cautious, fearful, and introverted. Physical symptoms in children include nausea, stomach aches, diarrhea, and headaches. In adolescents, health care providers may see the opposite behavior, that is, emotionally labile or unstable behavior with angry outbursts, frequent fighting, substance abuse, or acting out sexually. Note the similarity of some of these signs of anxiety with those for depression in adolescents. Often these signs are linked by common roots in childhood trauma, such as physical or sexual abuse. Hence, follow-up questions should probe for early trauma, and if it is suspected, the protocols for handling child maltreatment should be instituted as presented in Chapter 11. When nothing in the psychosocial history of a child or adolescent seems to justify impulsive, risk-taking, or acting-out behaviors, the health care provider should consider the possibility of attention deficit disorder with or without hyperactivity (ADD/ADHD).[49]

ANXIETY IN THE ELDERLY

The medical and organic causes of anxiety in the elderly are for the most part the same as for anyone else. In addition, because of the fragility of their autonomic nervous system, older persons may be more susceptible to anxiety disorders after the occurrence of a major stressor. Also, if there is a concurrent physical disability, older persons may have more severe symptoms of PTSD.[50] Because many elderly patients are on multiple medications, often from different providers, you need to be vigilant about drug interaction. The problems created by multiple providers writing prescriptions for the same patient can be alleviated if one provider is designated as the primary care physician and all prescriptions are routed through that person. However, as a safety precaution, you should ask your elderly patients to bring into the office all prescription and over-the-counter medications and any food supplements or herbal remedies once every 2 or 3 months. Often a provider will be able to spot several compounds that should not be mixed.

Many older persons develop fears and anxiety disorders caused by psychosocial factors. For example, living alone in a high-crime inner-city neighborhood can trigger agoraphobia and other anxiety disorders. Some older persons who fear dying or dying alone may become anxious. Also about 10% of frail elderly persons are subjected to **elder abuse**. This is defined by the American Medical Association as "an act or omission that results in harm or threatened harm to the health or welfare of an elderly person."[51] Depending on the severity, elder abuse can cause psychoemotional symptoms ranging from resignation, depression, mental confusion, insomnia, fear, agitation, and anxiety attacks to PTSD.[52] Anxiety disorders in elderly persons in dependent living

environments may be signs of abuse by a caretaker or a relative.

Treatment and Referral

Many mental disorders occur as a result of or in combination with a wide range of organic, somatic, and psychosocial conditions. This is true especially of mood and anxiety disorders. Boxes 12-8 and 12-10 illustrate the large number of medical and neurologic conditions that can cause or be comorbid with depressive and anxiety disorders, respectively. In cases of genetic or lifelong conditions, such as recurrent major depression, you may have to address the deficits of neurotransmitters with an appropriate psychotropic medication. If you can identify psychosocial stressors from the distant past or in the present as causative factors for the patient's mental disorder or disorders, you may have to take a combination approach. The patient may need pharmacological relief for the mental and emotional anguish. The patient also may need psychotherapy to address maladaptive behavioral patterns and to explore and resolve psychological issues.

Sometimes the screening process reveals complex long-term comorbid substance abuse and/or other mental disorders. In such cases, the primary health care provider should consult with or refer the patient to a mental health or substance abuse specialist for more comprehensive assessment and recommendations on treatment options. Such options may include hospitalization in a mental health emergency (suicide risk, severe substance dependence, or loss of functioning ability as determined by a GAF score of less than 30). However, what might be the ideal or even required treatment option from a combined professional perspective may not always be acceptable to the patient. For example, patients may refuse appropriate treatment for a variety of reasons ranging from denial of the problem (as in substance abuse) and fear of financial costs, to the inability to recognize and act in their own best interest. In the case of suicide planning or attempts, it is mandatory that you proceed with involuntary hospitalization. Most states require that a complete psychiatric evaluation be performed by a mental health specialist (psychiatrist, psychologist, or clinical social worker) before permitting such involuntary commitment. Sometimes a patient refuses a recommendation for hospitalization when the situation is considered urgent but not life threatening, such as in substance abuse, a major depressive episode, a manic episode, or severe anxiety or panic disorders. In such instances, you may wish to form an assessment team comprising a mental health specialist and a social worker brought in on a consulting or referral basis. The mental health specialist conducts a comprehensive mental assessment, and the social worker assesses the patient's functioning in the psychosocial environment. If both assessments agree that the patient's level of functioning in the cognitive, social, and/or professional spheres is seriously impaired (GAF score of 50 or less), you can make a collaborative effort to persuade the patient that it would be in his or her best interest to be hospitalized. If the patient's family was involved in bringing the patient in for assessment and treatment, you might ask the social worker to convene a family conference. The purpose of this process is similar to the purpose described in Chapter 8 for deciding the level of care for an older person or the confrontation of a substance abuser described in Chapter 9. Each participant would be asked to come from a caring perspective and state how the patient's behaviors and functioning have changed or have adversely affected the person speaking. The primary care provider, mental health specialist, social worker, and possibly a clergy person each give a professional assessment and recommendations for treatment. If all goes well, the patient will be persuaded to enter the hospital. If the patient refuses or is cognitively impaired to the point of not being able to understand the full import of the impairment or to render an informed decision, the family and the health care team can initiate proceedings for an involuntary commitment.

In less urgent situations, partial hospitalization may be appropriate. This usually entails daytime attendance for treatment activities, such as individual and group psychotherapy. In other instances, a combination of psychotherapy and regular appointments with the primary care provider to monitor and adjust psychotropic medications will be sufficient. In cases of adjustment disorders with either depressive or anxious features, short-term pharmacological treatment may be sufficient. Because of the multiplicity of psychoactive drugs and rapid innovations in pharmacological remedies for mental disorders, this book does not contain a discussion of specific medications. However, antidepressants are conveniently classified into three groups: 1) the antidepressants, including the serotonin-selective reuptake inhibitors (SSRIs), such as fluoxetine and sertraline; 2) the tricyclic antidepressants (TCAs), such as amitriptyline and desipramine, and 3) monoamine oxidase inhibitors, such as phenelzine and tranylcypromine.[53] Before choosing an appropriate psychotropic medication and deciding on a dosage regimen, you must evaluate the patient for any possible adverse interactions with other prescription drugs, over-the-counter medications, and herbal remedies the patient might be taking. After a patient begins the regimen, it is critical that you closely monitor both effectiveness and side effects. You need feedback from the patient (and possibly family members) on whether the medication is having the desired effect or is producing intolerable or dangerous side effects. You may find that patients metabolize mood-altering medication in highly individual ways, depending on neurologic tolerance developed by previous use or abuse of prescription drugs or other substances, tissue-retained neurotoxins, or idiosyncratic biochemical sensitivity. In some instances, patients may have paradoxical effects from a class of drugs. For example, certain SSRIs, rather than lift depression, can cause obsessive rumination about suicide or violence.[54] In addition, fluoxetine has been known to cause life-threatening ventricular arrhythmias in depressed patients with heart disease.[55] In such cases, you must be prompt and flexible to switch to another class of antidepressant drugs. In the elderly, decreased hepatic and renal clearance and decreased gastrointestinal absorption rates necessitate special attention when you prescribe drugs of any kind. For older persons, it is recommended that the lowest possible dose is prescribed to achieve the desired therapeutic effect.[56] In general, health care providers should be aware that assessment for symptomatic changes as well as for side effects needs to be pursued after pharmacological treatment has begun.

CONTINUITY OF CARE

Any decision about referral and/or treatment must take into account the principle of continuity of care. Arrangements for aftercare are especially critical after psychiatric hospitalization. Patients may need supportive counseling and other assistance as they come out of the hospital and make the transition back into their communities. Such aftercare plans should include periodic review conferences or contacts between treatment team members. In cases of patients with severe mental disorders, such a team may include a case manager, family members, a primary care team member, and possibly a community advocacy representative. Each member of this treatment team plays a vital role in at least one of the essential components of treatment: medication compliance, focused counseling, and social and living support.

Continuity of care is especially important for those with serious mental disorders, many of whom become homeless.[57] There is a reciprocal relationship between mental illness and substance abuse and homelessness. A person who becomes socially and occupationally dysfunctional through mental illness or substance abuse tends to lapse into poverty and become homeless unless that person has a strong and dedicated family or social support network.[58] In fact, surveys show that 66% to 84% of the homeless report having mental illness and/or substance abuse problems.[59]

Ensuring that patients receive continuity of care regardless of ability to pay is an ethical obligation of all health care professionals. However, arranging such care becomes easier if you are familiar with the range of publicly financed services available in your area. Federal and state programs finance a wide range of services for persons with chronic mental disorders or mental retardation.[60] For example, under Medicaid funding, community mental health clinics and private companies offer **assisted living** services and adult day care programs designed to normalize the functioning of persons with mental retardation or developmental disabilities. Such programs teach daily living skills and offer **supported** or **sheltered employment** programs to help such persons maintain semi-independent or group living. **Habilitation aides**, assigned either part time or around the clock, assist in providing good nutrition and personal hygiene. They also ensure that the persons are compliant with their medication regimens and get to their appointments with health care providers for monitoring blood levels of key medications and for periodic assessments of their functional abilities. Well-functioning assisted living programs in combination with effective psychotropic medications are the best way to keep persons with chronic mental disorders functional in the community and out of the ranks of the homeless.[61]

● ●

PATIENT PROFILE 12.3

WHAT ARE THEY DOING WITH MY BLOOD?

Setting: Paul is a 45-year-old single man with chronic schizophrenia. He is generally physically healthy but often becomes noncompliant with his medications around the holidays. His behavior deteriorates; his paranoia increases; and sometimes he requires hospitalization. He recently was hospitalized, during which he stabilized on medication. After 2 weeks he was discharged. He has an appointment at the mental health clinic today for follow-up with his nurse practitioner, Carol. She has been managing his mental illness for 7 years now.

Carol: Hello, Paul. How are you today?

Paul: So-so. I don't like that hospital. They're mean. They don't let you smoke but twice a day.

Carol: Hmmmm. That must be hard for you. It's probably because a staff person is required to go outside with you when you smoke. You know the routine and the importance of supervision.

Paul: Yeah, I know, but it is irritating.

Carol: I am sure it is. Let's talk about your medications now. I understand you are back on Clozaril. How are you doing now that you are taking Clozaril?

Paul: OK, but I don't like getting weekly blood taken out. What do they do with all my blood anyway? *(Oh, boy. That sure sounds paranoid. But I think Carol knows me well enough not to put me back into the hospital for what I said.)* You understand that I am not just being paranoid.

Carol: (Smiles to relieve his concern about his statement.) Yes, I understand that you have a normal concern about the blood being taken. We take blood samples to be sure you are receiving the right amount of Clozaril for it to help you. It can also cause changes in your blood cells, so we check for that too. That is all we do with your blood.

Paul: Oh yes, I remember that now.

Carol: Have you gone back to your partial hospitalization program?

Paul: Not yet, but I will, starting Monday next week.

Carol: Good.

Points to Consider

- Carol reconnects with Paul knowing how important continued rapport is for him and his abilities to trust her.
- Carol realizes that Paul's medication regimen is an essential aspect for maintaining his stability. Asking about how he is doing on the Clozaril is important for Carol to identify.
- When Carol explains why she is taking his blood, she reaffirms the logic and importance of regular blood checkups.

- Carol realizes the importance of the partial hospitalization program for Paul and by asking him about it, reinforces its importance to Paul.

● ●

Conclusion

This chapter focuses mainly on depression and anxiety because these disorders are common in the general population and in primary care practice. This chapter does not provide detail on the wide variety of mental disorders described in DSM-IV. Unless you have received extended training in psychiatry, diagnosis and treatment of many of the other mental disorders will be beyond your level of clinical expertise. However, some of the less common mental disorders will present in your practice. When you recognize the unknown and/or are uncertain of the correct diagnosis, the right next step is to seek consultation or referral.

In keeping with the holistic orientation of the mind–body connection, it is important to reiterate that psychosocial stressors not only may cause mental disorders but also can produce a wide range of physical symptoms known as somatization. With awareness that the body is often the battleground for struggles within the mind, the health care provider will find that a whole host of physical symptoms can stem from mental problems that are being played out in the body. Somatization is at the intersection of mental and physical problems. Because of the mind–body connection, psychological distress often manifests as physical symptoms (somatization). Conversely, frequently physical symptoms or behaviors are produced either consciously or unconsciously by a chronic mental disorder. This connection is dealt with in the next chapter.

REFERENCES

1. Ballweg R, Stolberg S, Sullivan ME (1999). *Physician Assistant: A Guide to Clinical Practice* (2nd ed). Philadelphia: Saunders.
2. American Association of Family Physicians (1996). Position Paper on the Provisions of

Mental Health Care Services by Family Physicians. Available at: http://www.aafp.org/practice/mentalhe.thtml.

3. Staab JP et al. (2001). Detection and diagnosis of psychiatric disorders in primary care settings. *Med Clin North Am*, 3:579–596.

4. US Public Health Service (1999). *Mental Health: A Report of the Surgeon General*. Washington: US Dept of Health and Human Services. Chapter 1.

5. Skaer TL, Robison LM et al. (2000). Anxiety Disorders in the USA 1990–1997: Trend in Complaint, Diagnosis, Use of Pharmacotherapy and Diagnosis of Comorbid Depression. *Clin Drug Investing*. 20,4:237–244.

6. Sartorium N, Ustun TB, Lecrubier Y, et al. (1996). Depression comorbid with anxiety: results from the WHO study on psychological disorders in primary health care. *Br J Psychiatry*, 169 (suppl 30):38–43.

7. Kaplan HI, Sadock BJ (1998). *Synopsis of Psychiatry* (8th ed). Philadelphia: Lippincott, Williams & Wilkins, p 2.

8. MacDonald S (2001). Court grants confidentiality to EAP records. *EAP Assoc Exchange* 31:24.

9. Kaplan & Sadock (1998). *Synopsis of Psychiatry*, 8th ed. Philadelphia: Lippincott, Williams & Wilkins, 629.

10. Dossey L (1999). *Reinventing Medicine: Beyond Mind-Body to a New Era of Healing*. San Francisco: Harper Collins, 91–95.

11. Platt FW, Gordon GH (1999). Common Problems in Interviewing. In *Field Guide to the Difficult Patient Interview*. Philadelphia: Lippincott, 12–15.

12. American Psychiatric Association (1994) Diagnostic and Statistical Manual of Mental Disorders, Fourth Edition. (Hereafter cited as *DSM-IV*). Washington, DC: APA Press, xxi.

13. *DSM-IV*, p 25.

14. *DSM-IV*, p xxi.

15. *DSM-IV*, p xxi.

16. *DSM-IV*, pp xxi–xxii.

17. *DSM-IV*, p 25.

18. *DSM-IV*, p 26.

19. *DSM-IV*, p 29.

20. Kaplan HI, Sadock BJ (1998) *Synopsis of Psychiatry*, 8th ed. Philadelphia: Lippincott, Williams & Wilkins, 275.

21. Kaplan HI, Sadock BJ (1998) *Synopsis of Psychiatry*, 8th ed. Philadelphia: Lippincott, Williams & Wilkins, 250.

22. Folstein MF, Folstein S, McHugh PR (1975): Mini-mental state: A practical method for grading the cognitive state of patients for the clinician. *J Psychiatr Res* 12:89, 1975.

23. Kaplan HI, Sadock BJ (1998) *Synopsis of Psychiatry*, 8th ed. Philadelphia: Lippincott, Williams & Wilkins, 318.

24. Staab JP, Evans DL (2001). A streamlined method for diagnosing common psychiatric disorders in primary care. *Clin Cornerstone* 3:1–9.

25. American Psychiatric Association (1995). *Diagnostic and Statistical Manual of Mental Disorders: Primary Care Version*. Washington: American Psychiatric Association.

26. Staab JP, et al (2001) Detection and diagnosis of psychiatric disorders in primary care settings. *Med Clin North America*, 85(3):581.

27. Shedler J, Beck A, Bensen S (2000). Practical mental health assessment in primary care: Validity and utility of the PsychoDiagnostics Panel. *J Family Pract* 49:614–621.

28. Spitzer RL et al. (1994). Utility of a procedure For diagnosing in primary care: The PRIME-MD 1000 study. *JAMA* 272:1794.

29. Spitzer RL, Kroenke K, Williams JB (1999). Validation and utility of a self-report version of PRIME-MD: The PHQ Primary Care Study. *JAMA* 282:1737.

30. Shedler J, Beck A, Bensen S (2000). Practical mental health assessment in primary care: Validity and utility of the PsychoDiagnostics Panel. *J Family Pract* 49:614–621.

31. The QPD is available from Digital Diagnostics, Inc. 225 N. Mill St., Aspen, CO 81611.

32. *DSM-IV*, 317–392.

33. *DSM-IV*, 393–426.

34. Shoemaker RC, Hudnell HK (2001). Possible estuary-associated syndrome: Symptoms, vision, and treatment. *Environ Health Perspect*, 109:539–545.

35. Morris JG (2201). Human health effects and Pfiesteria exposure: a synthesis of available data. *Environ Health Persp*, 109 (Suppl 5):787–790.

36. Psychological Corporation. Beck Depression Inventory (BDI), available from Psychological Corporation, 555 Academic Court, San Antonio, TX 78204.

37. Feldman MD, Christensen JF (1997). *Behavioral Medicine in Primary Care: A Practical Guide* Stamford CT: Appleton and Lange. 181.

38. Kaplan HI, Sadock BJ (1998) *Synopsis of Psychiatry*, 8th ed. Philadelphia: Lippincott, Williams & Wilkins, 870.
39. Merck, Sharp & Dohme (2000). *The Merck Manual of Geriatrics*. Rahway, NJ: Merck Research Laboratories. 311, 313.
40. Kaplan HI, Sadock BJ (1998) *Synopsis of Psychiatry*, 8th ed. Philadelphia: Lippincott, Williams & Wilkins, 1295.
41. Feldman MD, Christensen JF (1997). *Behavioral Medicine in Primary Care: A Practical Guide*. Stamford CT: Appleton & Lange, p 182.
42. Feldman MD, Christensen JF (1997). *Behavioral Medicine in Primary Care: A Practical Guide*. Stamford CT: Appleton & Lange, p 178.
43. Feldman MD, Christensen JF (1997). *Behavioral Medicine in Primary Care: A Practical Guide*. Stamford CT: Appleton & Lange, p 182.
44. *DSM-IV*, 212–214.
45. Knesper DJ, Riba MB, Schwenk TL (1997). *Primary Care Psychiatry*. Philadelphia: Saunders, p 166.
46. Beck Anxiety Inventory (BAI), available from Psychological Corporation, 555 Academic Court, San Antonio, TX 78204.
47. Twenge JM (2000). The Age of Anxiety? Birth Cohort Change in Anxiety and Neuroticism, 1952–1993. *J Personality and Social Psych*, 79, (6): 1007–1021.
48. Stossel S (1997). The Man Who Counts the Killings, *Atlantic Monthly* 274:86–104.
49. Barkley RA (1997). *ADHD and the Nature of Self Control*. New York: Guilford, 3.
50. Kaplan HI, Sadock BJ (1998) *Synopsis of Psychiatry*, 8th ed. Philadelphia: Lippincott, Williams & Wilkins, 1297.
51. Kaplan HI, Sadock BJ (1998) *Synopsis of Psychiatry*, 8th ed. Philadelphia: Lippincott, Williams & Wilkins, 1299.
52. Kaplan HI, Sadock BJ (1998) *Synopsis of Psychiatry*, 8th ed. Philadelphia: Lippincott, Williams & Wilkins, 1299.
53. Tierney LM , McPhee SJ, Papadakis MA (eds) (2002). *Current Medical Diagnosis and Treatment* (41st ed). Stamford, CT: Lange Medical Books/McGraw-Hill, 1089.
54. Gaby AR (2001). Why All the Violence? Prozac and other selective serotonin-reuptake inhibitors (SSRIs). *Townsend Letter for Doctors and Patients*, May 2001:125.
55. Roose SP, Glassman AH, et al. (1998). Cardiovascular effects of fluoxetine in depressed patients with heart disease. *Am J Psychiatry*, 155:660–665.
56. Kaplan HI, Sadock BJ (1998) *Synopsis of Psychiatry*, 8th ed. Philadelphia: Lippincott, Williams & Wilkins, 1299.
57. Drake RE, Wallach MA (1999, May). Homelessness and mental illness: A story of failure [editorial] *Psychiatr Serv* 50(5):589.
58. Dixon L, Stewart B, Krauss N, Robbins et al. (1998). The participation of families of homeless persons with severe mental illness in an outreach intervention. *Community Ment Health J*, 34(3):251–259.
59. Martha RB, Laudan YA, et al. (1999). *Homelessness: Programs and the People They Serve, Summary Report*, Findings of the National Survey of Homeless Assistance Providers and Clients. Washington: Urban Institute, Table 2.4.
60. Randolph F, Blasinsky M, Leginski W, et al. (1997, March). Creating integrated service systems for homeless persons with mental illness: The ACCESS Program. Access to community care and effective services and supports. *Psychiatr Serv* 48(3):369–73.
61. National Center for Homeless Education. 800-308-2145 or www.serve.org/nche

CHAPTER 13

Challenging Patients

This chapter focuses on treating patients whose diagnoses may require additional scrutiny from the health care provider. It highlights the differences between somatoform disorders, which are unconscious and unintentional, and factitious disorders, which are conscious and intentional. It discusses how to identify malingering, particularly focusing on the drug-seeking and disability-seeking patient. Attention is also given to the patient with borderline personality disorder. The chapter offers suggestions for specific management procedures and protocols to provide clear treatment objectives and regimens.

Introduction

Certain types of patients with mental or behavioral disorders require supplemental skills in assessment, diagnosis, and treatment. Among these patients are those with somatoform disorders, including somatization disorder, hypochondriasis, conversion disorders and pain disorders. Also requiring supplemental skills are the factitious disorders, which include factitious disorder by proxy. Every health care practice encounters patients who want to obtain prescription medications to abuse, trade, or sell. Patients known as malingerers present themselves primarily to become certified for disability or to evade some other obligation. The crisis-prone patients with borderline personality disorder are often considered the most challenging to treat or manage.

The common thread in patients with somatoform or factitious disorders is that they present with signs and symptoms of medical conditions that usually are not verifiable with medical diag-

nostic procedures. Thus, diagnosing and treating patients from these categories is often frustrating. Over time, health care providers may lose empathy for them as persons. Instead, they begin to apply such stereotypes as liars, freeloaders, or malingerers to patients. Such labels can create negative feelings toward other patients. For example, resentment over having been misled or tricked by drug-seeking patients to prescribe opioids for what may be feigned back pain may make the health care provider suspicious about the next patient who complains of back pain. To prevent losing objectivity and respect and to protect yourself from liability problems that such patients can engender, you need to understand these disorders and know how to manage them effectively and objectively. Although the prevalence of each of these disorders is low—generally 5% or less—the cases you will encounter are likely to be memorable because they test your skills, patience, and professionalism. This chapter describes and explains these disorders and/or behaviors, ways to identify them, and management strategies for working with such patients.

Somatoform Disorders

Somatoform disorders are characterized by patients' reports of physical symptoms that suggest a medical disorder but that cannot be fully explained by that medical disorder, by substance abuse, or by any other mental disorder.[1] Managed care studies have noted that as many as 50% of patients walking into primary care settings are the *worried well*, who have some physical symptom or symptoms that they want checked out medically. Generally these patients are reassured if the findings of a physical examination and/or medical tests reveal no pathology.[2] However, when standard physical examinations and diagnostic procedures do not reveal a bona fide medical condition, such patients may insist that the condition is real and may demand more tests. Indeed some with symptoms that are seemingly unverifiable may have any of the wide range of symptoms shown in Box 13-1, which can be caused by endogenous or exogenous toxins.[3] Neurotoxins are particularly insidious because they prefer the lipid environment to the bloodstream. As such, they may persist or accumulate in a variety of tissues, escaping detection by standard medical tests. The number of biotoxins that can cause these symptoms is expanding rapidly, and so is the potential for exposure. Lyme disease, cylindrospermopsis, ciguatera, pfiesteria, and Stachybotrys mold are but a few of the agents that produce proinflammatory cytokines on numerous pathways.[4-6] Neurotoxins in the body degrade the functioning of the highly sensitive optic nerve.[7] A simple test measuring the degradation of visual acuity and contrast sensitivity can quickly determine whether and to what extent a person's physical systems have been affected by neurotoxins. One test is the Visual Contrast Sensitivity (VCS) examination, which detects the effects of neurotoxins on the optic nerve. A relatively simple but effective 10-day treatment uses the cholesterol-lowering drug cholestyramine to target the neurotoxins by binding them in the bile and then excreting them from the body.[8]

This short digression reinforces the principle that medical conditions must be ruled out before making a diagnosis of somatoform disorder. The multiple, changing, and persistent symptoms of patients with neurotoxic poisoning can easily be confused with either somatization disorder or possibly malingering.[9] Using a quick and inexpensive VCS test to rule out neurotoxic involvement can often relieve anxiety and frustration in both the patient and the provider. It is estimated that after those with seemingly hidden physiological or neurochemical causes are ruled out, 5% to 10% of patients in primary care settings do meet the criteria for somatoform disorders.[10]

A distinguishing characteristic of somatoform disorders (as contrasted with factitious disorders) is that they are *unintentional*. Patients with somatoform disorders *truly* believe that they have medical problems.[11] The fact that these patients usually present in medical care settings emphasizes that these patients do not see themselves as mental health clients. Instead they tend

---

Box13-1 Symptoms of Chronic Neurotoxin-Mediated Illnesses
(Can be transient, recurrent or persistent, generally appear in clusters.)

Gastrointestinal
  Irritable bowel syndrome
  Gastroenteritis
  Diarrhea
  Nausea
Sensorium
  Reduced visual acuity
  Painful to touch
Neurological
  Headaches
  Short-term memory problems
  Attention deficit disorder
  Attention deficit hyperactivity disorder

Musculoskeletal
  Aching joints
  Muscle aches
  Muscle weakness
Sleep
  Insomnia
  Fatigue
Systemic
  Persistent fevers
Respiratory, Pulmonary
  Chronic sinus congestion
  Asthma
Endocrine
  Decreased sexual drive

Psychological
  Depression
  Anxiety
  Confusion
  Inability to concentrate

Adapted with permission from Shoemaker RS. *Desperation Medicine*. Baltimore: Gateway Press, 2001.

to present repeatedly to make persistent requests for medical investigation of their physical symptoms. In cases of somatization, such investigations usually do not produce substantiating physical evidence.[12] Believing their symptoms to be real, such patients often get frustrated or even angry when informed of negative findings of physical examinations and laboratory tests. They are likely to seek out another health care provider, and if not satisfied, another and another. Because of the time, effort, and resources spent to diagnose, alleviate, or treat such conditions, patients with somatoform disorders are recognized in the medical care system as presenting special management problems.[13,14]

There are several somatoform disorders: somatization disorder, undifferentiated somatoform disorder, conversion disorder, pain disorder, hypochondriasis, body dysmorphic disorder, and somatoform disorder not otherwise specified (NOS).

SOMATIZATION DISORDER

Somatization disorder is a polysymptomatic disorder that usually sets in before age 30 and extends over years. It is characterized by pain along with gastrointestinal, sexual, and pseudoneurological symptoms. These symptoms can cause clinically significant distress or impairment in personal, social, and/or occupational areas of functioning. These symptoms are *unintentional and involuntary*. In the United States, this disorder is more common among women than men, and the incidence is higher in African-Americans than other ethnic groups. It occurs most often in patients from low socioeconomic backgrounds and low education levels. Some estimates of its prevalence are 0.13% in the general population, 5% of patients seen in family practice, 9% in hospitals, and 12% of patients with chronic pain.[15]

Etiology

Research on etiology has yielded several overlapping explanations. One psychodynamic hypothesis is that *anxious avoidant* infant attachment patterns, coupled with an early illness, can produce **illness beliefs**,[16] that is, a learned pattern of using illness to communicate or fulfill their need for personal attention.[17] Most such patients have a negative sense of self and poor interpersonal communication skills.[18] Unaware of or unable to express inner feelings, they unconsciously choose to respond to feelings of alienation, depression, anxiety, or panic by unintentionally developing and maintaining disease symptoms. Even though the production of these symptoms may be unconscious, some brain imaging studies seem to validate neurological involvement, pointing to deficits or interference with neurotransmitters in key areas of the cortex.[19] Specifically, it is suggested that faulty perception and assessment of body sensations is caused by attentional and cognitive impairments.[20] These neurological aberrations may also be genetic, as indicated by family studies.[21] Somatization disorder is usually comorbid with other psychiatric conditions, including major depressive disorder, personality disorders (antisocial, histrionic), substance-abuse–related disorders, generalized anxiety disorder, and phobias.[22]

ASSESSMENT

The attention deficits and poor interpersonal communication that are characteristic of this condition can make it difficult to obtain comprehensible data from patients. The combination of a lack of awareness of inner psychological processes and resistance to suggestions that multiple physical symptoms may be caused by mental stresses or a psychological disorder often increases the determination of these patients to prove that their problems are physical and medical.[23] For a positive diagnosis of somatization disorder, DSM-IV requires that the patient in the course of the disorder have complained of at least four pain symptoms, two gastrointestinal symptoms, one sexual symptom, and one pseudo-neurological symptom, none of which can be completely explained by physical examination or laboratory testing.[24] With such a wide range of symptoms, somatization disorder can overlap with a number of general medical conditions. To distinguish between medical conditions and somatization, DSM-IV says the following three features need to be apparent: 1) involvement of multiple organ systems, 2) early onset *without* development of physical signs or structural abnormalities, and 3) no laboratory evidence confirming the suggested medical condition.[25] Taking a complete and thorough psychosocial history ensures that a definitive differential diagnosis can be made. Of particular interest should be normative and nonnormative events in the patient's early childhood and in family of origin. Many patients with somatization disorder have close family members and other relatives with serious psychiatric disorders, such as avoidant, paranoid, self-defeating, and obsessive-compulsive features, or antisocial personality disorder. Childhood maltreatment is also common among this population, as it is with factitious disorders. Children may learn a pattern in which unexpressed and unresolved emotional distress is played out in the body without conscious knowledge of the process because they are often prevented by the abuse or dysfunctional family from developing a viable mode for voicing their emotions or developing a healthy self. As they grow into adults, some enter into violent marriages or partnerships, in which the body again becomes the battleground for the psyche.[26]

• •

PATIENT PROFILE 13.1

I JUST DON'T FEEL GOOD

Setting: *Mary is a 24-year-old married woman with two children aged 18 months and 3 years. Dr. Winter has been treating her for minor complaints over the past 2 years in his suburban office. However, in the past 3 months she has been complaining of unspecified aches and pains for which he can find no organic causes.*

Dr. Winter: Good morning, Mary. How are those two great kids you have?

Mary: Oh, they are terrific but a handful! Some days I feel like I am running after them all day.

Dr. Winter: I know how that is. So how can I help you today? *(That indeed is a good question. This is her third time in to see me this month.)*

Mary: Well, my stomach is acting up again. I have avoided the foods you told me to, but I still seem to have a lot of pain. I get headaches all the time now, and sometimes my legs feel odd—numb. I haven't been visiting my sister and her kids as much as I used to. I just don't feel like it. *(He must be tired of me coming in and complaining so much.)*

Dr. Winter: *(There is that whining tone again. I must be careful not to let it get to me.)* I am glad to hear that you avoid those spicy and gas-producing foods. First, tell me a little more about the stomach pain, and then we'll talk about your other symptoms.

Mary: Well, it starts here and then spreads to over here (moving her hand from the center of her abdomen to the left side).

Dr. Winter: Does it start at any particular time—before or after meals?

Mary: No.

Dr. Winter: How long does it last?

Mary: About half an hour.

Dr. Winter: Well, Mary, we've done about every appropriate test as necessary to evaluate your pain and nothing shows up. *(I remember her saying that her husband was picky about how she keeps house. I wonder if there is something more here, maybe domestic violence.)* How are things at home? Are you and your husband getting along all right? Sometimes when there are young children in the home, the marriage can be stressed.

Mary: *(Oh, dear, I am so embarrassed to tell him but maybe it is now or never.)* My husband, you know, uhhhh, is kind of picky about my housekeeping. I'm not a very good housekeeper. I can never seem to please him. And the two kids run around and play all day, and it's hard to clean up before he comes home in the evening.

Dr. Winter: You certainly have your hands full. Has anything particularly happened lately?

Mary: Last night when dinner wasn't ready on time, he really got mad and well, got rough.

Dr. Winter: What do you mean, rough?

Mary: He sort of pushed me.

Dr. Winter: Pushed you? How did he push you?

Mary: Here, on my chest against the wall.

Dr. Winter: That doesn't sound good. No matter what kind of a housekeeper you are, there is no excuse for violence. How long has this been going on?

Mary: Oh, ever since my second baby was born. He's also under a lot of stress at work now. These last 3 months have been worse.

Dr. Winter: *(Three months ago was when she started coming in with these aches and pains. I wonder if she and her children are safe.)* Mary, sometimes when we are under a lot of stress, the body takes on aches and pains to express how badly it feels. Do you think that might be happening here?

Mary: I don't know. I just don't feel good.

Dr. Winter: I know we also need to talk some more about the headaches and that odd feeling in your legs, but first tell me more about his behavior. *(I knew something else was going on here. I am so glad I asked her about her home situation. At least she was willing to answer my question honestly today. She may be psychosomatizing. Now we can begin to get somewhere with these other symptoms. I will need to talk more with her about assessing the safety of the children and put her in touch with the local domestic violence shelter if the violence continues or escalates.)*

Points to Consider

- Doctor reestablishes rapport with Mary by asking her about her children.
- Dr. Winter notices the tone of her voice and guards himself against a possible negative reaction.
- Dr. Winter praises her dietary changes and asks for information about her stomach complaint.
- Following his intuition, Dr. Winter pursues details about domestic violence, which is crucial, since Mary has opened up and responded to the questions.

- He identifies one possible psychosocial cause of her complaints and tells Mary how the domestic violence situation may be causing her symptoms.

• •

Other somatoform disorders to be ruled out include **hypochondriasis, conversion disorder,** and **pain disorder** (discussed later). In these disorders the symptoms are usually related to *one specific area or disease.* For example, persons with hypochondriasis are prone to magnify and misinterpret a physical symptom and assume they have a deadly disease. In conversion disorder a disturbance of bodily functioning simulates acute neurological pathology but does not conform to underlying neurological anatomy. Rather the signs and symptoms of conversion disorder tend to conform to the patient's imagined concept of the condition. Conversion disorder often appears after severe psychic stress and may manifest as stroke, blindness, deafness, a paralyzed limb, anesthesias, or paresthesias.[27] By contrast, in somatization disorder, the symptoms usually start in childhood or adolescence, or at any rate before age 30; tend to recur lifelong; and include symptoms affecting several systems. Because pain disorder is relatively common and presents special medical management problems, it is treated separately.

Treatment and Management

Patients with somatization disorder tend to consume an inordinate amount of medical resources, up to 6 times the national average in hospital costs and 14 times the national average in costs for physicians' services.[28] Coordination and continuity of care are essential for appropriate treatment to prevent patients from using multiple providers.[29] It is crucial that one person be the identified primary health care provider to coordinate consultations, referrals, and tests and to ensure that all progress notes, reports, and laboratory results are returned and integrated into the patient's medical record. It may be difficult to review such reports and notes sufficiently, but it is essential for long-term effective treatment of patients with the propensity to make use of multiple providers for their imagined medical conditions.

In cases of somatization disorder, it is crucial to understand that medical treatment of the purported condition is *not* likely to make the patient well. Since the production of symptoms is driven by unconscious psychological motivations to get attention and nurturance, patients tend to replace "successfully" treated conditions with new symptoms affecting other body systems. To prevent this cycle, an eclectic management approach based on three principles gleaned from the literature has been suggested.[30] The first is for one community-based care provider to establish a trusting therapeutic alliance.[31] This is best done by empathic acknowledgment of the patient's pain and suffering, thus communicating compassionate caring. Smith et al suggest scheduling regular appointments for such patients to eliminate the need to fall ill to get attention.[32] Scheduling regular appointments also keeps the health care provider informed about events and changes in the patient's life, about attempts to self-medicate (including remedies from complementary and alternative medicine), and also about whether the patient is seeing other providers. Second, Cloninger sees education as another treatment and management technique for somatization disorder. He suggests informing the patient of the diagnosis, explaining that somatization disorder is a medically recognized illness and that the patient is not going crazy, also pointing out that the symptoms are known to be linked to stress. Using information gained from a thorough psychosocial history, the health care provider and the patient can then jointly identify the stressors in the intrapsychic, interpersonal, social, and/or occupation spheres. Only after discussion of stress problems and their association with the production of symptoms is it likely that such patients will accept referral to mental health counseling. Third, the patient should be reassured that the health care provider will furnish continuity of care and perform appropriate assessments of new complaints. This last principle is designed to maintain the therapeutic alliance and discourage the patient from seeking out other providers. Other strategies include using low dosages of anxiolytics to address both depression and the tendency toward obsessive-compulsive behaviors. Careful monitoring is advised to prevent abuse. The medical care provider or mental health professional should steer the patient into having nurturance needs met outside the medical setting. Thus, some have suggested encouraging such patients to join and become active in community-based organizations or volunteer activities.

PAIN DISORDER

Chronic pain syndromes are among the most frustrating and most expensive conditions in health care.[33] Estimates show that pain is the major presenting problem in an estimated 8 million physician office visits annually at an annual level of $60 billion in health care costs.[34] Pain disorder is usually characterized by severe pain that is the predominant focus of clinical attention and *not fully explained by any nonpsychiatric medical or neurological disorder.* Pain is highly subjective; it is not easy to measure. Wilder Penfield's guidance for the clinician is that if the patient is not a malingerer (more fully discussed later), the patient's report about the pain should be believed. Thus, if the pain is subjectively real, the questions to explore are 1) how disabling the pain is and 2) how emotional factors or comorbid psychiatric conditions contribute to the pain.[35] Indeed there is a high frequency of comorbidity with depressive disorders, and dependent or histrionic personality disorder. To distinguish psychosomatic pain from pain associated with medical conditions, such terms as **atypical pain** and **psychogenic pain** have been used.

The somatized pain can be seen as a reaction to inner psychic pressures or repressed trauma.[36] As in somatization disorder, most individuals with pain disorder have early childhood histories of physical and emotional maltreatment to the point of trauma. Such individuals may react to stressors by unconsciously recreating the repressed pain experience of the earlier trauma.[37]

Current stressors may include a chaotic or neglectful family or a dysfunctional marriage. In such situations, pain becomes a manipulative tool to attract attention and nurturance. If the afflicted person is successful in obtaining attention as a **primary gain**, the pain experience is reinforced. When repeated or prolonged use of pain disorder in addition to getting sympathy also yields **secondary gains**, such as monetary benefits or avoidance of distasteful activities, the patient may come to regard seeking medical care for pain as a positive life pattern. However, when others perceive that secondary gains predominate, they often stop being supportive and instead apply the negative label of **malingerer**. Indeed, if the pain symptoms are deliberately feigned, the diagnosis of pain disorder is inaccurate; the patient has factitious disorder.

Because the experience of pain is so subjective, it is critical to rule out neurological or orthopedic conditions to arrive at an accurate differential diagnosis. For example, one study showed that 40% of patients initially referred to a pain clinic as having psychogenic or somatized pain were upon further investigation found to have organic conditions such as myofascial disease, facet disease, peripheral nerve entrapment, temporomandibular joint disease (TMJ), thoracic outlet syndrome, or herniated disc problems.[38] Once organic causes have been ruled out, Guggenheim suggests using the MADISON Scale (Box 13-2) to determine the amount of emotional overlay in the patient's pain.[39]

In treating pain disorder, comorbid psychiatric disorders and current psychosocial family or relationship stressors need to be addressed with a coordinated multidisciplinary response, similar to that in somatization disorder.[40] The impairment of the patient's functioning and the role of psychosocial stressors, family dysfunction, and depression must be determined. Suicide rates among pain sufferers is 9 times that of the general population. Pharmacological treatment of psychogenic pain is difficult with analgesics and problematical with opioids. However, it has been noted that 25% to 50% of those with pain disorder have analgesic effects with antide-

---

Box 13-2 MADISON Scale for Determining Emotional Markers in Pain Disorder

M **Multiplicity:** Pain is either in more than one place or of more than one variety; when treated, may recur elsewhere.

A **Authenticity:** More interested in clinician's acceptance of pain as genuine than in a cure.

D **Denial:** Especially exaggerated marital bliss or family harmony; when admits to being depressed or anxious, will refuse to see connection to pain.

I **Interpersonal relationship:** May deny connection to presence of particular person as affecting pain. However, close observation of patient's nonverbal and interactive behavior may reveal worsening pain in that person's company.

S **Singularity:** The pain is described as unlike that of anyone else, ever.

O **"Only you":** The patient immediately idealizes the health care provider as *savior,* despite numerous failures by other competent experts.

N **Nothing helps, no change:** Patient claims that there is no relief whatsoever from any type of intervention, including opioids, and there is no temporal fluctuation in the pain under a variety of circumstances.

Adapted from Guggenheim FG. (2000) Somatoform disorders. In Sadock BJ, Sadock VA, eds. *Kaplan and Sadock's Comprehensive Textbook of Psychiatry* 7th ed. Philadelphia: Lippincott Williams & Wilkins, 2000:1616.

---

pressants.[41] Behavioral therapies also seem to diminish the experience of chronic pain and reduce the number of pain episodes.

When working with pain disorder patients, you can easily develop positive countertransference during the initial diagnostic process, when you feel sympathy for the person who appears to have singularly acute pain. Once you discover that there is no physical basis to the pain or that it keeps shifting, that sympathy can quickly turn into anger over having been deceived. In subsequent interviews, you are likely to have negative countertransference, which can obstruct treatment. Because treating such patients is often difficult and time-consuming, you may subconsciously rate such patients low in treatability, manageability, or likability.

Factitious Disorders

The incidence of patients with factitious disorders is estimated at less than 1%,[42] although specific conditions such as fever of unknown origin may have rates as high as 3.5%.[43] Perhaps because they are so rare, patients who intentionally fabricate signs and symptoms of illness present health care providers with challenging problems in diagnosis and treatment management Box 13-3). The DSM-IV diagnostic criteria for factitious disorder specify intentional production or feigning of physical or psychological signs and symptoms of illness for the purpose of being identified as sick or as a patient.[44] Those who intentionally feign signs and symptoms of physical and/or psychological disorders to avoid unpleasant work, avoid legal responsibility, or obtain financial reward, such as a disability pension, are termed **malingerers**.[45] Those who feign illness to assume the sick role are said to be motivated by internal reasons. Malingerers are said to be motivated by external reasons. The term **Munchausen syndrome** was first applied by Ascher to those who want to assume the sick role (See Sidebar below).[46] Such persons make up only about 10% of patients with factitious disorders.[47] Patients with Munchausen Syndrome tend to be memorable because their elaborate and skillful fabrication of stories backing up their physical or psychological signs and symptoms fool so many health care providers. Their seemingly senseless self-harming behaviors and sometimes multiple unnecessary surgeries are also troubling.[48] Those with predominantly psychological signs and symptoms generally can produce behavioral symptoms and feign neurological signs that are consistent with a known mental disorder. Such patients may elicit considerable sympathy for the fabricated stories of traumatic stress induced in wartime or from witnessing gruesome deaths of loved ones. They may also feign mood disorders, such as depression, bipolar disorders, dissociative disorders, eating disorders, sexual paraphilias, hypersomnia, or amnesia.[49] Even though patients with factitious disorders present with pseudo-medical conditions, it is important to remain open to the possibility that they may contract a genuine medical disorder, possibly as a consequence of self-inflicted procedures.

The more florid version of Munchausen syndrome, also known as **prototypical Munchausen syndrome**,[50] is characterized by multiple presentations at hospitals, either with dramatic and frequently life-threatening physical symptoms or with equally serious psychological

---

Box13-3 Clues for Recognizing a Patient with Factitious Disorder

1. Presents personal medical history as high drama, fantastic tales (pseudologia fantastica).
2. Disrupts ward and breaks hospital rules.
3. Argues continually with medical staff.
4. Shows off medical jargon and knowledge.
5. Demands narcotic pain medications.
6. Advertises or brags about previous medical treatment and surgeries. Shows off scars.
7. Gives contradictory histories.
8. Develops frequent or inexplicable medical complications.
9. Presents new symptoms after negative workups.
10. Becomes hostile when closely questioned about inconsistencies in history.

Adapted from Maxmen JS, Ward NG. *Essential Psychopathology and Its Treatment* 2nd ed. New York: WW Norton, 1995;308.

BARON VON MÜNCHHAUSEN (1720–1791) — This German cavalry officer, after retiring from military service, told fantastic tales of his improbable battle exploits, which were immortalized in 1785 in a satirical book that is still popular today.

symptoms that seem to require psychiatric hospitalization.[51] A subgroup of those with factitious disorder feign combined psychological and physical symptoms. For example, a person claims complicated bereavement due to trauma and also produces complaints of incapacitating pain associated with metastatic cancer. Because such persons tend to go from hospital to hospital feigning various illnesses and often demanding invasive procedures, they have also been called *hospital hoboes*,[52] *hospital addicts*,[53] and *metabolic malingerers*.[54] Such adverse labels illustrate the animosity such patients can arouse in health care providers, who discover they have been tricked into providing unnecessary medical treatment.

Nonprototypical Munchausen patients tend to have single-system complaints, wander less from provider to provider, and be less florid in the fabrication of their history.[55] Instead they rely on manipulating diagnostic instruments, tampering with laboratory specimens, or actually inflicting cellular tissue damage on themselves. Nonprototypical patients may simulate fevers with an oral thermometer, get a reading of arrhythmias by switching leads on an electrocardiogram, or add blood to urine or sputum specimens. They appear to be indifferent to pain and painful procedures. They may infect themselves by smearing bacteria on self-inflicted wounds or produce some metabolic disturbance by injecting themselves with insulin, thyroid hormones, or blood thinners.[56] A typical profile is a woman under 36 who appears as passive, immature, and hypochondriacal.[57] Many of them have health-related jobs or significant knowledge about illness and the medical environment. Their medical knowledge and access to medications and instruments allows them to produce textbook symptoms for the illness they have chosen.[58]

Munchausen by Proxy

A more disturbing disorder is that of individuals who fabricate or induce signs and symptoms of illness in another, usually a child but sometimes also a closely related adult (Box 13-4). Factitious disorder by proxy, better known as **Munchausen by proxy**, typically involves a mother who, having induced medical illness in her child, presents the sick child for medical care.[59] Often the mother asks for painful, invasive diagnostic procedures or even surgeries. Through repeated episodes, she may expose the child to mortal danger.[60] A telltale sign is when the parent or caregiver seems overly caring and attentive and/or overinvolved in the child's medical care or with the medical staff.[61] As in the case of nonprototypical Munchausen's, many individuals perpetrating Munchausen by proxy have worked in health care and seem to want to impress health care staff with their knowledge of medical procedures.[62] They may resort to poisoning, injecting insulin, central nervous system stimulants or depressants, or suffocation to produce serious medical disorders in the child. Estimates of the prevalence of Munchausen by proxy are 2.8 cases per 100,000 children age 1 year and younger and 0.5 cases per 100,00 in children 16 and younger. The typical victim is 2 to 3 years old at diagnosis[63] and is likely to have been abused in this fashion for an average of 15 months.[64] The longer the abuse goes undetected, the greater the danger to the child's siblings, including death by suffocation, which the perpetrator presents as sudden infant death syndrome (**SIDS**).[65]

ETIOLOGY

Written speculation on the paradoxical behavior of persons going to such great lengths to play a sick role and to subject themselves or others to great discomfort and pain dates to the second century.[66] Many persons with factitious disorder were abused and neglected as children, and many of them had early childhood illnesses or extended hospitalizations.[67] As adults they seek nurturance in an approach–avoidance fashion by becoming both victim and victimizer. Through skillful manipulation, the individual becomes the object of care and concern, meanwhile defying and devaluing those who provide that care. Authors looking at the psychosocial context of the high prevalence of chronicity note that new

Box13-4 A Sick Child: When Is It Munchausen by Proxy?

SITUATION	NORMAL PATTERN	MUNCHAUSEN PATTERN
A. Parent brings in child for evaluation and treatment of illness	A. Signs and symptoms not exotic Predictable response to medical intervention Parent relieved when symptoms resolved	A. Exotic signs and symptoms. Parent *only* source of information. Parent insists that child is sick. Child does not respond predictably. Symptoms worsen or change.
B. Parent of formerly premature infant alarmed at even mild symptoms.	B. Usually well-documented antecedents Mother usually reassured when resolved	B. Parent only source of crisis episodes. Not replicated if infant separated.
C. Parent discontinues child's prescription	C. Concern over adverse effects. Compliance after discussion or more explicit about reservations.	C. Parent vague on claims about medication not working or aggravating condition.
D. Exaggeration of child's symptoms	D. To assure immediate medical attention Welcomes recovery. Stops behavior.	D. Parent wants personal attention. Recovery greeted by disbelief. New symptoms invented.
E. Shifting symptoms	E. Parent confused or alarmed over previous distress episodes (e.g., asthma) Relieved when satisfactory explanation given; antecedents verified by other sources.	E. Carefully constructed fabrication. Will not accept medical explanation. Symptoms continue to shift. Parent sole "authenticator" of shifting symptoms.
F. Older child reports illness symptoms not supported by medical evidence	F. May be case of child malingering When identified, parent takes action. Later reports all is well or that child needs counseling.	F. Child may have been coached by parent. Internal contradictions when story retold. Parent does not accept disconfirming evidence. Symptoms worsen.
G. Sleep apnea in infant	G. Parent cooperative, follows instructions. If medication prescribed, blood levels constant.	G. Mother overinvolved with staff and child. Episodes more frequent. Blood level fluctuations. Mother makes threats about ineffective intervention.

episodes tend to occur after severe sexual or relationship distress.[68,69] On the Minnesota Multiphasic Personality Inventory (MMPI), such persons have been shown to have a poor sense of identity, poor sexual adjustment, poor frustration tolerance, strong dependency needs, and narcissism.[70]

The causation of Munchausen by proxy has also been the subject of active speculation.[71] Feldman cites evidence from covert video surveillance of perpetrators to support one psychodynamic view of its cause.[72] According to this theory, an unsatisfactory childhood relationship with a desired but unavailable father can later lead to "perverse relationships with physicians and hospital staff members." The abusing mother uses her child as a manipulative object in an intensely ambivalent relationship with the medical establishment to pursue and punish the surrogate parents, that is, health care providers, who can give or withhold attention. The pattern revealed by hidden cameras typically showed a mother who in one moment exhibited devotion and care in the presence of hospital staff but became instantly indifferent to her child when she thought herself to be no longer observed.[73]

> **Box13-5 Ideal Membership of Interdisciplinary Team for Managing Challenging Patients**
>
> - Emergency room admitting physician
> - Attending or prescribing physicians for current and previous episodes
> - Surgeon or surgeons if patient has had surgery
> - One or more hospital floor nurses
> - Social worker
> - Ethicist if available

DIAGNOSIS AND TREATMENT MANAGEMENT

It is the duty of a health care provider to do his or her best to authenticate signs and symptoms of physical illness with any patient. However, persons with factitious disorder can be very deceptive, so that a correct diagnosis often is not made until several health care practitioners note a pattern in hospital admissions, invasive diagnostic procedures, or surgeries. If the clinical history indicates a possibility of factitious disorder, the immediate formation of an interdisciplinary task force is recommended.[74] Members should include any health care providers who have had opportunity to observe and interact with a patient who is suspected of inducing signs or symptoms in himself or herself or in another (Box 13-5). Assembling such a task force may not be easy or seem cost efficient, but it is in practice *the most efficient and resource-sparing* method to diagnose and manage persons with factitious disorders. Having a joint discussion of the case can also defuse any interpersonal tensions among team members, which such patients tend to foster by setting one health care provider against another in process called **splitting** (also discussed in the section on borderline personality disorder). Such patients can arouse intense negative countertransference in caregivers. Indeed, Plassman[75] sees the ability to induce countertransference as the key to the success of individuals who mislead so many health care providers over a number of episodes of feigned illness. Countertransference may start with overidentification with the "suffering" of a patient or with the "distress" of a mother with a "sick" child. Such strong feelings of empathy can lead the health care provider to overlook clear evidence of inconsistency between symptoms and medical evidence or disconfirming behavior. This is an especially difficult issue in the case of Munchausen by proxy. Pondering this dilemma, one pediatrician said, "As a physician, one of the things you learn early on is to listen to the parents. And what makes Munchausen by proxy so difficult to deal with is that your ally in the child's health care is really not your ally. I don't want to use the word 'adversary,' but in fact I guess it is an adversarial relationship, because they are playing a game with you, except you don't know you're playing a game."[76] Such well-intentioned trust in cases of Munchausen by proxy can have fatal consequences for the child. A forensic pathologist, testifying at a trial in which a mother was convicted of serially killing five of her children answered the question why such cases are not discovered earlier, "Doctors don't want to think that parents harm children."[77]

Such cases of faked SIDS have demonstrated that sometimes the health care provider needs a healthy case of suspicion or even wear the hat of a forensic investigator. If it is suspected that the mother may be smothering the infant to induce serious crises, covert video surveillance of the hospital room is very effective in providing direct evidence of the malfeasance. Similarly, in cases of suspected self-injection with insulin or stimulants, a surreptitious room search may yield the evidence to prove that someone is inducing crisis symptoms. Since both covert surveillance and room searches raise legal and ethical questions, it is prudent to involve both the legal system and a medical ethics committee.

The anger, aversion, or disgust following the realization that health care providers have been duped into responding to faked medical crises may produce **therapeutic nihilism**.[78] This term describes the hostile attitude and actions of health care providers who suspect that a patient has feigned medical or psychiatric disorders. Therapeutic nihilism may come in the form of refusing to provide subsequent medical or psychiatric services on the assumption that the patient will produce fraudulent signs and symptoms. Another response has been to circulate the name of the "pseudo-patient" to hospitals and professional colleagues in the area, to warn them not to provide medical services for such persons.[79] Such practices raise serious ethical and legal concerns.

Treatment and Management

Firm confrontation of patients with factitious disorders is counterproductive. Patients confronted with their contradictory stories or inconsistent findings, instead of recanting or displaying embarrassment, become indignant, question medical competence of attending staff, or even threaten litigation. If this bluff fails, they may abruptly leave (against medical advice) and wander off to another health facility to recycle the same factitious behaviors. To prevent a chronic continuation of factitious disorder, most authorities recommend a supportive approach.[80] This entails that the clinician gently redefine the problem as one caused by some underlying stress and offer ongoing psychotherapy for those. Another is to treat identified comorbid psychiatric disorders, in the hope that this will reduce the compulsion to continue to produce such attention-seeking behaviors.

Malingering and the Drug-Seeking Patient

Malingering is the *intentional* "production of false or grossly exaggerated physical or psychological symptoms, motivated by external incentives such as avoiding military duty, avoiding work, obtaining financial compensation, evading criminal prosecution, or obtaining drugs."[81] There are two types of malingerers: 1) passive deception, in which the person feigns inability to perform tasks or cope with life and 2) active deception, in which the person intentionally produces a cluster of symptoms. This diagnosis may be indicated if 1) the patient is referred for health care by an attorney, 2) there is a large difference between the claims of disability and the objective findings, 3) the patient is uncooperative or noncompliant with treatment regimen, and 4) the patient also has antisocial personality disorder. A preponderance of malingerers are men seeking drugs. The two most challenging subgroups of people with this disorder are the drug-seeking patient and the patient inappropriately seeking some form of disability compensation. One aspect of this challenging group is that by the nature of their requests, they pressure you into changing your role. Partly to protect yourself against charges of being a drug supplier, you may find yourself having to assume the role of detective, using a forensic approach to your physical examinations, clinical history interviews, and the precautions you take in the collection of laboratory specimens.

Treatment and Management

The challenge of treating patients who are seeking drugs is complicated and often long term. They mostly ask for prescriptions for pain medication or sedatives. Because there is high comorbidity with substance abuse disorder, an additional diagnosis of polysubstance-related disorder or other (or unknown) substance-related disorders may be indicated. The patient may also be abusing over-the-counter (OTC) or prescription drugs, illicit drugs, and herbal preparations. Of course, the health care provider must always look for signs that alcohol is being abused in conjunction with OTC and prescription medications. Because treating drug-seeking patients can be confusing and challenging, Box 13-6 lists red flags suggesting that the patient's main goal is to get drug prescriptions for abuse rather than for a real medical problem.

Such patients also generally resist suggestions about alternatives for reducing stress or for alternative ways of reducing their pain. The phrase "Yes, but. . ." is a clue that they do not really want such help; they just want you to prescribe drugs for them. When in doubt, prescribe medications, *but* only in small amounts. This will also ensure proper medical management and protect your name and reputation under regulations for restricted drugs. Another safeguard is to alert the pharmacy to the possibility of forgery and changes in the prescription. Because drug-seeking patients tend to be polysubstance abusers, ask the patient to bring in all medication bottles and have staff verify them with the pharmacies and/or physicians' offices. If possible, ask someone to observe the patient moving around when the patient does not know he or she is being watched. These observations may yield evidence about whether the patient is feigning symptoms.

● ●

PATIENT PROFILE 13.2

THIS OLD WAR INJURY REALLY HURTS

Setting: *Rodney is a 38-year-old single man, a military veteran who is a frequent patient at a health clinic. He is being managed by Chris, a physician assistant, who was a medic in the war Rodney fought in. Today, Rodney wants to be seen because one of the pieces of shrapnel lodged in his right thigh is working its way out,*

Box13-6 Red Flags for Drug-Seeking Patients

- Tend to ask for specific drugs rather than focusing on symptoms first. Do not have time for diagnostic tests. Getting drugs is more important than finding causes or getting well.
- Extraordinarily knowledgeable about names, doses, side effects, cost, and availability of medications.
- Push to escalate the dosage.
- Ask for samples, often of the latest type or most potent pain killer. Do not present as typical patients. May be alternately manipulative, argumentative, threatening, whining, ingratiating, dishonest.
- Attempts to steer patient to another less addictive drug meet strong objections. May claim to be allergic to anything other than desired drug.
- Frequent visits to emergency rooms and walk-in clinics or have multiple physicians.
- Claim to have an obviously chronic condition but deny treatment by anyone else for it.
- Medical history inconsistent. Classic textbook symptoms or elaborate stories with possible inconsistencies or very vague on details.

- History of drug abuse or a criminal history of multiple charges of driving under the influence, selling drugs, or other illegal activities.
- May have out-of-town home address or old identification with invalid address.
- Previous prescribing physician not available. Out-of-town physician, retired, or died.
- Supply vanished. The dog ate the pills, neighbors stole them, accidentally thrown away with the garbage or flushed down the toilet.
- Abrupt changes in symptoms when laws or regulations related to disability change.
- Claim urgent need for drug before leaving town on an emergency (relative is ill or dying).
- Appeal to your vanity: "You were so great with my friend when he was ill. I am sure you can help me."
- Other family members come in with factitious complaints, all wanting the same drug.
- History of hospital discharges against medical advice right after obtaining drugs.

causing additional pain. His medical record from the Veterans Administration Medical Center documents the injury as such: Rodney was walking several yards behind the point man when a booby trap went off and pieces of metal flew at him, with several pieces of shrapnel lodging in his left arm, chest, and right thigh.

Chris, knowing that Rodney has an appointment with him at 11 AM, stations himself at a window, where he observes Rodney getting off his motorcycle. Chris thinks, *If he is riding his motorcycle today, he must not be in much pain.* Rodney gingerly jumps off his motorcycle, adjusts the kick stand easily with his right foot, and starts walking in an almost normal gait toward the clinic. As he gets closer to the clinic, he starts limping more obviously.

Chris: Hello, Rodney. I see you came in because of your old injury. *(I am glad I watched him, because now I suspect that he's malingering.)*

Rodney: Hi, Dr. Chris. Yeah (moaning as he shifts his right leg), I just can't seem to get any relief from one of those painkillers. Can you double the dosage? *(I had better not seem too eager, or he'll get wise that I'm selling them.)*

Chris: First let me remind you I am a physician assistant, not a doctor.

Rodney: Yeah, I knew that.

Chris: What exactly happens when you say you can't get any relief? *(It is probably a good idea to get a little more detail.)*

Rodney: Well, I take one in the morning when I first get up, then one about 6 hours later. Then by afternoon I'm feeling pretty rotten. Sometimes I take them more frequently and still I'm in pain. (Grimaces and grins at the same time.)

Chris: Hmmmm. *(I see in the chart that this is his third increase in dosage of this narcotic painkiller in 6 months. I wonder if he's addicted or maybe selling them.)* You have had three increases in the past 6 months, and you are on the maximum dosage. Before I make a decision about your medication, I want an x-ray of your right thigh to see the depth of the shrapnel position. If it is superficial, perhaps we can remove it with a simple incision. Remember, we did that with the one in your left arm.

Rodney: Hey Chris, old buddy, you and me were in the same war together. *(Maybe if I pull on his guilt strings about him not getting wounded.)* I got wounded and you were left sitting pretty. Don't leave me in pain like this, old buddy. Shall I send some of my motorcycle buddies after you? (He laughs snidely.) How about it, old buddy? *(I'd like to see my old motorcycle gang after him. He'd holler "uncle" for sure. Or maybe he is getting suspicious of me?)*

Chris: *(Oh great, now he's calling me "old buddy," trying to ally himself with me because we were in the same war and he got wounded and I didn't. His gang? That's a threat. But I have to stick to what I think is right.)* I'm reluctant to do that until we see how deep the shrapnel is. How about taking it easy for a while, you know, no wild motorcycle rides?

Rodney: Sure, you're the expert. *(I'd better let this one go for now and maybe after they do the x-ray, I can push again for increasing the dosage. Anyway, I can always buy some on the street.)*

Points to Consider

- Chris makes a thorough review of Rodney's medical record from the Veterans Administration Medical Center to confirm his combat history and his injuries.

- By observing Rodney's behavior prior to entering the clinic, Chris gains more information about Rodney's true motion capabilities.

- Chris seeks details about Rodney's use of the medication and reviews documentation of medications prescribed when patient requests a stronger dose.

- Chris recognizes Rodney's manipulative behavior and holds his ground.

- Chris mentions a surgical option because it is considered better management of the problem.

- Chris did not comply with Rodney's request but did acknowledge a genuine reality to the complaint of pain and recommended non-prescriptive treatment.

• •

Disability Certification

Because you are in the health care profession, you will encounter people who seek out assistance from you for disability certification. Most of them are genuine, honest, and in need of help. They may qualify for benefits under one or more programs. Types of disability include worker's compensation, Veterans Administration disabilities (service related and not), Social Security disability, supplemental disability income (SSI), and long-term disability through an employer. Long-term disability related to employment may arise from organic diseases, such as black lung disease and brown lung disease; asbestos poisoning; long-term exposure to toxic fumes or chemicals; back problems; carpal tunnel syndrome; and psychological disorders, such as posttraumatic stress disorder (PTSD), depression, or anxiety.

Often it is not easy to distinguish between a person genuinely seeking assistance for disability compensation and one who is inappropriately seeking some form of disability certification or drugs. When in doubt, you may wish to request a psychiatric consultation or some psychological testing. If you find yourself having a negative response to patients who seek disability, you may need to identify your own values and attitudes that may cloud an objective assessment of such a patient. Having been successfully manipulated by a malingerer may leave a bitter taste of resentment and may prejudice you against patients who claim disability, real or not. If you see a great number of these patients, you may wish to have an assortment of assessment tools available to apply to the situation.[82,83]

Borderline Personality Disorder

Rather than reviewing the entire realm of personality disorders, this particular disorder has been chosen because patients with borderline personality disorder (BPD) are usually challenging and absorb large amounts of health care providers' time and energy. As with factitious

SPLITTING — First identified by Freud, splitting is an unconscious process that actively separates contradictory self-representations, contradictory object representations, or contradictory feelings from one another. It is a useful defense mechanism that helps the developing child to separate the "good" nurturing mother from the "bad" neglectful mother. Splitting can be projected onto health care providers, who are seen as alternately all good and nurturing or all bad and rejecting.

Adapted with permission from Gabbard GO. Psychoanalysis. In Sadock BJ, Sadock VA, Eds. *Kaplan and Sadock's Comprehensive Textbook of Psychiatry.* 7th ed, vol 2. Philadelphia: Lippincott Williams & Wilkins, 2000;591, 603.

disorders, patients with BPD make excessive use of health care for personal attention. Persons with this disorder often are so demanding, bizarre and unpredictable that they forfeit the good will of their providers. Their behaviors are characterized by the following: 1) impulsivity, 2) unstable and intense interpersonal relationships, 3) inappropriate and intense anger 4) identity confusion, 5) affective instability, 6) problems being alone, 7) physically self-harming or suicidal behaviors, 8) chronic feelings of emptiness and boredom, 9) transient stress-related paranoid ideation and 10) dissociative symptoms.[84] BPD occurs twice as often in women as men.[85] Its prevalence in the general population is 2% to 4%. Its prevalence in the psychiatric population is 20%,[86] and it usually appears in conjunction with other mental disorders, such as mood disorders, factitious disorders, or ADHD.[87]

ETIOLOGY

It is assumed that in persons with BPD the major developmental drive for individuation has been severely damaged. Thus, instead of autonomy, the child develops doubt and fear of abandonment. Such feelings may be induced by severe abuse and neglect or by a mother who resisted the individuation attempts of the child.[88] In either case, the child may get mixed messages of being wanted or loved and being rejected. In response to internal separation anxiety, the child learns the defense mechanism of **splitting**, that is, both loving and hating the caregiver (see Sidebar above).[89] As such children grow into adolescence and adulthood, they develop an approach–avoidance pattern in their interpersonal relations. Their relationships are subject to extreme fluctuations, as they tend to characterize people as either good or bad, often switching people suddenly from one category to the other on the basis of a perceived slight or rejection.

The constant need to be reassured and the fear of rejection, which often manifest as paranoid thoughts about being slighted or abandoned, can create havoc in health care settings. Such patients often are very needy and ingratiating one moment and then switch to hostility or intense anger if they feel you are not instantly available at all times, or if they perceive that you are annoyed with them. Because they are chronically bored and feel empty inside, persons with BPD tend to seek stimulation desperately, often in risky or self-harming behaviors. These may be gambling, frequent intense (unsafe) sexual encounters, drug abuse, instigating fights, self-mutilation, and/or suicide attempts. They often require short-term hospitalization, typically after a suicide attempt. While in the hospital they may exhibit splitting behaviors, needy one moment and dissatisfied and angry with their treatment the next, often to the point of abruptly leaving against medical advice.[90] When they show up in regular health care settings after minor crises, they may exhibit transient paranoid thoughts, dissociation, or psychotic symptoms. They frequently abuse prescription medications, and they will doctor-shop for prescriptions if they cannot get them from their regular provider.

● ●

PATIENT PROFILE 13.3

HELP ME (I HATE YOU)

Setting: Susan is a 38-year-old divorced woman who has been coming to this mental health clinic for 15 years. She has a long history of multiple complaints, usually related to intense emotional episodes, suicidal behaviors, and the need for medication. She sometimes leaves the clinic to go sampling other doctors. She usually returns to this clinic after some minor disagreement with the other doctor. Martin, a physician assistant, has been her case coordinator for most of the past 9 years. She is here today because her relationship with her female lover of a year has ended and she is despondent.

Martin: Hello, Susan. How are you?

Susan: You want to know the truth? Shitty, that's what. How would you feel if the love of your life just left you? Oh, I just don't know if I can take this again. (*She juts her chin out aggressively and then starts to cry. She looks up at Martin to check out how he is taking her news.*) I have had thoughts about cutting myself again.

Martin: (*Here we go again. She's making passive suicidal statements and then checks me out to see how I am responding. I remember that a year ago, when she broke up with her last lover, she also got suicidal and self-destructive.*) It must be a tough time for you. Will you agree not to hurt yourself until we can get you some help?

Susan: Maybe, but I really need help now. (*I really need more Xanax.*) Why can't you understand me? (*Men. I hate them.*) You don't know what tough is.

Martin: I do understand how bad you can feel when you've broken up with someone you've been close to. Briefly tell me what happened. (*I hope this isn't too long.*)

Susan proceeds to tell Martin a medium-length version of what happened, during which he asks her to summarize what happened.

Martin: I can see why you feel so low.

Susan: Low? That's an understatement. I've bottomed out. Totally.

Martin: Yes, I understand that you feel that way. Remember last year when this happened with your last lover? You came out of it all right. *(This is taking longer than I have today. She needs to get back into her behavior management program.)* Tell me, when did you last see your therapist?

Susan: A couple of months ago. But if I can't see her, maybe you and I could meet for a drink somewhere?

Martin: You know that as your physician assistant, I cannot have a social relationship with you. First I'll call and find out if you can see your therapist today. I know that talking this out with her could help you.

Susan: Yeah, she's OK. *(I can talk with her easier than I can with this jerk.)*

Martin: Let's check with the receptionist up front and maybe she can fit you in today. *(Then her therapist can assess the seriousness of the suicidal and self-destructive statements and set up a safety plan.)*

Points to Consider

- Martin normalizes Susan's feelings by assuring her that the end of a relationship is stressful for anyone.

- Martin picks up on the pattern of aggression and neediness.

- Martin identifies her phrasing as passively suicidal and remembers some of her history related to suicidal behavior.

- Martin takes the time to hear about the breakup but is alert to the time frame as well.

- Martin clarifies his role with Susan and makes an appropriate referral to her therapist.

• •

Treatment and Management

Effective treatment in the medical setting often means well-coordinated management. The problems in treating such persons come from their appeal to your nurturing qualities. Their very neediness often triggers intense countertransference. To manipulate you into feeling guilty, patients with BPD may make legal threats about your so-called failure to treat them promptly or properly.[91] The ultimate escalation of attention getting or punishing techniques by such patients may be attempted or successful suicide. Such manipulative behaviors make objectivity difficult for everyone involved in the person's care. Thus, as with the other disorders discussed here, it is absolutely essential that one person coordinate a team approach to medical treatment and prescriptions. Second, to limit the divisive effect such patients can have on a multi-provider practice or in a hospital setting, it is important that all team members agree to set limits on who such patients must deal with to get medical services. It is important that such limits be agreed on and clearly communicated to the patient as soon as the manipulative pattern of pitting providers against each other becomes apparent. Having periodic team meetings to debrief each other, especially after a crisis with a suicidal BPD patient, can be helpful to defuse countertransference issues of anger and frustration in health care providers. Consistency and refusal to allow the patient to distort boundaries and professional roles are cornerstones in working with these patients.

Despite good and vigilant management efforts, the unpredictable and sometimes tragic behaviors of BPD patients tend to persist. For treatment of the psychiatric disorder itself, referral to psychotherapy or even psychiatric hospitalization is indicated. Cognitive behavior therapy, especially when conducted in groups or in a hospital settings, seems to be moderately effective in modifying the underlying character structure.[92] Ongoing supportive psychotherapy oriented toward problem solving and teaching coping skills may diminish their flights into risky or suicidal behaviors.[93] Pharmacological therapies should be oriented toward specific dysfunctional features of their disorder. Thus, to control intense anger, hostility, or psychotic episodes, antipsychotic medication may be useful. Anti-convulsants have been found to reduce impulsivity and thus improve global functioning. Antidepressants are used to deal with the feelings of emptiness and depression. Combined anxiolytics and antidepressants must be carefully monitored both for abuse and for possible paradoxical effects.[94,95]

In general, working with patients with BPD is fraught with problems. There is a fine line between giving support and rescuing, and between encouraging independence and signaling abandonment. Maxmen and Ward suggest that structured and consistent contact through regularly scheduled appointments may be more productive than responding to crisis-induced emergencies. They also suggest that only experienced clinicians should attempt to provide psychotherapy for "these most difficult of patients."[96]

Conclusion

The common thread that runs through somatization and factitious disorders is that they are psychiatric rather than medical conditions. Thus a primary concern must be to address the psychological aspects of these disorders. This includes identifying the comorbid psychiatric disorders. To begin with, you will need a complete psychosocial history, including information about and *from* the rest of their family, a complete medical history with details from other physicians who have treated them, and reports from their hospitalizations. Ordering reports from other health care professionals and hospitals and reading them is a time-consuming and laborious task. However, reports and consultations are prerequisites to an accurate differential diagnosis. Taking the time up front to familiarize yourself with the patient's history will save you a great deal of time and energy in the end. Once a patient is identified as falling into one of the categories discussed in this chapter, ongoing consultation and forming a treatment team with other professionals are essential tools for managing such patients.

Throughout your professional career you will encounter patients who are particularly challenging for you. They may evoke strong feelings or negative reactions from you. If this happens, you can use the opportunity to become aware of elements within yourself about which you may not be familiar. Being duped by such patients is not a personal failure. Rather it is an episode from which to learn.

REFERENCES

1. American Psychiatric Association (1994) Diagnostic and Statistical Manual of Mental Disorders, Fourth Edition. (Hereafter cited as DSM-IV). Washington, DC: APA Press, 445–469.
2. Anonymous (1997, Feb). When it's all in their heads: managing the somatizing patient. *Healthcare Demand Discharge Manag*, 3:21–24.
3. Shoemaker RS (2001). *Desperation Medicine*. Baltimore: Gateway Press.
4. Farstad DJ, Chow T (2001). A brief case report and review of ciguatera poisoning. *Wildern Environ Med*, 12:263–269.
5. El-Nabawi A, Quesenberry M, Saito K, et al. (2000). The N-methyl-D-aspartate neurotransmitter receptor is a mammalian brain target for the dinoflagellate Pfiesteria piscicida toxin. *Toxicol Appl Pharmacol*, 169:84–93.
6. Grattan LM, Oldach D, Perl TM, et al. (1998). Learning and memory difficulties after environmental exposure to waterways containing toxin-producing Pfiesteria or Pfiesteria-like dinoflagellates. *Lancet*, 352: 532–539.
7. Shoemaker RC (2001). Residential and recreational acquisition of possible estuary-associated syndrome: a new approach to successful diagnosis and treatment [In Process Citation] *Environ Health Perspect*, 109, Suppl 5:791–2.
8. Shoemaker RC (1998). Treatment of persistent Pfiesteria-human illness syndrome. *Md Med J*, 47: 64–66.
9. Tracy JK, Oldach D, Greenberg DR, et al. (1998). Psychologic adjustment of watermen with exposure of Pfiesteria piscicida. *Md Med J*, 47:130–232.
10. Escobar JI (1996). Overview of somatization: diagnosis, epidemiology, and management. *Psychopharm Bull*, 32:589–596.
11. Kapfhammer HP (2001). Somatoforme Stoerungen. Historische Entwicklung und

moderne diagnostische Konzeptualisierung. *Nervenarzt*, 72:487–500.

12. Margo KL, Margo GM (2000). Early diagnosis and empathy in managing somatization. *Am Fam Physician*, 61:1281–1285.

13. Smith GC, Clarke DM, Handrinos D, et al. (2000). Consultation-liaison psychiatrists' management of somatoform disorders. *Psychosomatics*, 41:481–489.

14. Hoffmann DE (2000). Managing the persistent patient with chronic pain. How can we help a patient with a psychiatric illness who persistently demands medical appointments? *HEC Forum*, 9:365–372.

15. Guggenheim FG (2000). Somatoform disorders. In Sadock BJ, Sadock VA (Eds). Kaplan and Sadock's *Comprehensive Textbook of Psychiatry* (7th Ed). Philadelphia: Lippincott Williams & Wilkins 1515.

16. Avia MD (1999). The development of illness beliefs. *J Psychsom Res* 47:199–204.

17. Stuart S, Noyes R (1999). Attachment and interpersonal communication in somatization. *Psychosomatics* 40:34–43.

18. Hollifield M, Tuttle L, Paine S, Kellner, R (1999). Hypochondriasis and somatization related to personality and attitudes toward self. *Psychosomatics*, 40:387–395.

19. Guggenheim FG (2000). Somatoform disorders. In Sadock BJ, Sadock VA, Eds. Kaplan and Sadock's *Comprehensive Textbook of Psychiatry* (7th Ed). Philadelphia: Lippincott Williams & Wilkins 1529.

20. Kaplan HI, Sadock BJ (1998). *Synopsis of Psychiatry* (8th Ed). Philadelphia: Lippincott Williams & Wilkins 632.

21. Noyes R, Happel RL, Yagla SJ (1999). Correlates of hypochondriasis in a nonclinical population. *Psychosomatics*, 40:461–469.

22. DSM-IV 448–249.

23. Righter EL, Sansone RA (1999). Managing somatic preoccupation. *Am Fam Physician* 59:311–312.

24. *DSM-IV* 449.

25. *DSM-IV* 448.

26. Guggenheim (2000). Somatoform Disorders. In Sadock BJ, Sadock VA, Eds. Kaplan and Sadock's *Comprehensive Textbook of Psychiatry,* 7th Ed. Philadelphia: Lippincott Williams & Wilkins, 1515–1516, 1524.

27. Guggenheim (2000). Somatoform Disorders. In Sadock BJ, Sadock VA, Eds. Kaplan and Sadock's *Comprehensive Textbook of Psychiatry,* 7th Ed. Philadelphia: Lippincott Williams & Wilkins, 1505.

28. Guggenheim (2000). Somatoform Disorders. In Sadock BJ, Sadock VA, Eds. Kaplan and Sadock's *Comprehensive Textbook of Psychiatry,* 7th Ed. Philadelphia: Lippincott Williams & Wilkins, 1515.

29. Guggenheim (2000). Somatoform Disorders. In Sadock BJ, Sadock VA, Eds. Kaplan and Sadock's *Comprehensive Textbook of Psychiatry,* 7th Ed. Philadelphia: Lippincott Williams & Wilkins, 1518.

30. Martin RL, Yutzy SH (1999). Somatoform disorders. In Hales RE, Yudofsky SC, Talbott JA (Eds). *American Psychiatric Press Textbook of Psychiatry* (3d Ed). Washington: American Psychiatric Press. 674–675.

31. Cloninger CR (1994). Somatoform and dissociative disorders. In Winokur G, Clayton P (Eds). *Medical Basis of Psychiatry* (2nd Ed). 169–192.

32. Smith GR, Monson RA, Ray DC (1986). Psychiatric consultation in somatization disorder: a randomized controlled study. *N Engl J Med*, 314:1407–1413.

33. Aronoff GM, Tota-Faucette M, Phillips L, Lawrence CN (2000). Are pain disorder and somatization disorder valid diagnostic entities? *Curr Rev Pain*, 4:309–312.

34. Guggenheim (2000). Somatoform Disorders. In Sadock BJ, Sadock VA, Eds. Kaplan and Sadock's *Comprehensive Textbook of Psychiatry,* 7th Ed. Philadelphia: Lippincott Williams & Wilkins, 1523.

35. Cited in Guggenheim (2000). Somatoform Disorders. In Sadock BJ, Sadock VA, Eds. *Kaplan and Sadock's Comprehensive Textbook of Psychiatry,* 7th Ed. Philadelphia: Lippincott Williams & Wilkins, 1522.

36. Birket-Smith M (2001). Somatization and chronic pain. *Acta Anaesthesiol Scand*, 45:1114–2120.

37. Kulich RJ, Mencher P, Bertrand C, Maciewicz R (2000). Comorbidity of post-traumatic stress disorder and chronic pain: implications for clinical and forensic assessment. *Curr Rev Pain.* 4:36–48.

38. Guggenheim (2000). Somatoform Disorders. In Sadock BJ, Sadock VA, Eds. *Kaplan and Sadock's*

Comprehensive Textbook of Psychiatry, 7th Ed. Philadelphia: Lippincott Williams & Wilkins, 1525.

39. Guggenheim (2000). Somatoform Disorders. In Sadock BJ, Sadock VA, Eds. *Kaplan and Sadock's Comprehensive Textbook of Psychiatry,* 7th Ed. Philadelphia: Lippincott Williams & Wilkins, 1523.

40. Lebovits AH (2000). The psychological assessment of patients with chronic pain. *Curr Rev Pain,* 4:122–126.

41. Fishbain DA, Cutler RB, Rosomoff HL, Rosomoff RS (1998). Do antidepressants have an analgesic effect in psychogenic pain and somatoform pain disorder? A meta-analysis. *Psychosom Med,* 60:503–509.

42. Leamon MH, Plewes J (1999). Factitious disorders and malingering. In Hales RE, Yudofsky SC, Talbott JA (Eds). *American Psychiatric Press Textbook of Psychiatry* (3d Ed). Washington: American Psychiatric Press 698–699.

43. Feldman MD, Ford CV (2000). Factitious disorders. In Sadock BJ, Sadock VA, Eds. Kaplan and Sadock's *Comprehensive Textbook of Psychiatry* (7th Ed). Philadelphia: Lippincott Williams & Wilkins 1535.

44. *DSM-IV* 474.

45. *DSM-IV* 474.

46. Asher R (1951). Münchhausen syndrome. *Lancet,* 1:339–341.

47. Eisendrath SJ (1996). Current overview of factitious physical disorders. In Feldman MD, Eisendrath SJ (Eds). *The Spectrum of Factitious Disorders.* Washington: American Psychiatric Press 21–36.

48. Leamon MH, Plewes J (1999). Factitious Disorders and Malingering. In Hales RE, Yudofsky SC, Talbott JA, Eds. *American Psychiatric Press Textbook of Psychiatry* (3rd Ed). Washington: American Psychiatric Press. 695.

49. Feldman MD, Ford CV (2000). Factitious Disorders. In Sadock BJ, Sadock VA (Eds). Kaplan and Sadock's *Comprehensive Textbook of Psychiatry* (7th Ed). Philadelphia: Lippincott Williams & Wilkins. 1537.

50. Nadelson T (1985). The false patient: chronic factitious disease, Münchhausen syndrome and malingering. In Cavenar JO (Ed). *Psychiatry,* Vol 2. Philadelphia: Lippincott.

51. Feldman MD, Ford CV (1994). *Patient or Pretender: Inside the Strange World of Factitious Disorders.* New York: Wiley, 83–106.

52. Clark EJ, Melnich SC (1958). Munchausen's syndrome or the problem of hospital hoboes. *Am J Med,* 25:6–12.

53. Barker JP (1962). The syndrome of hospital addiction (Münchhausen syndrome): A report on the investigation of seven cases. *J Mental Sci,* 108:107–182.

54. Gorman CA, Wahner HW, Tauxe WN (1970). Metabolic malingerers: Patients who deliberately induce or perpetuate a hypermetabolic or hypometabolic state. *Am J Med,* 48:708–714.

55. Sutherland AJ, Rodin GM (1990). Factitious disorders in a general hospital setting: clinical features and a review of the literature. *Psychosomatics,* 36:392–399.

56. Leamon MH, Plewes J (1999). Factitious disorders and malingering. In Hales RE, Yudofsky SC, Talbott JA (Eds). *American Psychiatric Press Textbook of Psychiatry* (3rd Ed). Washington: American Psychiatric Press. 697.

57. Plassmann R (1994). Münchhausen syndromes and factitious diseases. *Psychother Psychosom,* 62:2–26.

58. Guziec J, Lazarus A, Harding JJ (1994). Case of a 29-year-old nurse with factitious disorder: the utility of psychiatric intervention on a general medical floor. *Gen Hosp Psychiatry,* 16:47–53.

59. Schreier HA (1992). The perversion of mothering: Münchhausen syndrome by proxy. *Bull Menninger Clin,* 56:421–437.

60. Rosenberg DA (1987).Web of deceit: a literature review of Münchhausen by proxy. *Child Abuse Neglect,* 11:547.

61. Leamon MH, Plewes J (1999). Factitious disorders and malingering. In Hales RE, Yudofsky SC, Talbott JA (Eds). *American Psychiatric Press Textbook of Psychiatry* (3rd Ed). Washington: American Psychiatric Press. 702.

62. Repper J (1995). Munchausen syndrome by proxy in health care workers. *J Adv Nursing,* 21:299–304.

63. Donald T, Jueidini J (1996). Munchausen syndrome by proxy: child abuse in the medical system. *Arch Pediatr Adolesc Medicine,* 150:753–758.

64. Rosenberg DA (1987). Web of deceit: a literature review of Münchhausen by proxy. *Child Abuse Neglect,* 11:547–563.

65. Meadow R (1999). Unnatural sudden infant death infant syndrome. *Arch Dis Child,* 80:7.

66. Feldman MD, Ford CV (2000). Factitious disorders. In Sadock BJ, Sadock VA (Eds). Kaplan

and Sadock's *Comprehensive Textbook of Psychiatry* (7th Ed). Philadelphia: Lippincott Williams & Wilkins. 1533.

67. Nadelson T (1985). The false patient: chronic factitious disease, Munchausen syndrome and malingering. In Cavenar JO (Ed). *Psychiatry*, vol 2. Philadelphia: Lippincott Williams & Wilkins.

68. Songer DA (1995). Factitious AIDS: a case report and literature review. *Psychosomatics* 36:406–411.

69. Carney MWP (1980). Artefactual illness to attract medical attention. *Br J Psychiatry* 136:542–547.

70. Feldman MD, Ford CV (2000). Factitious disorders. In Sadock BJ, Sadock VA, Eds. Kaplan and Sadock's *Comprehensive Textbook of Psychiatry* (7th Ed). Philadelphia: Lippincott Williams & Wilkins. 1537.

71. Schreier HA, Libow JA (1993). *Hurting for Love: The Munchausen by Proxy Syndrome.* New York: Guilford Press.

72. Feldman MD, Ford CV (2000). Factitious disorders. In Sadock BJ, Sadock VA (Eds). Kaplan and Sadock's *Comprehensive Textbook of Psychiatry* (7th Ed). Philadelphia: Lippincott Williams & Wilkins. 1536–37.

73. Byard RW, Burnell RH (1994). Covert video surveillance in Munchausen by proxy. *Med J Austral* 160:352.

74. Feldman MD, Eisenrath SJ (Eds) (1996). *The Spectrum of Factitious Disorders.* Washington: American Psychiatric Press.

75. Plassmann R (1994). Münchhausen syndromes and factitious diseases. *Psychother Psychosom,* 62:91–94.

76. Schreier HA, Libow JA (1993). *Hurting for Love: The Munchausen by Proxy Syndrome.* New York: Guilford.

77. Firstman R, Talan J (1997). *The Death of Innocents.* New York: Bantam Books.

78. Bhugra D (1988). Psychiatric Munchausen syndrome: literature review with case reports. *Acta Scand,* 77:497–503.

79. Powell R, Boast N (1993). The million dollar man: resource implications for chronic Munchausen syndrome. *Br J Psychiatry,* 162:253–256.

80. Maxmen JS, Ward NG (1995). *Essential Psychopathology and Its Treatment* (2nd Ed). New York: Norton. 306.

81. *DSM IV* 683.

82. Hall HV, Pritchard DA (1996). *Detecting Malingering and Deception: Forensic Distortion Analysis (FDA).* Delray Beach, FL: St. Lucie Press.

83. Rogers R (1988). *Clinical Assessment of malingering and deception.* New York: Guilford Press.

84. *DSM-IV* 654.

85. *DSM-IV* 652.

86. Fornari VM, Pelcovitz D (2000). Identity problem and borderline disorders. In Sadock BJ, Sadock VA (Eds). *Kaplan and Sadock's Comprehensive Textbook of Psychiatry* (7th Ed). Vol 2. Philadelphia: Lippincott Williams & Wilkins. 2926–2927.

87. Cloninger CR, Svarkic DM (2000). Personality disorders. In Sadock BJ, Sadock VA (Eds). *Kaplan and Sadock's Comprehensive Textbook of Psychiatry* (7th Ed). Vol 2. Philadelphia: Lippincott Williams & Wilkins. 1746–2747.

88. Masterson JF (1976). *Psychotherapy of the Borderline Adult: A Developmental Approach.* New York: Brunner/Mazel.

89. Kernberg O (1975). *Borderline Conditions and Pathological Narcissism.* New York: Jason Aronsons.

90. Maxmen JS, Ward NG (1995). *Essential Psychopathology and Its Treatment* (2nd Ed). New York: Norton. 407.

91. Phillips KA, Gunderson JG (1999). Personality disorders. In Hales RE, Yudofsky SC, Talbott JA (Eds). *American Psychiatric Press Textbook of Psychiatry* (3d Ed). Washington: American Psychiatric Press. 809.

92. Linehan MM (1993). *Cognitive-Behavioral Treatment of Borderline Personality Disorder.* New York: Guilford Press.

93. Linehan MM, Armstrong HE, Surarez A (1991). Cognitive behavioral treatment of chronically parasuicidal borderline patients. *Arch Gen Psychiatry* 48:1060–1064.

94. Kaplan and Sadock (1998). *Synopsis of Psychiatry,* 8th Ed. Philadelphia: Lippincott, Williams & Wilkins, 787.

95. Markovitz PJ, Schulz SC (1993). Drug treatment of personality disorders. *Br J Psychiatry,* 162:122.

96. Maxmen JS, Ward NG (1995). *Essential Psychopathology and Its Treatment* (2nd Ed). New York: Norton. 412.

CHAPTER 14

Sociopolitical and Ethical Issues

Health care providers live in a world consisting of a personal sphere, a professional sphere, and the wider sociopolitical sphere. This final chapter examines the American dilemma of rising health care costs and the problem of the uninsured and the underinsured. There is a brief discussion of the response of the federal government and the insurance industry to manage use and financing of health care. The chapter also discusses moral and ethical issues in reproductive rights and end-of-life decisions that may present you with personal dilemmas. The last section explains the major categories of complementary and alternative medicine and how to respond to and integrate such practices into standard health care.

American Health Care in Crisis?

The World Health Organization in its assessment of the world's 195 national health systems ranked the United States 37th in overall performance and 55th in fairness of access of the American health care system.[1] Part of the explanation for this ranking is that health care coverage in America, in contrast to that of other developed countries, is not provided by government, but rather is a unique mix of a single payer system (i.e., Medicare, Medicaid, and other federal health programs) with private health insurance. As one analyst described the pros and cons of the American system:[2] it provides "advanced medical interventions and high access to care (i.e., little queuing and early treatment)." However, our health care costs are a higher percentage of our gross domestic product than in other developed countries, and "the current system has also resulted in the greatest percentage of uninsured or underin-

sured of any industrialized nation, and access to health care by the poor remains a problem."

There are many reasons for the high costs. Technological advances have made available to the general practitioner a wide battery of effective but expensive diagnostic tests. Replacing worn-out parts, such as hips, clogged arteries, and even organs, are miraculous ways to enhance the quality of life. Indeed the availability of heart–lung machines and kidney dialysis has allowed us to postpone what in earlier times would have been certain death. However, these new procedures came at great cost. One consequence of the rising costs of medical care is that the insurance premiums for group coverage became too expensive for most small or even medium-sized employers to offer as an employee benefit. Costs for individual health insurance coverage quickly spiraled out of reach for many self-employed persons. As a result, the number of uninsured has been rising steadily, so that by the turn of the millennium there were by various estimates between 38 million and 44 million uninsured,[3] 11 million of whom were children under 18.[4] Having such large numbers of uninsured has impaired public health and disrupted the American health care system. Up to two-thirds of persons without insurance and those with high deductibles and copayments tend to avoid routine medical checkups and care for minor health problems.[5] Because they are not monitored and do not receive treatment for chronic illnesses or routine screening for various types of cancer, they tend to die earlier, often of complications from medical conditions that would not have been fatal if diagnosed and treated earlier.[6] Unable to afford preventive care, the uninsured and underinsured tend to use the emergency room of the nearest hospital when a health condition has become too serious to ignore.

Emergency room medicine is expensive. The sheer numbers of uninsured persons showing up for emergency medical care has thrown many community and private hospitals into financial crisis, because they cannot recover the true costs of treating patients who do not have insurance.[7] To recoup these losses, most hospitals have had to raise the prices for hospital services and tests charged to those with insurance coverage: This is known as **cost shifting**. The problem was that the more hospitals charge their insured patients, the higher the costs for employer-provided health benefit plans. As large insurers raised their premiums, more medium-sized and small business enterprises dropped or reduced health insurance as a benefit for their employees.[8] As more people joined the ranks of the uninsured, they swelled the ranks of those using emergency rooms for health problems. The vicious circle kept getting worse as the proportion of insured to uninsured decreased, and a declining number of insured, along with Medicare and Medicaid, were carrying the burgeoning costs of the uninsured, pushing up insurance premiums, leading to more cancellations of employer based benefits.[9]

FEDERAL REFORM EFFORTS

The federal government's response to the problem of the uninsured was Medicare (1965) to finance health care for the elderly,[10] Medicaid to cover those on welfare,[11] and in 1997 the Children's Health Initiative Program (CHIP), administered by the states to provide coverage for children of the working poor.[12,13] Concerned with the rising costs of Medicare, the federal government had a three-part response to cost shifting. One was the diagnosis-related groups, or **DRGs**. Under this system the federal Health Care Finance Administration, or **HCFA**, created a statistical system of classifying any inpatient stay into groups for purposes of payment and length

of stay in a hospital. One goal of the DRG system was to prevent cost shifting in the form of medical tests or procedures not deemed necessary for a particular condition. Another goal was to set fixed reimbursement fees for authorized procedures and limit the length of stay for each DRG.[14] A second federal response was recognition that the traditional fee-for-services system, which rewarded health care providers according to the volume of services, used the wrong incentives.[15] This came in the form of the HMO Act of 1973 and in 1982 the extension of the principle of **capitation** to HMOs providing services to Medicare.[16] The HMO Act was designed to encourage movement to managed care. The final implementation of the concept of capitation payments under Medicare risk contracts in 1985 rounded out the major federal response to the pressures of cost control. With Medicare and Medicaid accounting for 40% of health care spending in the United States, these changes set the stage for a major restructuring of the American health care system (Box 14-1).[17]

MANAGED CARE

Managed care has become the dominant feature of the American health care system. By 1999, enrollment in various managed-care organizations by Americans covered by health care benefits was estimated at close to 90%.[18] Originally the different types of managed-care organizations (**MCOs**) were easily distinguished by either the enrolled population, that is, HMOs, or the participating providers, that is, preferred provider organizations, or **PPOs**. However, over time most MCOs evolved into hybrids with common features. Rather than looking at the labels, HMO or PPO, it is more instructive to categorize an MCO by examining where along a continuum of managing payments and delivery of services they fall. On one end is the old indemnity system, which simply manages payment for services, and on the other end are closed panel provider plans that tightly control cost, usage, and quality.[19]

Box14-1 Managed Care: The Land of Acronyms

HMO (health maintenance organization) originally designated a prepaid group practice that provided medical care to a group of voluntarily enrolled members in return for a preset per month per member fee. With an increase in self-insured businesses, and arrangements that no longer rely on prepayment, that definition is no longer accurate. Although the term HMO is still used due to licensing laws, it now also includes 1) health plans that place at least some of the health care providers at risk for medical expenses, and 2) plans that use primary care physicians as gate keepers.

MCO (managed care organization) is now a generic term that applies to any managed care plan, including a licensed HMO, **PPO** or **PPA** (preferred provider organization or arrangement), **EPO** (exclusive provider organization), **IDS** or **IDN** (integrated delivery system or network), also known as **IDFS** or **IFDN** (integrated delivery and financing system or network). An **IPA** (independent practice association) is an organization that has contracted with a managed care plan to deliver services in return for a single capitation rate. A **PHO** (physician–hospital organization) is formed to contract with managed care plans.

There are many variations of arrangements within each of the above.

Finally, there is **OWA**, which stands for other weird arrangements.

Adapted from Glossary of Terms and Acronyms. In Kongstvedt PR (Editor) *Essentials of Managed Health Care*, 4th Ed. Gaithersburg, MD: Aspen Publishers, 833-853.

Common to most managed care systems now are controls on usage. These can include limits on medical procedures that can be used without justification or precertification and/or limits on which provider or specialist the enrolled patient can choose for treatment. One cost saving was to be gained from requiring benefit members to use a designated primary care provider as an entry point for all health care. The emphasis on primary care providers versus the more expensive specialist was not only to save money but also to create incentives for the provider group to treat the problem without referring to a specialist.[20] In some plans, the primary care physician justifies treatment and referrals. In others, nonlocal case or care managers decide whether certain testing, treatments, or referrals are to be permitted. By requiring strict justifications, the MCOs tried to keep down the number of expensive diagnostic tests as well as referrals to specialists.

A second cost savings was to be realized from the greater bargaining power of the MCOs vis-à-vis the care providing institutions. Having large numbers of members gave the MCOs bargaining power to negotiate the fees for services. Similar to Medicare and Medicaid, the large MCOs had enough clout to set reimbursement fees for hospital care, surgery, and screening and diagnostic testing.[21] Another progression in the concerted efforts by government and insurers to control both costs and services was the introduction of the **capitation system**.

> *Capitation is a prospective payment system that prepays a fixed dollar amount to contracting physicians or groups of physicians, typically on a monthly basis. A physician or group accepting capitated payment commits to providing the agreed-upon primary care or specialty services for individual members of the MCO. The amount is based on the MCO's determination of the cost of providing covered care to each individual of the total membership pool. If a member uses no services in a given month, the physician or group is still paid the capitated amount. On the other hand, when a member patient needs an unusually high level of services in a month, the provider receives no additional payment.*[22]

This system encourages health care providers to hold down costs per patient and per visit. Capitation agreements can create significant financial risk if members use the services more frequently or if many enrolled patients have high-cost chronic needs. Unless the agreement includes separate payments for specialists (called subcapitation), the provider group can lose money if patients need frequent referrals to specialists.[23] In some plans (e.g., Kaiser Permanente) the physicians are paid employees of the HMO. Some plans offer financial incentives to physicians who hold down costs.[24] Making the patient responsible for higher copay costs for out-of-network health care providers or specialists gave incentives to the patients to use approved network providers, who were either under fixed reimbursement schedules or under capitation.

In general, there was initial success in cost containment as health care costs rose more slowly up to 1997. Some of the savings were due to the fierce competition among MCOs to sign contracts with large employers. In part it was also successful because hospitals initially thought they had no choice but to accept capitation or lower reimbursement rates to become approved provider institutions for the MCOs. By 1998 many Medicare-licensed HMOs were caught in the crunch of low reimbursements from Medicare and Medicaid under capitation arrangements.[25] Some responded by canceling their Medicare contracts.[26] Lower Medicare and Medicaid payments also limited the ability of hospitals to shift the costs of obligatory emergency room care for the uninsured.[27] As these financial pressures mounted, some MCOs tried to implement additional cost containment practices.[28] Among these practices was the implementation of rigid rules to inhibit referrals to specialists or emergency services, which brought about negative publicity and Congressional investigations.[29]

One of the unintended consequences of managed care is that it has undermined the financial viability of community mental health centers[30] and public hospitals.[31] The charity care that private physicians used to provide to uninsured patients almost disappeared in a system that uses capitation to reimburse providers.[32] Because providers in HMOs provide care only for members, uninsured persons are forced to seek care from publicly funded institutions via emergency care. In some locations with high concentrations of uninsured, the cost of maintaining public clinics and hospitals has put pressure on local governments to raise local taxes.[33]

IMPACT ON THE HEALTH CARE PROVIDER

Managed care appears to be continually evolving in response to both public and legislative pressures. It is essential that you stay current on the changes in federal and state regulations that affect your ability to refer for consultations or for specialized treatments. You may have to devote a portion of your continuing education to workshops to stay abreast of the constantly shifting economics of the managed-care industry and how changes may affect your practice and your personal financial liability under capitation. You may also want to participate in the political process to help shape the state and federal regulatory process. While you need to stay on top of the policy changes, it essential that you not get overwhelmed by day-to-day financial and administrative details. A smoothly running clinic or practice needs a good business administrator–manager to attend to these details. Much care should go into the selection of such a qualified individual, because in the constantly evolving world of managed care, the expertise of such a person can make the difference between success and failure of a health care enterprise.[34]

Moral and Political Issues

Some issues in health care evoke strong moral and political responses. One category centers on reproductive issues, such as eugenics, abortion, birth control, and genetics counseling. The other category concerns end-of-life decisions, such as assisted suicide, euthanasia, and voluntary discontinuation of treatment. Each presents ethical dilemmas for the health care provider. It is within the larger social context that each health care provider forms a personal response. Your own beliefs, values, and personal experiences may create strong feelings on each of these issues. Such feelings or experiences can make it difficult to be objective when a patient asks for advice or assistance. You need to be informed on the legal and professional obligations governing each issue. Often the ethical dilemma arises when you are faced with the acute anguish of patients in these situations.

REPRODUCTIVE ISSUES

In every primary care setting providers periodically encounter an adult or adolescent who has just learned that she is pregnant. She may be seeking help from the provider to end the pregnancy, either pharmacologically or through surgical abortion. Advising a woman who faces a decision about an unexpected and perhaps unwanted pregnancy can be challenging. The process is generally highly charged with emotion for both you and your patient. Your own ambivalence between empathy with her suffering and moral judgment may make it difficult for you to be objective. Some practitioners have strong beliefs that may lead them to push the patient in one direction or another without fully exploring the situation or respecting the woman's right to base her decision on her perception of the psychosocial implications for her future. It is important to remember that it is not your role to make the decision for the pregnant woman. A woman facing such a decision needs an empathic listener to help her sort out her feelings and lead her objectively through the likely consequences of each of the various options.

• •

PATIENT PROFILE 14.1

I DON'T KNOW WHAT TO DO

SETTING: Melinda, a 17-year-old single girl, has called in to make an emergency appointment with Patti, a nurse practitioner at a suburban county health department whom she has seen twice for reproductive health counseling.

When Melinda first saw Patti, she said she was sexually active. She assured Patti that she did not need to go on the pill, that she would increase condom use to protect herself. Concerned about Melinda's self-admitted drinking and partying,

Patti gave her the standard warnings about the need for consistent condom use to reduce the risk of pregnancy and STIs.

Now Melinda tells Patti over the phone that she has missed her period and that a home pregnancy test came up positive. Melinda's pregnancy test at the health department came out positive also. Patti has just told Melinda that she is pregnant.

Melinda: Oh my God, what am I going to do? I am so scared. (She starts to cry and Patti sits quietly for a few moments.)

Patti: Yes, I can understand that you'd feel scared. Maybe if we talk for a little while, it might help.

Melinda: Every time I think about what I should do, I start feeling panicky. I get confused and start crying.

Patti: I'd like to understand the situation better, so could I ask you some questions? You said you missed your period?

Melinda: Yes. Actually, it was confusing. I had a little bleeding about 10 days before my period was supposed to start, but it lasted only about a day.

Patti: That might have been implantation bleeding. That sometimes happens when the fertilized egg comes down from the Fallopian tubes and implants on the side of the uterus. So, let's try to pinpoint the time. When do you think you got pregnant?

Patti: A little over a month ago, I think. I went to an all-night party and everyone was there and I got drunk and pretty stoned, and I think I might have had sex with a couple of the guys there that night. I don't really remember, but that's what some of my girl friends have told me since.

(Melinda continues to be tearful.)

Patti: Hmmmm. It's probably a good idea to check you for sexually transmitted infections now, too.

Melinda: Oh my God, I hadn't even thought about that. (Melinda slumps in her chair.)

Patti: Let's do a pelvic examination.

After the Examination

Patti: I see no direct evidence of any infections. You seem about 6 weeks along. Have you told your parents?

Melinda: Oh no. They'd kill me.

Patti: Tell me what you mean.

Melinda: They would just be so disappointed. They still see me as their little baby. I don't think they ever think of me as having sex.

Patti: Well, let's talk about that some more in a few minutes. Have you thought about what you want to do?

Melinda: Yes, I've thought about it, but I just don't know what to do.

Patti: There are three choices. Letting the pregnancy go full term and keeping the baby is one choice. Allowing the baby to be adopted is another choice. The third choice is to terminate the pregnancy. Let's talk about each one of them—the pros and cons—and then see if you are clearer about a decision. (*I must remember to include the risk factor here with her drinking alcohol and doing drugs.*)

Melinda: OK.

Patti: You know I can't make this decision for you. You have to make it, but I can help you understand the consequences of each of the choices.

Melinda: Yeah, I know, but I am glad I can talk with you about it. (*At least I am not alone and can talk it out with her.*)

Points to Consider

- Patti knows that Melinda needs emotional support at this time so she gives her a kind and comforting touch and understanding statements.
- Patti starts questioning Melinda to get more information about the pregnancy.
- After hearing the circumstances, Patti tells Melinda they need to check for STIs as well.
- With Melinda being a minor, Patti raises the subject of involving her parents, but leaves it for further exploration until after explaining all the options to her.

- Patti notes that she needs to explore Melinda's alcohol and drug use as one of the factors putting the fetus at risk.
- Patti lets Melinda know that she must make the decision of what to do about the pregnancy herself; Patti cannot make it for her.

• •

A careful joint evaluation of the psychosocial context is key to her reaching a sound decision. What level of family, social, or financial support will the woman have for keeping the child, giving it up for adoption, or ending the pregnancy? A real concern for the health care provider is the woman's physical and emotional health. A full-term pregnancy may be dangerous or even life threatening if the patient is too young or if there are complicating health problems, such as diabetes. It is the duty of the clinician to inform the patient of the possible adverse effects of a full-term pregnancy on her physical and/or mental health. Since the U. S. Food and Drug Administration in November 2000 approved **mifepristone** (Mifeprex) for use in **medical abortion** regimens, primary care practitioners who provide reproductive health care can now offer a private procedure for early abortions.[35] Although it takes more time than a surgical abortion and entails some cramping and bleeding, it appears to be more acceptable to women, especially minors, than surgery.[36] Clinical trials in the United States and Europe have proven mifepristone to be safe and 95% effective if administered within 63 days of last menstruation.[37] It is expected that usage in the United States will rise rapidly as providers become more familiar with it and restrictions on its use are eased. In the near term providers need to determine their state's restrictions, if any, on dispensing this drug.[38]

ABORTIONS FOR M INORS

If the patient is an adolescent, the health care provider needs to know and discuss with her the state laws on abortion for minors. A constitutional right to privacy in reproductive health matters was first recognized be the U. S. Supreme Court in 1965[39] and was extended in 1976 by the Supreme Court to "mature minors" in *Planned Parenthood of Central Missouri versus Danforth.*[40] In 1979 in *Bellotti versus Baird*, the court said that the maturity of the minor had to be determined expeditiously and kept confidential.[41] However, under pressure from religious groups and antiabortion groups, the absolute right to privacy for minors has been whittled away. In the 1992 decision *Planned Parenthood of Southeastern Pennsylvania versus Casey*, the Supreme Court upheld the right of states to require **parental notification**, a 24-hour waiting period, and informed consent.[42] Many states have laws modeled on that decision requiring health care providers to supply the minor with detailed information regarding fetal development, assistance for childbirth, legal responsibilities of the father to support the child, and agencies that assist with adoption. It has been argued that such laws are intended not to inform the patient of the risks and benefits of abortion but rather to discourage them from having one.[43] Most laws recognize that in cases of severely dysfunctional or separated families or a history of familial physical or sexual abuse, parental notification or consent may not be safe, advisable, or possible.[44] As an alternative to parental notification, a waiver from a judge or the adolescent's physician can state that it would be in her best interest that the parent or parents of the underage girl not be notified. The waiver would also declare the minor patient to be mentally competent to make her own decision. However in actual practice, you will find that in most situations a parent or guardian accompanies the minor to the clinic.

To be on the safe side in almost all cases of unaccompanied minors seeking advice on what to do about an unplanned pregnancy, it is suggested that an immediate referral to a counselor be arranged to explore all the options. Such a referral may be to an experienced nurse, social worker, or mental health counselor assigned to the clinic, or it may be to someone from the nearest family shelter or women's center.[45] If the unaccompanied minor is younger than 14, the health care provider may rightfully be reluctant to state that the patient is competent to make such a weighty decision on her own. The provider might first wish to explore whether the pregnant adolescent's fears of being beaten or severely punished by unforgiving parents corresponds with reality. This approach is not recommended if the interview with the patient reveals previous parental physical or sexual abuse. Instead the clinician might inquire if the adolescent has a trusted relative (mother, grandmother, aunt, uncle), girlfriend, or even neighbor who can help her make the decision and/or help her get a judicial waiver letter.

Facing an unwanted pregnancy is a momentous decision point with long-range internal and external consequences. The woman usually has an intense inner struggle with her conscience over the alternatives of ending the pregnancy, keeping the baby, or seeking adoption. Factors weighing on her mind may include personal moral apprehension about abortion, concerns about her future, the reactions of friends and family, concerns about her ability to provide for the child if she has to abandon her education, and concerns about another mouth to feed if she is already living in poverty.[46] Your task is to help her clarify her own values and then support the decision she makes. It would be wise to have in place a protocol for pregnancy counseling, including referral procedures and counseling resources, so that decisions can be made promptly. If ultimately the woman makes a decision that conflicts with your beliefs, it is still incumbent upon you to provide her with professional service, including appropriate referrals.

EUGENICS

The successful mapping of the human genome has raised the possibility of manipulating genes to improve human beings. According to the National Academy of Sciences, errors in our DNA, our genetic material, "are responsible for an estimated 3,000 to 4,000 hereditary diseases."[47] Some of these hereditary diseases are relatively common; others tend to be specific to certain ethnic groups, such as sickle cell disease in African Americans, Tay-Sachs disease in Ashkenazi Jews, and thalassemias primarily in populations of Mediterranean, Chinese, and Asian origins.[48] Altered genes are now known to play a part in cancer, heart disease, diabetes, and many other common diseases. Genetic flaws increase a person's risk of developing these relatively common and other complex disorders. The diseases themselves stem from interactions between genetic predispositions and environmental factors, including diet and lifestyle.

Rapid advances in gene technology have sparked excitement, concern, and a vigorous and often emotional debate between scientists, legal scholars, and ethicists over policy implications.[49] Some hail the genomic breakthroughs as bringing many benefits to humanity and to health care. They predict that gene research and gene therapy will lend great accuracy and certainty to efforts to identify and understand the etiology and pathophysiology of many diseases. Such knowledge can be used in the design of medications that specifically target areas of the brain or body. Some scientists and entrepreneurs cheerfully predict that gene insertion or gene manipulation in utero will permit us to "correct" genetic aberrations responsible not only for various birth defects but also for later-onset diseases such as cancer.[50] Some scientists predict that such gene manipulations will allow us to eliminate whole categories of diseases linked to genetic defects, just as we have eliminated smallpox through vaccinations. Optimists predict that the new knowledge will usher in a whole new era of improved health care in which decisions regarding prevention, treatment, lifestyle recommendations, and nutrition, and even reproduction will be guided by the knowledge of specific gene-related proclivities.

Others look with alarm at the many potential legal, and ethical consequences in the use or misuse of genomic information. It is likely that new discoveries will allow us to identify more genes linked to susceptibility to a wide range of physical diseases and mental and behavioral disorders. Civil libertarians, among others, fear that such information could be used by employers or health insurers to discriminate against a person whose blood test revealed a genetic propensity for a costly condition like cancer or addiction.[51] In the forefront of concern is the issue of privacy. This is an especially serious problem unless health records can be secured against remote electronic access.[52] (A White House executive order protecting federal workers against employment discrimination, issued at the height of a partisan political battle over patients' rights, was designed to be a model for the states.)[53] Another concern is that the use of such information to label a person could also profoundly damage one's self-concept. Having an adverse label linked to genome information could lead to persons seeing themselves (and their family) as flawed or defective. [54]

Moral objections to research on human genes center on the possibility of manipulating genes for creating superior human beings, that is, eugenics. Some fear that using stem cell tissue for gene therapy or genetic engineering is "playing God."[55] Many prominent leaders in the medical and scientific community argue equally strongly that a ban on research on therapeutic cloning of stem cells "would impede progress on some of the most debilitating diseases known to man." Those ailments include Parkinson's disease, Alzheimer's disease, diabetes, cardiovascular diseases, spinal cord injuries, and various cancers and neurological diseases, among others.[56]

The technology using DNA analysis of genetic markers is already producing positive results via prenatal screening. The use of amniocentesis and chorionic villi sampling is likely to increase as the list of genetically transmitted defects grows longer. These procedures can also detect whether certain infections like HIV or hepatitis in the mother have crossed the placental barrier. They can reveal fetal damage from alcoholism, drug abuse, or exposure to other toxins. Also, persons exposed to radioactive or other mutagenic toxins may choose to be screened to see if their reproductive chromosomes were damaged. In all cases of evidence of fetal damage or of a fetus carrying a potentially lethal gene, the parents may need genetic counseling on the risks of carrying the fetus to term or about having children. However, genetic screening is not without legal or ethical challenges. For example, if a prenatal screen reveals Down's syndrome or a more serious birth defect, the parents may need counseling to decide whether to proceed with the pregnancy. Also, some parents who are known carriers of genes for hemophilia and certain other genetically transmitted conditions that affect only males may wish to use prenatal testing for gender selection of a child. In each such case referral to genetic counseling is indicated. "Genetic counseling provides nondirective communication of medical information and options, as well as psychosocial support for the individual couple making these difficult decisions."[57] In addition, knowing that a genetic disorder is present allows for planning and for delivery at a center that is equipped to deal with perinatal complications. Genetic evaluation and counseling are also indicated whenever a baby is born with a birth defect. Although sometimes genetic tests come back showing normal findings, it is important to remember that new genetic syndromes are being discovered that might explain such defects. In addition to taking family histories, a professional geneticist can through a physical examination detect minor anomalies, such as fingerprints, eye spacing, and skin changes, to aid in the identification of genetic syndromes.[58] Cytogenetic and metabolic testing, cranial imaging, and behavioral assessment can be used to rule out genetic disorders when there are no obviously unusual physical features.

DIFFICULT POSTNATAL DECISIONS

Advances in medical technology have created dilemmas in postnatal care. Sometimes an infant born with serious birth defects or with a medical complication, such as oxygen deprivation in the birth canal, may severely compromise chances of surviving and thriving. Such situations present parents and health care providers with pressing and difficult decisions about whether to undertake heroic efforts to preserve life or to take no measures and let the infant die (Box 14-2)[59] In such situations, parents who one moment were flush with the joy of a happy event may be shocked and angry the next, when they find out that the healthy baby they expected is impaired or imperiled. It may be difficult for them to make a decision under such emotional stress. In despair some may just tell the attending physician "Whatever you say."[60]

Affleck[61] suggests that some dialog be conducted. The parents after hearing the news must be given a chance to express their feelings and concerns and ask questions. If the defect is genetic, parents need to be told whether surgical or stem cell therapy to repair the defect is available. The care team members should share their own concerns and provide realistic appraisals about the chances and definitions of success for such interventions. The parents need to know that reparative therapy can be long and expensive. The time and energy required of the parent(s) for the intensive care of such a child can lead to neglect of older siblings. Such care may devolve to social service agencies later, when parents have neither the resources nor the emotional energy to maintain that level of care for the growing child.

Box 14-2 The Baby Doe Rule

Issued by the Reagan Administration, it mandates treatment of impaired newborns unless (1) the infant is permanently comatose, (2) treatment would merely prolong the onset of death, or (3) treatment would not be effective. These criteria have been criticized as being unrealistic or ineffective in light of what goes on in the critical moments after birth when decisions need to be made rapidly by parents and the attending physician(s). Some argue that the rules discriminate against infants who may never have the chance to become competent adults.

Sources: Jones GE (1990) Do the Baby Doe rules discriminate against infants? *Pediatrician* 17:87–91; Moskop JC, Saldanha RL (1986) The Baby Doe rule: still a threat. *Hastings Cent Rep.* 16:8–14.

As can be seen from this short overview of eugenics, there are numerous issues. Work with the new technologies has created new ethical dilemmas. Discussion about ethical guidelines for the use of gene technologies is ongoing. Your task is to keep current on these efforts and to participate in such discussions among your colleagues on the local level. With such discourse, health care providers can forge therapeutic alliances with patients and their families to make the difficult decisions made possible by the new technologies.

End-of-Life Issues

The **right-to-die issue** has spurred an intense ongoing debate in the medical professions and professional journals.[62] The controversy surrounding the notion of health care providers legally helping patients die is seen by some as the successor to the abortion issue.[63] It is an emotional issue that has inflamed politics, religion, and the medical profession.[64] Thirty-nine states prohibit **doctor-assisted suicide**, sometimes called **physician aid-in-dying**, or hastened death. Others seeking assistance also refer to this issue as **rational suicide**. Proponents have put the issue on the ballot in referendums in Oregon, Michigan, California, Washington, and Maine in recent years. Only in Oregon did voters approve the ballot measure. In fact, they did so twice. The *Oregon Death with Dignity Act* first passed in 1994 and was reaffirmed in another referendum in 1997, making Oregon the first state to permit assisted suicide. Interestingly enough, the words "assisted suicide" are not to be found in the Oregon law. Instead, it talks about allowing physicians to respond to an "informed decision by a qualified patient to obtain a prescription to end that patient's life in a humane and dignified manner and that is based on the patient's appreciation of the relevant facts after being fully informed by the attending physician." [65]

Proponents of the right-to-die see assisted suicide as a civil rights issue in which the right to die is the ultimate right to self-determination.[66] According to supporters of this position, each person has an inalienable right to end his or her own suffering if there is no hope of recovery.[67] Supporters of this philosophy propose that autonomy and relief of suffering are paramount and that dying patients have the right to make the process of dying as painless and dignified as possible and to control the time and manner of their death.[68] Patients who wish to avail themselves of this option often talk about assisted suicide as a way to maintain some semblance of control and dignity before they lose physical and mental functions.

The right-to-die concept is bitterly opposed by the right-to-life activists. They have worked tirelessly to convince the public that doctor-assisted suicide should not be legalized.[69] Their argument is that all life is sacred and no one should be in the position of ending a life either by assisted suicide or by discontinuing a life-support system. They see either of those as murder. The medical profession itself is deeply divided over the issue. Some opponents note that the Hippocratic Oath prohibits the hastening of death.[70] Others point out that health care providers by lack of any formal training are unprepared to end life. Pointing to data from the Netherlands revealing clinical problems with assisted suicide—such as the patient being unable to swallow enough medication to make it a lethal dose—some opponents charge that assisted suicide could easily turn into active euthanasia. They seize upon this evidence to invoke the slippery slope argument, saying that if the patient cannot participate, assisted suicide could easily turn into a nightmare in which health care providers decide who should live and who should die. Some opponents of the right-to-die even see advance directives as part of that slippery slope.

A position that has long been held quietly by physicians involved in terminal care is that in certain carefully controlled situations, providing assistance with suicide to a suffering terminally ill patient is an extension of palliative care and thereby fulfills the ethical responsibility to choose "the least harmful alternative."[71] They argue that the ancient aphorisms of the Hippocratic Oath should not be used to avoid personal responsibility inherent in the practice of medicine. Rather, decisions on care should be made on the basis of each situation, taking into account the patient's wishes, the family's wishes, the health care provider's own experience and history with the patient, and the patient's prognosis. Thus, to accede to the request for medication to end life by a patient who is terminally ill might be regarded as an individual act of conscience responding to a higher call to duty than the Hippocratic Oath. As one respected medical authority put it, providing help to a patient, whose suffering cannot otherwise be relieved, to die in a serene and merciful way can be seen as more compassionate care than to prolong life that is devoid of any quality.[72]

● ●

PATIENT PROFILE 14.2

PLEASE HELP ME DIE

SETTING: Tomoko, a 78-year-old married woman born in Japan, has been living in the United States since she was a young woman. She is in the last stage of amyotrophic lateral sclerosis (ALS) and is being cared for at home by her husband Joshua under hospice care. Her hospice worker, Prudence, a registered nurse, is making a home visit. Prudence has been treating Tomoko for almost a year now, mostly through home visits. Tomoko, Joshua, and Prudence have become very close.

Prudence: Good morning, Joshua. *(He looks really tired.)* How is Tomoko today?

Joshua: It is getting harder and harder for her to write on her chalkboard. I am not sure how much long she will be able to communicate with us. *(How much longer can this go on? Well, Tomoko will talk with Prudence about what we talked about last night. Maybe she can help us.)*

Prudence: Yes, that is going to be another hard step for you and her. These losses just keep coming, don't they?

Joshua: Yes, we've all lost so much and now we are closer to losing her. *(And yet there is a place inside of me that will always be with her.)*

Prudence: You know, Joshua, you will always have her in your memories.

Joshua: *(That's why I really care about Prudence, she can almost read my mind.)* Yes, we've had some good ones. After the war, when I met her in Tokyo, I'll never forget that day.

Prudence: *(Patiently waits a few moments as Joshua goes into a reverie of memories and sighs.)* How is she doing on her medications?

Joshua: All right. Oh! I have to go to the store to fill a prescription. Is it all right if I go down there while you are seeing her? I have my cell phone and you have the number, so call me if anything happens.

Prudence: Sure, I'll go on in now.

Joshua: She has something she wants to talk with you about.

Prudence: *(Nods. As Joshua gets ready to go out, she goes into Tomoko's room, drops a tape in the player, and turns it on. Tomoko likes to hear her choir sing. Prudence is a member of a choir and she regularly tapes the rehearsals for Tomoko. Music softly fills the room.)* Hello, Tomoko. I brought you a tape of our last rehearsal. It was a little ragged at the beginning but our last run-through was passingly good. I see you've been writing on your chalkboard. Joshua said you had something you wanted to talk with me about?

(Tomoko nods and makes frustrating gestures with the chalkboard.)

Prudence: He also said you were having trouble writing now.

(Tomoko makes more frustrating gestures.)

Prudence: Yes, I know. Remember, we talked about that happening? *(Every time I see Tomoko, I feel the sadness in this house, and I get sad too. They have endured so much, first the aftermath of the war in Japan, then the adjustment of their in-laws to a cross-cultural marriage, followed by the teasing their children endured in school, and now this. At least they* *had some good years after the children went off to college and made their own lives. They are so proud of them and their grandchildren. Look at all those pictures Joshua has put up on the wall where she can see them. He is so thoughtful of her.)*

(Tomoko angles the chalkboard towards Prudence. She has written, "Please help me die.")

Prudence: *(I was wondering when this question would be asked. Could I be as brave?)*

Points to Consider

- Prudence realizes that her role has shifted from nursing to grief counselor.

- Prudence gives attention, support, and relief time to Joshua, Tomoko's main caregiver, because he needs it as much as or more than Tomoko.

- When Prudence gives Joshua time to listen internally to his own memories, she helps him cope with his own grief.

- Prudence remembers Tomoko's love of music and has brought a tape for her to enjoy, thus improving the quality of her life.

- Prudence acknowledges her own grief and feelings, which is the first step in taking care of herself and her stressors.

• •

The ongoing debate will be informed by the data now flowing from the two jurisdictions where death with dignity acts are in force—the Netherlands and Oregon.[73] Oregon has mandated annual reviews of the practice and has instituted strict reporting requirements. On receipt of some of the data from the first report, additional regulatory safeguards to prevent possible abuses were added.[74] Some see the fine-tuning of these social experiments as removing many of the ethical and legal objections to having physicians participate in such difficult end-of-life decisions.[75] However, because it is such an emotionally charged issue, it is unlikely that the political process will respond in a timely fashion to provide legal protection to physicians who do accede to

requests from terminally ill patient to assist in ending their suffering.

Whether you live in a jurisdiction that provides legal protection or not, you are likely to have to confront the right-to-die issue with a patient at some time. Medical ethicists predict that with the rapid increases of our aging population in the coming decades, the number of terminally ill patients requesting assistance from their health care provider to end unbearable pain and suffering will rise.[76] Thus, health care providers need to search out their conscience on how to respond to such requests. Each individual case is different and is between the patient, the family, and the health care provider. In general, as in the jurisdictions where such decisions are legal, assessment for such a decision should be shared with at least one other health care provider. This is not only a personal issue of conscience, but in jurisdictions where prohibited by law, it is also a legal issue.

Complementary and Alternative Medicine

In 1993 the *New England Journal of Medicine* published the results of a survey on **complementary and alternative medicine** (CAM). David Eisenberg and his colleagues from Harvard found that in 1990 about a third of American adults had used at least one unconventional therapy the previous year, had made 425 million office visits to providers of such therapies (exceeding the 388 million to primary care providers), and had paid 75% of the costs for alternative care out of pocket.[77] The federal government estimated that by the turn of the millennium, 42% of health care consumers annually spent $27 billion on CAM.[78] The holistic health movement has become big business with a large consumer demand for vitamins, herbal preparations, and self-help books on healing. A thriving literature advertises holistic healing practices including acupuncture and balancing body, mind, and spirit through meditation and yogic breathing. It also offers specific herbs to strengthen the

CHAPTER 14 SOCIOPOLITICAL AND ETHICAL ISSUES ▼ 277

immune system, alleviate depression, or fight cancer. Some of the modalities listed in this chapter are being practiced by persons who may have a certification from their own professional association but may not be regulated by state licensure. However, many licensed health care professionals are blending various CAM modalities into their regular practice in what has become known as **integrative medicine**.[79]

Many health care consumers turn to CAM because they feel that allopathic medicine has little to offer for many common complaints. Indeed, a number of those who came into contact with other systems of healing during their search for spirituality in the turbulent 1960s became prominent researchers and authors of influential books supporting CAM.[80-82]

Understandably, there has been official and professional concern about persons self-medicating with practices or herbal preparations for which rigorous testing or scientific evidence of efficacy was lacking. Amid cries that much of the CAM therapies were quackery and that the public was being swindled, the National Institutes of Health (NIH) in 1992 established the Office of Alternative Medicine (OAM) with a budget of $2 million. In 1998, under pressure from the American medical establishment and the pharmaceutical industry, NIH upgraded the OAM into the National Center for Complementary and Alternative Medicine (NCCAM), whose fiscal year 2003 budget is more than $100 million.[83] NCCAM research grants are dedicated to putting the various therapies under strict scientific scrutiny. While clinical studies have already validated short-range benefits of some therapies, NCCAM admits it will take years to get results from studies of long-range benefits or dangers.[84] Meanwhile, practitioners of traditional medicine need to look at how the use of CAM affects their relationship with, and treatment of their patients. Thus, we need to know what these alternative therapies are and how they attract health care consumers.

The NCCAM defines complementary and alternative medicine as "health care and medical practices that are not currently an integral part of conventional medicine."[85] It goes on to say that the list of CAM practices changes continually as new ones are added and as some CAM practices and therapies are proven effective and are accepted as mainstream health care practices. The NCCAM has devised a classification system of grouping the various CAM practices into five major domains:

1. **Alternative medical systems**

2. **Mind–body interventions**

3. **Biology-based treatment**

4. **Manipulative and body-based therapies**

5. **Energy therapies**

Within each of these categories are individual modalities too numerous to list in a broad overview. Instead we will focus on the major conceptual framework of each domain and give a few limited examples from each domain (Box 14-3).

ALTERNATIVE SYSTEMS

Some alternative medical systems predate Western systems by many centuries. They are the traditional systems of medicine practiced by individual cultures. Each generally has its own cultural and/or spiritual explanatory schema. Most are at great variance with Western scientific explanations of pathology. They rely instead on an internally consistent belief system, often involving concepts of subtle energy. For example, **traditional Oriental medicine** emphasizes that proper balance of the vital energy, also known as **qi**, or chi, is necessary for good health and that disturbances in the qi energy cause disease. The practitioner of traditional Oriental medicine may use one or more techniques from acupuncture, herbal medicine, cupping, scraping, massage, or even qi gong movement. Traditionally the task of the Oriental healer was to keep patients healthy by using some of these techniques for maintaining the proper flow of qi and a balance of the **yin** and **yang** energies.[86]

Box 14-3 Complementary and Alternative Medicine Modalities

I. Alternative Medical Systems

Ayurvedic medicine, feng shui, folk medicine, herbal medicine, homeopathy, iridology, naturopathic medicine, shamanism, traditional Chinese (Oriental) medicine

II. Mind–Body Interventions

Aromatherapy, art therapy, autogenic training, biofeedback, dance/movement therapy, do-in, gestalt therapy, qi gong, guided imagery, hypnotherapy, meditation, music therapy, postural therapy, prayer, relaxation techniques, sound therapy, speech therapy, spiritual healing, yoga

III. Biology-Based Therapies

Chelation therapy, herbs, home remedies, neural therapy, nutritional therapy, orthomolecular therapy, ozone therapy, supplements

IV. Manipulative and Body-Based Therapies

Alexander work, body work, chiropractic, colon therapy, cranial sacral therapy, enzyme therapy, Feldenkrais' Awareness Through Movement, Hellerwork, Hydrotherapy, kinesiology, massage therapy, metamorphic technique, osteopathic manipulation, reflexology, Aston-Patterning, shiatsu, strain-counter strain, Structural Integration, Trager.

V. Energy Therapies

Auric healing, Bach flower remedy, Bioenergetics/radix, color therapy, crystals/gem therapy, electromagnetic therapy, Hands of Light Healing, magnet therapy, polarity therapy, radionics, Reiki, Therapeutic Touch, Thought Field Therapy, vibrational medicine

Source: nccam.nih.gov/nccam/fep/classify. This web site contains specific information on each modality.

There is an old myth that in ancient China, the healing practitioners were on retainer by wealthy families as long they kept their clients healthy, and when a client fell ill, payments stopped until health was restored again.

Ayurveda is the traditional system of medicine of Hindu cultures. Deepak Chopra, a medical doctor from India, has popularized in the West this holistic approach, which emphasizes the essential unity of body, mind, and spirit.[87]

Ayurvedic medicine strives to restore the innate harmony within the individual through a balanced use of diet, exercise, meditation with special breathing exercises, herbs, colonic cleansing, and massage.

According to NCCAM, **shamanism**, or indigenous healing, has been and still is the most widely practiced type of healing throughout the nonindustrialized world and among native Americans in America. It is a system that predates Oriental and Ayurvedic medicine and has been used especially for serious illness in almost all ancient cultures. The shamans, sometimes wise or healing women,[88] are said to understand in a spiritual sense the nexus of the mind, the body, and the soul. The most distinguishing feature of shamanic healing is the ability to heal with the imagination. The practices include using ritual to induce altered states of consciousness, in which deep levels of the unconscious are accessed and mobilized to fight the affliction, injury, or disease.[89] Effectiveness of shamanic healing has usually been associated with the heightened sense of expectancy on the part of the sick or injured person after a guided journey into the realm of the imagination.[90]

Another major system dating to the early 1800s is **homeopathy**. Developed by the German physician Samuel Hahnemann, it is based on the principle that "like cures like," that is, the same substance that in large doses produces the symptoms of an illness in very minute doses will cure it. The homeopathic pharmacopoeia includes more than 2,000 specific medications, usually prepared as tinctures or as pills with lactose fillers. The substances, which can come from plants, minerals, or even animals, are dispersed in infinitesimal dilute solutions, such as $1:10^{20,000}$, which makes them impossible to detect by standard chemical analysis. Although homeopathic medical schools no longer exist in the United States, homeopathic remedies have continued to remain popular, especially in Europe.

Naturopathy views disease as a manifestation of disturbances in the processes by which the body heals itself. It emphasizes health restoration rather than treatment of symptoms.

Naturopathic physicians employ a wide array of techniques taken from other CAM systems. Thus, a naturopath may choose a combination of nutrition and special diets, homeopathy, herbal medicine, contrasting-temperature hydrotherapy (Kneipp), spinal and soft tissue manipulation, physical therapies using low-voltage electrical currents, ultrasound, light therapy, a pharmacology based on "natural" remedies such as flowers and aromatherapy, and therapeutic counseling.

MIND–BODY INTERVENTIONS

The second major domain in the NCCAM classification system is **mind–body interventions**. The principle in this domain is that the mind on a conscious or unconscious level can have a powerful influence on bodily functions and symptoms. Thus, a wide range of techniques, some of which have been integrated into standard medical practice, fall into this category. For example, patient education and cognitive-behavioral therapy to create awareness and bring about changes in dysfunctional personal habits or to enhance coping skills for handling stressors in the psychosocial environment have become part of accepted practice. Guided imagery and hypnotherapy, which have been shown to be effective in treating serious disease conditions, have found acceptance among some practitioners of standard medicine[91,92] but are still regarded with suspicion by others. Other mind–body interventions employing meditation, humor, light, color, sound, music, art, movement, or dance as therapeutic techniques have their ardent proponents and followers[93] but are still regarded as falling outside the mainstream. Some therapies from this last group are generally considered appropriate for people with diagnoses such as autism, stroke, or mental retardation.[94]

BIOLOGY-BASED TREATMENTS

The **biology-based treatment** domain is divided into herbal, special dietary, orthomolecular, and individual biological therapies. This domain has undergone a major image shift in the past 10 years. What was once relegated to the specialty magazines associated with health food fads has increasingly made its way into a broad array of the periodical literature appealing to the general public. An ever-expanding arsenal of herbs is being advertised and touted for treating depression, strengthening the immune system, preventing Alzheimer's dementia, relieving arthritis, and improving sexual potency. Widespread publicity has been given to a number of special nutritional approaches believed to be effective for controlling degenerative diseases and promoting health and vitality. Among these are macrobiotic[95] and vegetarian diets[96] and the specialty diets by successful authors like Atkins,[97] Ornish,[98] Pritikin,[99] and Weil.[100]

Proponents of orthomolecular therapy argue that the processing of food, environmental pollution, and stress reduce the amount of vitamins and minerals available to our bodies for optimal functioning. Accordingly, we need to supplement our inadequate intake or compensate for stress with a variety of vitamins and minerals, often in megadoses, as a preventive measure to enhance the body's disease fighting ability, to retard the aging process, and to promote physical and neurological health. Some specific pathologies caused by specific orthomolecular deficiencies are also said to respond well to treatment with vitamins, minerals, or hormones, sometimes derived from herbal preparations. Examples of such biological therapies include ingesting capsules of ground shark cartilage to treat cancer and arthritis or bee pollen to treat allergies.

MANIPULATIVE AND BODY-BASED METHODS

The fourth domain identified by NCCAM are the **manipulative and body-based methods**. Typical of these, **osteopathy** and **chiropractic medicine** have long held that disturbances and misalignments in the musculoskeletal structure can have far-reaching effects on other systems of the body. Chiropractic and osteopathic manipulation are no longer considered CAM, at least judging by the insurance industry's acceptance of these therapies. Other body therapies focus more on soft tissue manipulation to reduce stress, trauma-induced tension, or energy "blockages" and thereby normalize or enhance physical and mental functioning. Among these are massage, Structural Integration (Rolfing), Awareness Through Movement (Feldenkrais), Trager, trigger point release therapy, shiatsu, and foot reflexology.

ENERGY THERAPIES

The final NCCAM category is **energy therapies**. One type, known as the biofield, focuses on energy fields originating from within the body and surrounding it. Another, known as the electromagnetic field, involves the use of magnets, magnetic fields, or low-level electrical currents to treat specific conditions, such as asthma, cancer, or pain. In the biofield realm, proponents of **Reiki** or **Therapeutic Touch** believe that the practitioner can channel healing energy to balance the patient's energy field. In Reiki there is direct laying on of hands to do the healing. In Therapeutic Touch, practitioners scan for imbalances by passing their hands over the patient's body and then work to create balance.

INTEGRATIVE MEDICINE

This brief overview of the more common therapies in the NCCAM classification system provides a glimpse of the principles which underlie each category. Those mentioned in passing are described in greater detail in other sources, including standard textbooks.[101] With almost half the American public using some form of CAM at least once a year and spending about 40% of their health care dollars on it,[102] the medical profession has had to take notice. A 1998 *Journal of the American Medical Association* article presenting the results of a second national health consumer survey on the use alternative medicine, found that:

Users of alternative health care are more likely to report having had a transformational experience that changed the way they saw the world. . . . They find in [CAM] an acknowledgment of the importance of treating illness within a larger context of spirituality and life meaning. . . . The use of alternative care is part of a broader value orientation and set of cultural beliefs, one that embraces a holistic spiritual orientation to life.[103]

The widespread public acceptance of these principles and a growing body of research supporting them have forced even ardent science-oriented medical researchers to acknowledge that health and disease are not merely the results of the interactions of mechanical and physiological processes within the body and that psychosocial and spiritual factors play a major role in the genesis and progression of disease and in healing. Indeed this is the position of the authors of this book.

For example, counseling and guided imagery have been successfully integrated into the conventional treatment of a variety of conditions like cancer,[104,105] vascular problems,[106] even HIV.[107] Similarly, stress management and diet counseling are becoming standard adjuncts to the treatment of many diseases. Most challenging to the Western scientific tradition are large controlled studies by some of the most respected research institutions that appear to confirm the principle that healing can occur without physical contact.[108–111] Larry Dossey, a pioneering medical researcher, concludes that "healing can be achieved at a distance by directing loving and compassionate thoughts, intentions, and prayers to others, who may even be unaware these efforts are being extended to them."[112] Dossey asserts that integrating spirituality into the healing process can enrich the way you practice medicine. However, barriers still abound. While some clinicians already pray with or for their patients, others feel uncomfortable even bringing up the topic with the patient. Many patients feel inhibited from mentioning their spiritual faith in a medical environment to anyone other than a pastor. If spiritual practices such as prayer can be acknowledged to promote healing, speed recovery from surgery, and shorten hospital stays, it follows that practitioners should explore the patient's comfort level about it. If the patient and the family respond positively, your encouragement and endorsement of such practice can have an empowering effect on the patient and lower the stress levels of all concerned, including the provider.[113] Dossey argues persuasively that the integration of such practices would lead to a paradigm shift in the practice of Western medicine.[114]

Whether as a clinician you believe in some or all of the CAM approaches is less important than how you relate to your patients who do believe in them. Overall, we suggest that you stay open, receptive, and supportive of any of the efforts of the patient to bring other modalities to bear on their recovery. It is essential that you respect each person's beliefs about the efficacy about a specific CAM technique. When you show interest and respect, you are much more likely to get patients to give you information about what else they are doing, whether that be seeing faith healers or taking herbal extracts that were recommended by their grandmother. For example, for the latter you may need to consult the new desk references for herbal medicines[115] or for nonprescription drugs and dietary supplements[116] to check for adverse interactions with standard pharmacological preparations (See Patient Profile 14.3). Your effort should be directed to use as much of the alternative technique as feasible to complement the standard medical regimen you prescribe. To build your competence in integrative medicine, you will need to keep up with the research findings by NCCAM on the CAM modalities. You may also find it personally stimulating to read some of the writings of the pioneers in this field.

• •

PATIENT PROFILE 14.3

JUST A LITTLE SOMETHING FOR MORE ENERGY

SETTING: Daniel is a 47-year-old divorced man with high blood pressure and depression. He is being followed by his physician assistant, Carrie.

Carrie has been treating him in a small clinic in a rural township for 3 years. He had a nasty divorce 2 years ago and is depressed, for which he receives Prozac 30 mg. His presenting problem is that he sometimes has a racing heartbeat. Carrie takes a few minutes to review Daniel's chart before entering the examination room.

Carrie: Hello, Daniel. I see that you are in today because you said your heart races sometimes. Your blood pressure is a little high today. What is going on?

Daniel: Sometimes my heart just seems to pound fast and hard. It isn't connected to anything I've done. It just sort of comes out of the blue. I've also been feeling sluggish lately. I'm getting ready for a big presentation at work and really need to be up for it.

Carrie: Hmmm. *(We'll need to check out his heart again. I wonder if this sluggishness is a signal of an increase in the depression.)* Daniel, let's check out your heart again and schedule you for some tests, but do you know that lowered energy level is one of the signs of depression? How are you sleeping?

Daniel: OK, but every so often I get up in the middle of the night with ideas for the presentation. I get up, write them down, and go back to bed. I usually fall asleep right away.

Carrie: How about your appetite?

Daniel: Fine. I eat a good breakfast, have lunch at work, and then I usually fix up something myself or nuke one of those "healthy" dinners you suggested I buy.

Carrie: Are you still getting out regularly to walk your dogs?

Daniel: You bet. Although it seems they walk me more than me walking them. And I have to admit that sometimes if the weather is bad I make it a short run.

Carrie: Have there been any other changes in your lifestyle lately?

Daniel: No.

Carrie: *(Well, let's see what kind of results we get from these tests. What else could be going on?)* Daniel, are you taking any over-the-counter drugs I don't know about? The last time we talked about that was a month ago.

Daniel: No... oh... well, yes. I mean, not a drug but an herbal preparation my sister gave me. She said it was just a little something for more energy. Actually I brought the bottle because I thought you might like to know about it so you can recommend it to your other patients. It does give me a boost in energy. (He hands her the bottle and she looks at the label.)

Carrie: Daniel, this contains a very potent stimulant called ephedra, and you should not be taking it because it isn't good if you have any kind of heart problems. That's what's causing your heart to race. *(I am so glad he brought the bottle!)*

Daniel: Oops! Wow. I didn't know herbs could be harmful. I thought they were natural.

Carrie: Yes, they can be harmful, especially when you have other problems for which you take medications. Some herbal and drug interactions can be harmful, as you've just found out. I think if you stop taking this, your heart will calm down, but we should do some tests anyway just to confirm that was the reason your heart was racing. We need to rule out any additional development anyway. Also, let's talk some more about your sluggish feeling. I am so glad you brought the bottle with you.

Daniel: Me too, and I am so glad you read the label.

Carrie: And Daniel, before you take anything else, please bring it in and we can talk about it.

Daniel: I sure will. Thanks.

Points to Consider

- When Carrie wonders if the sluggishness is connected with his depression, she is paying attention to the importance of the effects of depression on energy levels.

- When Carrie asks Daniel about his sleep, appetite and interest levels, she is monitoring vegetative signs of depression in Daniel.

- Checking on any lifestyle changes every so often can often reveal details that might influence their symptoms.

- Carrie asks Daniel to bring in any bottles of over-the-counter herbal preparations because that request can assist in the identification of substances that may interact negatively with Daniel's symptoms and medications.

- Carrie knows that heart conditions can change and it is a good idea to update testing to make sure the herbal preparation did not hurt his heart.

- Carrie knows that continued education of Daniel can assist him in being more responsible for and compliant in his treatment.

Conclusion

This chapter briefly covers a number of disparate moral, social, legal, and political issues that affect you on a personal and professional level. You will inevitably face the issues mentioned here—as well as some not covered, such as malpractice insurance. All of us in the health care professions need to be informed about them, examine our own values and attitudes on each, and be prepared to act in the highest professional manner when relating to a patient. Thus, whether that patient is uninsured or underinsured, seeking an abortion, seeking advice on a malformed fetus or neonate, wants your help in ending their suffering, or wants you to endorse an alternative medical modality, you often face moral, and ethical decisions, some of which have legal ramifications. Whether you provide primary care or a medical specialty, you will encounter one or more of these issues repeatedly. We view the exploration of the issues presented in this chapter as an introductory preparation for actual practice. Throughout your career, you will need to stay aware of the political and social changes relating to health care, because they will affect the way you practice your profession and the way you get reimbursed for your services. Most important, though, staying informed and exploring and sharing your thoughts and doubts on some of the difficult ethical decisions with your colleagues will give you a sense of participation, personal satisfaction with your work, and a sense of pride of belonging to your profession.

REFERENCES

1. World Health Organization (2000). Annex: Table 1, Table 7. In *World Health Report 2000*. Geneva: WHO.

2. Kongstvedt PR (ed) (2001). *Essentials of Managed Health Care* (4th Ed). Gaithersburg, MD: Aspen. p xxi.

3. Institute of Medicine (2000). *Coverage Matters: Insurance and Health Care*. Washington: National Academy Press.

4. Fronstein R (2000). Sources of Health Insurance and Characteristics of the Uninsured: Analysis of the March 1999 Current Population Survey. Washington, DC: Employee Benefit Research Institute.

5. Ayanian JZ et al. (2000). Unmet Health Needs of Uninsured Adults in the United States. *JAMA* 284 (16):2061–2069.

6. Baker DW, Shapiro MF, Schur CL (2000). Health insurance and access to care for symptomatic conditions. *Arch Intern Med* 160:1269–1274.

7. US Congress House Committee on Ways and Means, Subcommittee on Health. (1999). *Uninsured Americans: Hearing June 15, 1999*. Washington: US GPO.

8. Institute of Medicine (2000). Who goes without health insurance? Who is most likely to be uninsured. In *Coverage Matters: Insurance and Health Care*. Washington: National Academy Press.

9. US Census (2001). Health Care Revenues 1999. www.census.gov.

10. Starr P (1982). *The Social Transformation of American Medicine*. New York: Basic Books.

11. Stevens R, Stevens R (1974). *Welfare Medicine in America*. New York: Free Press.

12. Begley S, Hearn RP (2001). Children's Health Initiatives. In Isaacs SL, Knickman JR, Eds. *To Improve Health Care 2001: The Robert Wood Johnson Foundation Anthology*. San Francisco: Jossey Bass. 53–74.

13. Lewit EM (1998). The State Children's Health Insurance Program (CHIP). In *The Future of Children: Children and Managed Care*, 8 (2),152–158. Los Altos, CA: Packard Foundation.

14. Kongstvedt PR (2001). Negotiating and contracting with hospitals, institutions, and ancillary services. In Kongstvedt PR (ed). *Essentials of Managed Health Care* (4th Ed). Gaithersburg, MD: Aspen. 166–167.

15. Fox PD (2001). An overview of managed care. In Kongstvedt PR (ed). *Essentials of Managed Health Care* (4th Ed). Gaithersburg, MD: Aspen. 6.

16. Moon M (2001). Health Policy 2001: Medicare. *N Engl J Med* 344:928–931.

17. Zarabaso C, LeMasurier JD (2001). Medicare and managed care. In Kongstvedt PR (ed). *Essentials of Managed Health Care* (4th Ed). Gaithersburg, MD: Aspen, 657-682.

18. Wagner ER (2001). Types of managed care organizations. In Kongstvedt PR (ed). *Essentials of Managed Health Care* (4th Ed). Gaithersburg, MD: Aspen. 18.

19. Wagner ER (2001). Types of managed care organizations. In Kongstvedt PR (ed). *Essentials of Managed Health Care* (4th Ed). Gaithersburg, MD: Aspen. 19.

20. Kongstvedt PR (2001). Contracting and Reimbursement of Specialty Physicians. In Kongstvedt PR (ed). *Essentials of Managed Health Care* (4th Ed). Gaithersburg, MD: Aspen. 141–156.

21. Kongstvedt PR (2001). Negotiating and contracting with hospitals, institutions and ancillary services. In Kongstvedt PR (ed). *Essentials of Managed Health Care* (4th Ed). Gaithersburg, MD: Aspen. 157–176.

22. AMA (1996). Managing Managed Care, Washington, DC: AMA. 59.

23. AMA (1996). Managing Managed Care, Washington, DC: AMA. 65–70.

24. Kongstvedt PR (2001). Compensation of Primary Care Physicians in Managed Health Care. In Kongstvedt PR (ed). *Essentials of Managed Health Care* (4th Ed). Gaithersburg, MD: Aspen. 103–140.

25. Levit K, Cowan C, Lazenby H, et al. (2000). Health Spending in 1998: Signals of change. *Health Affairs*, 19:117–124.

26. Barents Group (1999). *How Medicare HMO withdrawals affect beneficiary benefits, costs, and continuity of care*. Menlo Park, CA: Henry J Kaiser Foundation.

27. Thorpe KE, Seiber EE, Florence, CS (2001). The impact of HMOs on hospital-based uncompensated care. *J Health Politics Policy Law*, 26:543–555.

28. Hurley R, Rawlings RB (2001). Who lost cost containment? A roster for recrimination. *Managed Care Q*, 9:23–32.

29. Plocher DW, Wilson WL, Lutz JA, Huston A (2001). Care management and clinical integration components. In Kongstvedt PR (ed). *Essentials of Managed Health Care* (4th Ed). Gaithersburg, MD: Aspen. 179–196.

30. Hawkins DR, Rosenbaum S (1998). The challenges facing health centers in a changing health care system. In Altman SH, Reinhardt UE, Shields AE (eds). *The Future US Healthcare System: Who Will Care for the Poor and Uninsured?* Chicago: Health Administration Press. p 99–122.

31. Gage LS (1998). The future of safety net hospitals. In Altman SH, Reinhardt UE, Shields AE (eds). *The Future US Healthcare System: Who Will Care for the Poor and Uninsured?* Chicago: Health Administration Press. 123–149.

32. Cunningham PJ et al. (1999). Managed care and physicians' provision of charity care. *JAMA*, 282:1087–1092.

33. Institute of Medicine (2001). Appendix A: A Conceptual Framework for Evaluating the Consequences of Uninsurance. In *Coverage Matters: Insurance and Health Care*. Washington: National Academy Press.

34. Plocher DW (2001). Fundamentals and core competencies of disease management. In Kongstvedt PR (ed). *Essentials of Managed Health Care* (4th Ed). Gaithersburg, MD: Aspen. 28–292.

35. Burke AE, Moore K, Blumenthal PD (2002). Mifepristone at one year: A forward look back. *Medscape Women's Health Journal*, 7(2), 2002.

36. Phelps RH, Schaff EA, Fielding SL (2001). Mifepristone abortion in minors. *Contraception*, 64:339–343.

37. Bjorge L, Johnsen SL, Midboe G, et al. (2001). Early pregnancy termination with mifepristone and misoprostol in Norway. *Acta Obstet Gynecol Scand*, 80(11):1056–1061.

38. Fielding SL, Lee SS, Schaff EA (2001). Professional considerations for providing mifepristone-induced abortion. *Nurse Pract*, 26:44–54.

39. Griswold v Connecticut, 381 US 479 (1965).

40. Planned Parenthood of Central Missouri v Danforth, 428 US 52 (1976).

41. Bellotti v Baird, 443 US 622 (known as Bellotti II) (1979).

42. Planned Parenthood of Southeastern Pennsylvania v Casey, 505 US 833 (1992).

43. Rocket LR (2000). Legal issues affecting confidentiality and informed consent in reproductive health. *J Am Med Womens Assoc*, 55:257–260.

44. Women's Health Center (1998). Parental Notification Law on Abortions: Q & A, Who it Affects, Exceptions, Procedures (Brochure). Charleston, WV: Women's Health Center.

45. Lambke MR, Kavanaugh K (1999). Nurses' Descriptions and Evaluations of Reproductive Counseling for Adolescent Females. *Health Care Women Int*, 20:147–162.

46. Brown SS, Eisenberg L (eds) (1995). *The Best Intentions: Unintended Pregnancy and the Well-Being of Children and Families.* Institute of Medicine, Div of Health Promotion and Disease Prevention. Washington, DC: National Academy Press.

47. NAS (2001). Genetic errors cause disease. In Beyond Discovery: The Path from Research to Human Benefit. Available at http://www4.nas.edu/beyond/beyonddiscovery.nsf/web/gene

48. McGinnis MJ, Kaback MM (1997). Carrier Screening. In Rimoin DL, Connor JM, Pyeritz RE. *Emery and Rimoin's Principles and Practice of Medical Genetics* (3d Ed). New York: Churchill Livingstone. 535–543.

49. Andrews LB et al. (eds) (1994). Assessing Genetic Risks: Implications for Health and Social Policy. Institute of Medicine, Div Health Science Policy. *Washington: National Academy Press.*

50. Gillis, J (2001, Feb 9). Big buildup to the genome: schools, companies constructing labs for research push. *Washington Post*, E-1.

51. Kite M (2001, Feb 8). Insurance firm admits using genetic screening. *The Times* (London).

52. Lewin T (2000, July 16). Boom in genetic testing raises questions on sharing results. *New York Times*, A1,16.

53. Clinton WJ (2000, Feb 8). Executive order to prohibit discrimination in federal employment based on genetic information. *US Fed Register* 65(28):6877–80.

54. Neilson J (1999). A patient's perspective on genetic counseling and predictive testing for Alzheimer's disease. *J Genet Couns*, 8(1):37–46.

55. Stolberg SG (2002, April 11). Bush makes fervent bid to get senate to ban cloning research. *New York Times*, A-28.

56. Goldstein A (2002, April 11). President presses senate on cloning. *Washington Post*, A-1.

57. Facher JJ, Robin NH (2000). Genetic counseling in primary care. *Postgrad Med*, 107:59–66.

58. Jones KL (1996). *Smith's Recognizable Patterns of Human Malformation* (5th Ed). Philadelphia: Saunders.

59. Fost N (1999). Decisions regarding treatment of seriously ill newborns. *JAMA*, 281:2041–2043.

60. Morrow J (2000). Making mortal decisions at the beginning of life: the case of impaired and imperiled infants. (Commentary). *JAMA*, 284 (9): 1146–1147.

61. Affleck G, Tennen H, Rowe J (1991). *Infants in Crisis: How Parents Cope with Newborn Intensive Care and its Aftermath.* New York: Springer Verlag.

62. Doctor-assisted suicide: a guide to journal and newspaper articles. Longwood College Library. http://web.lwc.edu/administrative/library/suiart .htm

63. Siegel B (1999, Nov 14). A legal way out. *Los Angeles Times*, U-1.

64. Knickerbocker B (1999, Sep 29). Doctor-aided suicide: shifting politics. Pro-life forces in House opt for backdoor strategy to try to curtail trend toward euthanasia. *Christian Science Monitor*. http://www.csmonitor.com/durable/ 1999/09/28/fp1s4-csm.shtml

65. Oregon Death with Dignity Act. Oregon Revised Statute 127.800–127.995. www.ohd.hr. state.or.us/chs/pas/ors.htm

66. Annas GJ (1997). The bell tolls for a constitutional right to physician-assisted suicide. *N Engl J Med*, 337: 1098.

67. Humphrey D, Clement M (1998). *Freedom to Die: People, Politics, and the Right-to-Die Movement.* New York: St. Martins Press.

68. Dworkin G, Frey RG, Bok S (1998). *Euthanasia and Physician-Assisted Suicide.* New York: Cambridge University Press.

69. Katz S (1998, April 27). Doctor assisted suicide: a bad oxymoron and a bad idea. *Connecticut Post* (editorial).

70. Groenewoud JH et al. (2000). Clinical problems with the performance of euthanasia and physician-assisted suicide in the Netherlands. *N Engl J Med*, 342: 551–556.

71. Quill TE (2000). Palliative treatments of last resort: choosing the least harmful alternative. *Ann Intern Med*, 132: 488–493.

72. Nuland SB (2000). Physician-assisted suicide and euthanasia in practice. *N Engl J Med*, 342: 583–584 (editorial).

73. Sullivan AD et al. (2000, Feb). *Oregon's Death with Dignity Act: The Second Year's Experience.* Portland: Oregon Department of Human Resources.

74. Reporting Requirements of the Oregon Death with Dignity Act, (1999). Amended rules. http://www.ohd.hr.state.or.us/chs/pas/oars.htm

75. Sullivan AD, Hedberg K, Hopkins D (2001). Legalized physician-assisted suicide in Oregon, 1998–2000. *N Engl J Med*, 344:605–607.

76. Alpers A, Lo B (1999). The Supreme Court addresses physician-assisted suicide: Can its rulings improve palliative care? *Arch Fam Med*, 8: 200–205.

77. Eisenberg DE et al. (1993). Unconventional medicine in the United States: prevalence, costs, and patterns of use. *N Engl J Med* 1993; 328:246–252.

78. Straus SE. (2000, June 7). Director, National Center for Complementary and Alternative Medicine speaking before the House Committee on Government Reform. http://nccam .nih.gov/nccam/ne/occam-testimony.html

79. Lambert C (2002). The new ancient trend in medicine: scientific scrutiny of alternative medicine. *Harvard Magazine*, 104:46.

80. Le Shan, L (1974). *The Medium, the Mystic and the Physicist.* New York: Viking.

81. Borysenko J (1987). *Minding the Body, Mending the Mind.* New York: Bantam Books.

82. Weil A (1995). *Spontaneous Healing.* New York: Knopf.

83. Budget Figures for FY 2003. http://nccam.nih./ about/ataglance/index.htm

84. NCCAM (2001) Expanding Horizons of Health Care: Five Year Strategic Plan (2001-2005). At http://nccam.nih.gov/about/plans/fiveyear.pdf

85. NCCAM (2001). Major Domains of Complementary and Alternative Medicine: National Center for Complementary and Alternative, National Institute of Health (NIH). http:// nccam.nih.gov/nccam/fcp/classify

86. NCCAM (2001). Major domains. http:// nccam.nih.gov/nccam/fcp/classify

87. Chopra D (1995). *Boundless Energy: The Complete Mind/Body Program for Overcoming Chronic Fatigue.* New York: Harmony Books.

88. Achterberg J (1990). *Woman as Healer.* Boston: Shambhala.

89. Achterberg J (1985). *Imagery in Healing: Shamanism and Modern Medicine.* Boston: Shambhala, New Science Library. 6, 11–12.

90. Frank J (1974). *Persuasion and Healing*. Baltimore: Johns Hopkins.

91. Simonton OC, Simonton S, Creighton J (1978). *Getting Well Again*. Los Angeles: JP Taracher.

92. Siegel BS (1986). *Love, Medicine, and Miracles*. New York: Harper Collins.

93. Castleman M (2000). *Blended medicine: the best choices in healing*. Emmaus, PA: Rodale Press.

94. NCCAM (2001). Major domains. http://nccam.nih.gov/nccam/fcp/classify.

95. Turner K (2000). *The Self Healing Cookbook: A Macrobiotic Primer for Healing Body, Mind, and Moods with Natural Foods* (9th Ed). New York: Regan Books.

96. Vesanto M, Davis B, Harrison V (2000). *Becoming Vegetarian: The Complete Guide to Adopting a Healthy Vegetarian Diet*. New York: Mass Paperbacks.

97. Atkins RC (2001). *Dr. Atkins' New Diet Revolution*, Revised Edition. Boston: Mass Paperbacks.

98. Ornish D (1983). *Stress, Diet and Your Heart*. New York: Holt, Rinehart & Winston.

99. Pritikin R. *The Pritikin Weight Loss Breakthrough: Five Easy Steps to Outsmart Your Fat Instinct*. New York: Mass Paperback.

100. Weil A (2000). *Eating Well for Optimum Health: The Essential Guide to Food, Diet and Nutrition*. New York: Knopf.

101. Kaplan HI, Sadock BJ (2001). Alternative Medicine and Psychiatry. In *Synopsis of Psychiatry*. Philadelphia: Lippincott Williams & Wilkins. 829–842.

102. Eisenberg DM et al. (1998). Trends in alternative medicine use in the United States, 1990–1997. *JAMA*, 280: 1569–75.

103. Astin JA (1998). Why patients use alternative medicine. *JAMA* 280: 1548–53.

104. Simonton OC, Simonton S, Creighton J (1978). *Getting Well Again*. Los Angeles: JP Tarcher.

105. Huddleston P (1996). *Prepare for Surgery, Heal Faster*. Cambridge, MA: Angel River.

106. Naperstak B (1991). *High Blood Pressure, Heart Disease* (audio tape). Cleveland: Health Journeys.

107. Naperstak B (1991). *HIV Spectrum, Including AIDS* (audio tape). Cleveland: Health Journeys.

108. Sicher F et al. (1998). A randomized double-blind study of the effect of distant healing in a population with advanced AIDS: Report of a small scale study. *West J Med*, 169(6):356–363.

109. Van Biema D (1998, Oct 12). A Test of the Healing Power of Prayer. *Time*, 72–73.

110. Horrigan B (1999). The MANTRA Study Project. *Altern Therap Health Med*, 5(3):75–82.

111. Dossey L (1997). *Healing Words: The Power of Prayer and the Practice of Medicine*. New York: Mass Paperbacks.

112. Dossey L (1999). *Reinventing Medicine: Beyond Mind-Body to a New Era of Healing*. San Francisco: Harper.

113. O'Loire S (1997). An experimental study of the effects of distant, intercessory prayer on self-esteem, anxiety, and depression. *Altern Therap* 3(6): 39–53.

114. Dossey L (1999). *Reinventing Medicine: Beyond Mind-Body to a New Era of Healing*. San Francisco: Harper. p 24.

115. Medical Economics (2001). *Physicians Desk Reference for Herbal Medicines* (2nd Ed). Medical Economics Data.

116. Medical Economics (2000). *Physicians Desk Reference for Non Prescription Drugs and Dietary Supplements*. Medical Economics.

INDEX

Page numbers in *italics* denote figures; those followed by a t denote table.

Abortion
  for minors, 270–271
  new drug for, 270
Abrazolam (Xanax), abuse of, 164
Abstinence Only programs, 113
Abuse (*See also* Addiction; Alcoholism; Substance abuse)
  child (*See* Child maltreatment)
  elder, 237
  in the family, 5 (*See also* Domestic violence)
  family secret rule and, *6*, 6–7
Activities of daily living (ADLs)
  defined, 137, *137*
  instrumental, 137
Acute crisis, in older adults, 136–137
Addiction, 155–177
  alcoholism, 155–157, 160
  behavioral, 155, 165–168
    addictive process in, 165–166
    affect on family system, 5–6
    eating disorders, 167–168
    exercise, 166–167
    Impulse-Control Disorders, 166
    sexual, 123
  behavioral symptoms of, 156–157
  correlation to Attention Deficit Disorder, 157–158
  cravings and, 155, 157
  defined, 155
  neurobiology of, 156–157
  psychosocial factors leading to, 157
  screening for, 155, 170–172, 176–177
    barriers to, 170, *170*
    CAGE questions, 170–171
    referral to treatment, 172
    TWEAK assessment, 171
  sexual, 123 (*See also* Sexual dysfunction, paraphilias)
  stages of, 168–170, *169*
    active quitting, 170

    adverse consequences, 169
    emergence, 168–169
    positive experiences, 169
    prevention of relapse, 170
    turning points, 169–170
  substance abuse
    alcohol, 160
    barbiturates, 164–165
    cannabis, 160
    club drugs, 162
    dissociative drugs, 162–163
    hallucinogens, 163–164
    heroin, 160–161
    sedatives, 164–165
    steroids, 165
    stimulants, 161–162
    tobacco, 159–160
  tolerance and, 155
  treatment, 173–176
    pharmacology, 176
    prevention of relapse, 175–176
    psychotherapy, 175
    therapeutic community, 175
    12 step programs, *173*, 173–174
  withdrawal and, 155
Adherence, treatment, 70–71
Adjustment disorders, 54, 225, 231
Adolescence, college and extended, 47–50
  defined, 47
  difficulties, 49
  task and challenges, 48–49
Adolescents
  abortion and, 270–271
  alcoholism in, 160
  anxiety disorders in, 236–237
  depressive disorders in, 232
  developmental tasks of, 44, *45*
  difficulties in, 46–47
  health care for, 46–47
  parenting of, 44, 46–47

Adolescents (continued)
  perceptions of death, 149
  pregnancy and, 269–270
  sexuality and, 111, 113
    date rape amongst, 213
    sex education, 126
    sexual abstinence, 113
    sexual abuse, 120
    sexually active, 113–114, 118
    survivors of sexual abuse, *214*
    taking sexual history, 118–119
  suicide in, 232
    reaction to, 149
Adult children, loss of parent and, 133–134
Adult survivors of sexual abuse, *214*
Adults
  in life course model, 50–52, *51*
  tasks and challenges of, 50–52, *51*
    factors affecting, 50–51
    poverty and, 51–52
Advance directives, 139–140
  Asian Americans and Pacific Islanders and, 25
  defined, 139
  health care provider role in, 140–142
  health care surrogate, 140
  living will, 139–140
  Medical Power of Attorney, 139–140
  misconceptions about, 140
Advertising
  sexuality and, 112
  view of older adults, 132
African Americans, 16–18
  black cultural values, 17–18
  continuum of cultural identification, 20–21
  effective communication with, 17–18
  historical perspective, 16–17
  prejudice of, 82–83
Age discrimination. 86–87
  barriers to, 170, *170*
  CAGE questions, 170–171
  referral to treatment, 172
  TWEAK assessment, 171
  sexual, 123 (*See also* Sexual dysfunction, paraphilias)
  stages of, 168–170, *169*
  active quitting, 170

Agoraphobia, 235
Alarm reaction, stress and, 96
Alcohol
  as coping mechanism, 104
  as gateway drug, 157, 159–160
Alcoholics Anonymous, 12 step program, 173–174
Alcoholism, 160
  in a colleague, 105–106
  pharmacological treatment, 176
  research on, 155–157
  type I, 157
  type II, 157
Alzheimer's disease, 134
Anabolic-androgenic steroids, 165
Anal retentive, 36
Androgen exposure, sexuality and, 115
Anhedonia, 232
Anorexia nervosa
  neurobiology of, 167–168
  steroids and, 165
Anxiety disorders, 230, 234–237
  in adults, 54
  assessment, 235–236
  Beck Anxiety Inventory (BAI), 235–236
  in children and adolescents, 236–237
  etiology, 230–231, 234
  health conditions associated with, 236
  low diagnosis rate for, 221
  in older adults, 237
  symptoms of, 235, *235*
  treatment, 237–239
    acute emergency, 238
    continuity of care, 239
    pharmacology, 238–239
    team approach, 238
Anxiety-related symptoms, family issues and, 8
Appraisal, of stress, 97–100
abortion and, 270–271
alcoholism in, 160
anxiety disorders in, 236–237
depressive disorders in, 232
developmental tasks of, 44, *45*
difficulties in, 46–47
health care for, 46–47
parenting of, 44, 46–47

diversity of, 23–24
effective communication with, 24–26, *26*
Attention Deficit Disorder (ADD), correlation
    to substance abuse, 157–158
Attitudes, in individual belief systems, 2
Atypical pain, 248

Baby boomers, aging of, 86–87
Baby Doe rule, 273
Balance
    between career and family, 52–53
    stress management and, 106–107
Barbiturates, abuse of, 164–165
Battering cycle, 186
Bayer Model of Complete Clinical Care,
    overview, 59, 62, *62*
Beck Anxiety Inventory (BAI), for anxiety dis-
    orders, 235–236
Beck Depression Scale, 231
Behavioral addiction, 155, 165–168
    addictive process in, 165–166
    affect on family system, 5–6
    eating disorders, 167–168
    exercise, 166–167
    Impulse-Control Disorders, 166
    sexual, 123
Behavioral therapy
    in addiction treatment, 175–176
    in borderline personality disorder, 259
Belief systems, 1–2, *2*
    attitudes, *2*
    core beliefs, 1, *2*
    spiritual beliefs, 1
    values, *2*
Benzodiazepines, abuse of, 164
Bereavement, 143–145
Bisexual (*See also* Gay, lesbian, bisexual, or
    transgendered (GLBT))
    in sexual continuum, 115, *115*
Black cultural values, 17–18 (*See also* African
    Americans)
Black English dialect, 17
Body image, health conditions that affect, 59
Borderline personality disorder, 257–260
    approach-avoidance pattern on, 258
    characteristics of, 257
    etiology, 257–258

treatment, 259–260
    cognitive behavioral therapy, 259
    psychotherapy, 259
    team approach, 259
Bottoming out, in addiction, 169–170
Boundary issues
    in family systems, 7–8
    maintaining, 72, 74
    between patient and physician, 71–74
    transference and, 72–74
"Bridge out of isolation," in domestic vio-
    lence, 193
Bulimia nervosa, neurobiology of, 167–168
Burnout, in physicians, 93–94

CAGE assessment, for addiction, 170–171
Cannabis, abuse of, 160
Capitation
    in managed care, 267
    role in health care crisis, 266
Career
    affects on health, 53–54
    balance between family and, 52–53
    difficulties with, 52
    socioeconomic status and, 51–52
    tasks and challenges of, 52–54
Caring, in end of life care, 150–151
Change
    core beliefs and, 1
    family system and, 3
Chemical addiction (*See* Substance abuse)
Chi, in traditional Oriental medicine, 277
Child abuse and neglect (*See* Child maltreat-
    ment)
Child maltreatment, 205–218
    adult survivors of
        pain disorder and, 248–249
        somatization disorder and, 246
    categories of, 206
    Child Protective Services, 210, 218
    defined, 206
    documentation, 217
    emotional maltreatment
        elements of, *207*
        incidence, 207t
    Endangerment Standard, 206
    Harm Standard in, 206

Child maltreatment (continued)
  identifying, 209–211
    barriers to, 209–210
    symptoms, 210–211
    team approach, 210
  incidence, 205, 206t
  medical neglect, 206–207, 207t
  Munchhausen syndrome by proxy, 251
    causation, 252–253
    incidence, 251
    symptoms, 252
    treatment, 253
  neglect
    elements of, 207
    incidence, 207t
  perpetrator in, 208
  physical abuse
    discipline vs., 208
    elements of, 207
    incidence, 207t
  reporting requirements, 217, 217–218
  risk factors in, 208–209
  sexual abuse, 211–217
    child interview, 213–216
    defined, 208
    developmental issues in, 213
    documentation, 217
    elements of, 207
    evaluation of severity in, 212, 212
    incidence, 207t
    indicators of, 213, 214
    medical examination, 216–217
    secrecy issue, 211–212
Child Protective Services, child maltreatment, 210, 218
Children (See also Adolescents)
  adult, loss of parent and, 133–134
  anxiety disorders in, 236–237
  domestic violence, affect on, 183
  factors for resilience of, 99, 103
  with learning disabilities, 43
  perceptions of death, 145–149, 147
  preschool and middle school, 42–44
Childrenization, of older adults, 132
Children's Health Initiative Program (CHIP), role in health care crisis, 266
Chiropractic medicine, 279–280

Chronic illness, sexuality and, 120–121
Closure of practice, 74–75
Club drugs, abuse of, 162
Cocaine, abuse of, 161–162
Cognitive behavioral therapy
  in addiction treatment, 175–176
  in borderline personality disorder, 259
Cognitive development, Piaget's model of, 36t, 37–38
Cohort factors, in life course model of human development, 50–51
Collectivist orientation, of Asian Americans and Pacific Islanders, 24
College, and extended adolescence, in life course model of human development, 47–50
Coming out, homosexuality and, 85, 116
Commitment, involuntary, 238
Communication
  with Asian Americans and Pacific Islanders, 24
  biomedical tasks and, 61–71
    boundary issues, 71–74
    educate, 68–69
    empathize, 65–66
    engaging patient, 61–65
    enlist patient, 70–71
    termination issues, 74–75
  Black English dialect, 17
  channels of, 61
  culture differences, 14
  in end of life care, 151
  factors affecting, 59–62
  first impressions, 63–65
  importance of, 59
  with Native Americans, 19–20
  non-heterosexual language, 85
  nonverbal, 61–62
    with Asian Americans and Pacific Islanders, 24
    culture differences, 14
    nonverbal leakage, 61
    nose rub, 61
    respiratory avoidance response, 61
  with older adults, 135–136
  paralanguage, 61
  trust and, 135, 136
  verbal, 61

Community
 as context, 8–10
  community ethos, 10
  education, 10
  health and social services, 9–10
  religion, 9
  social interaction, 9
 in family systems, 4, 5
Community ethos, 10
Complementary and alternative medicine
  (CAM), 276–281
 alternative systems, 277–279, 278
  Ayurveda, 278
  homeopathy, 278
  naturopathy, 278–279
  shamanism, 278
  traditional Oriental medicine, 277–278
 biology-based treatment, 278, 279
 defined, 277
 domains of, 277
 energy therapies, 278, 280
 integrative medicine and, 277, 280–281
 manipulative and body-based methods, 278,
  279–280
 mind-body interventions, 278, 279
Confidentiality
 in employee assistance programs (EAPs),
  222–223
 in genome information, 272
Conspiracy of silence, in end of life situations,
  139
Conversion disorder, vs. somatization disorder, 247
Coping
 alcohol and drug abuse in, 104
 barriers to, 104
 in the health care setting, 102–104
 stress management and, 102–106
 support networks, 102–104
Core beliefs, 1, 2
 in life course model of human development, 50
Cost shifting, in health care, 266
Countertransference, 72–74, 74
 in factitious disorders, 253–254
 with older adults, 136
 in pain disorder, 249–250

Couple, in life course model
 formation of, 39–42
 relationship difficulties, 40
 socioeconomic affects, 40
Cravings, in addiction, 155, 157
Crisis of care, in older adults, 136–137
Cultural influences
 affects on health care, 13–30
  historical perspective, 13–14
 in domestic violence, 184
 on sexuality, 111–114
Culture
 American subcultures, 15–30
  African Americans, 16–18
  Asian Americans and Pacific Islanders,
   23–26
  Hispanic Americans, 22–23
  Native Americans, 18–21
  rural, 26, 28
 defined, 13
 of health care, 94–96
 in life course model of human development, 51
 stress and, 99
Culture differences, 14–15
 in communication, 14
 in health care attitudes, 14–15
 implications of, 15
 taking medical history and, 68

Date rape, 164
 affect on victim, 213
 GHB (gamma hydroxybutyrate) in, 162
 Rohypnol (flunitrazepam) in, 162
 symptoms of, 216
Death (See also End of life care)
 of a child, 149
 impact of, 143–145
 perceptions of, 145–149
  adolescents, 149
  children, 145–149, 147
  parent loss of child, 149
Decision making, informed, 70
Dementia, 134–135
 Alzheimer's, 134
 multi-infarct, 134–135
 pseudo, 135

Denial
  aging and, 132, 135
  death and, 139, 145
  in mental disorders, 222
  sexuality and, 111
Depressive disorders, 231–234
  in adolescents, 232
  in adults, 54
  Beck Depression Scale, 231
  etiology, 230–231
  health conditions associated with, 233
  low diagnosis rate for, 221
  medication associated with, 233
  in older adults, 232–234
  substance abuse and, 157
  suicide and, 232
  vegetative signs of, 231, *231*
Descartes, 221
Designer drugs, abuse of, 162
Development (*See* Human development)
Developmental challenges, in Erikson's model,
    37
  for older adults, 133
Developmental tasks, 35
  of adolescence, 44, *45*
  of aging, 133–136
Dextromethorphan, abuse of, 163
Diagnostic and Statistical Manual of Mental
    Disorders (DSM-VI), 225–227
  addiction, defined, 155
  adjustment disorder, 225
  assessment short cuts for, 228–229
  differential diagnosis in, 226
  factitious disorders, 250
  Impulse-Control Disorders, 166
  major diagnostic categories, *226*
  mental disorder, defined, 225
  multiaxial system in, 225–227, *226*
    axis I, 225–226
    axis II, 226
    axis III, 226
    axis IV, 227
    axis V, 227, *228*
  somatization disorder, 245–246
  substance abuse, 155, *156*
  user friendly version, 228–229

Diagnostic-related groups (DRGs), role in
    health care crisis, 266
Differential diagnosis, Diagnostic and Statisti-
    cal Manual of Mental Disorders (DSM-
    VI), 226
Disability certification
  malingering and, 254, 257
  types of, 257
Disabled, sexuality in the, 121
Discipline, *vs.* physical abuse, 208
Disclosure, fear of, in mental disorders,
    221–222
Discrimination (*See also* Prejudice and dis-
    crimination)
  defined, 80
  fear of, in mental disorders, 222–223
Dissociative drugs, abuse of, 162–163
Distress
  beliefs that produce, 98
  characteristics of, *110*
  defined, 98
"Do Not Resuscitate" order, 140
Doctor-assisted suicide, 274
Domestic violence, 5, 183–202
  assessment, 191–196
    barriers to, 191–192
    breaking through isolation, 193–196
    detailed questions, *195*
    interviewing, 194–195
    PEACE questions, 194, *194*
    symptoms of, 192, *193*
  batterer profile, 186
  battering cycle, 186
    honeymoon phase, 186
    tension building phase, 186
    violent phase, 186
  cultural influences on, 184
  family secret rule and, *6*, 6–7
  incidence, 183
  isolation and, 190–191, 193–196
  legal issues in, 185–186
  long-term consequences
    on children, 183
    societal, 183–184
  obstacles to leaving relationships, 188–189,
    189

as silent epidemic, 183–184
training for professionals, 200–201
treatment, 196–200
 assurance, 198, *198*
 documentation, 199, *199*
 safety planning, 199–200, *200*
 stress on health care provider, 201–202
victim factors, 186–191
victimization progression, 189–191
 illness stage, 189–190
 injury stage, 189
 isolation stage, 190–191
Wheel of Non Violence and Equality, *201*
Wheel of Power and Control in, 186, *187*, 190
Dopamine, in addiction, 156
Drug abuse (*See* Substance abuse)
Dual diagnosis, in substance abuse, 157, 176
Dual relationships, 74
Durable Power of Attorney for Health Care, 139–140
Dyspareunia, 124

Eating disorders
 as behavioral addiction, 167–168
 gender differences in, 168, *168*
 symptoms of, 168
Ecstasy, abuse of, 162
Education (*See also* Patient education)
 as community context, 10
Ego, 35
 autonomous, 37
 strength, 37
Ego strengths, Erikson's model of, 35–37, 36t
Ejaculatory incompetence, 123
Elder abuse, 237
Elderly (*See* Older adults)
Electra complex, 36
Emotional distancing, in family systems, 7–8
Emotional maltreatment, of children
 elements of, *207*
 incidence, 207t
Empathy
 in communication, 65–66
 concerns about showing, 65–66

in end of life care, 150–151
Employee assistance programs (EAPs), for mental disorders, 222–223
End-of-life care, 131–152
 advance directives, 139–140
  health care provider role in, 140–142, *141*
 denial of family and, 139
 feeding issues, 141–142
 health care providers
  denial of, 142, 149–150
  role of, 149–152
 hospice, 142
 impact of death, 143–145
 moral issues related to, 274–276
 pain management, 142
 perceptions of death, 145–149
 post death arrangements, 142–143
 spirituality and, 151–152, *152*
Endangerment Standard, in child maltreatment, 206
Engagement, in communication, 61–65
 agenda, 64–65
 patient history and, 67–68
 rapport, 63–65
Enlistment
 in communication, 70–71
 decision making and, 70
 treatment adherence, 70–71
Enmeshment, in family systems, 7–8
Environmental issues, in Diagnostic and Statistical Manual of Mental Disorders (DSM-VI), 227
Erectile disorder
 acquired, 123–124
 lifelong, 123
Erikson's model of ego strengths, 35–37, 36t
 autonomy *vs.* shame, 37
 generativity *vs.* stagnation, 37
 identity *vs.* role confusion, 37
 industry *vs.* inferiority, 37
 initiative *vs.* guilt, 37
 integrity *vs.* despair, 37, 133
 for older adults, 133
 trust *vs.* mistrust, 37

Estate Recovery Laws, 139
 look back period, 139
 spend down, 139
Ethical issues (*See* Moral issues)
Ethnic groups (*See also* Culture)
 defined, 13
Ethnic prejudice, 82–83, *83*
Ethos, defined, 10
Eugenics, moral issues in, 271–273
Eustress, defined, 98
Euthanasia, 274
Evidence collection, in child sexual abuse,
 216–217
Excited utterances, in legal terminology, 199
Exclusive provider organizations (EPOs), 267
Exercise
 as behavioral addiction, 166
 in stress management, 102
Exhaustion, stress and, 96
Eye contact, in communication, 63

Factitious disorders, 250–254
 assessment, *250,* 250–251
 diagnosis, 253–254
 etiology, 251–253
 Munchhausen syndrome, 250
  nonprototypical, 251
  prototypical, 250–251
  by proxy, 251–253, *252*
 team approach for, 253, *253*
 treatment, 254
 vs. malingering, 250
False memories, in child sexual abuse, 215
Familism, in rural America, 29
Family
 balance between career and, 52–53
 in black culture, 18
 as context, in life course model, 39
 death in, 133
 death of a child, 149
 dysfunctional, 3, *4*
  causes of, 3, 5–6
  characteristics of, *6*
  factors for resilience in children, *99, 103*
  family "rules," 6
  family secret rule, *6,* 6–7
  health effects of, 8

 inappropriate boundaries, 7–8
 functional, 3, *4, 6*
 Hispanic Americans and, 22–23
 older adults in, 133
 sexuality and, 111
 as a system, 3–8
Family conference
 in caring for older adults, 137
 inclusion of client in, 137
 preparation for, 137
Family constellation, 7
Family secret rule, *6,* 6–7
Family structures
 affect on family system, 3
 diversity of, 7
Family support, stress and, 99
Fatalism, in rural America, 29
Fee-for-service system, role in health care crisis, 266
Fetishism, 125
 transvestic, 125
Fidelity, in end of life care, 151
Financial issues, in health care for the elderly,
 137, 139
First appointment, communication during,
 63–65
Flunitrazepam (Rohypnol), abuse of, 162
Freeze reaction, stress and, 97
Freudian theory of psychosexual develop-
 ment, 35–37, 36t
 genital stage, 37
 latency stage, 36–37
 oral stage, 36
 phallic stage, 36
Friendships, in rural America, 29
Frotteurism, 125
Funeral arrangements, 142–143

Gamma hydroxybutyrate (GHB), abuse of,
 162
Gastronomy tube, in end of life care, 141–142
Gateway drug, 157, 159–160
Gay, lesbian, bisexual, or transgendered
 (GLBT), 115–116
 biological aspects of, 115
 coming out, 85, 116
 improving health care for, 85–86

prejudice and, 84–86
psychological basis for, 115–116
situational homosexuality, 122
Gender differences
in eating disorders, 168, *168*
stress and, 99
in view of sexuality, 116
Gender identity disorder, 116
Gene mapping, 271–273
Genetic markers, prenatal screening and,
272–273
Geriatric care (*See* Older adults)
Geriatric care manager, role of, 138
GHB (gamma hydroxybutyrate), abuse of, 162
Global assessment of functioning, in Diagnostic and Statistical Manual of Mental
Disorders (DSM-VI), 227, *228*
Grief, 143–145
denied, 145
factors that affect, 144
stages of, 143, *143*
suicide and, 145
symptoms of, 145, *146*
traumatic, 144
Grief overload, 144

Habituation response, in addiction, 157
Hallucinogen Persisting Perception Disorder,
164
Hallucinogens, abuse of, 163–164
Harm Standard, in child maltreatment, 206
Hazelden treatment Model, 12 step program,
174–175
Healing, spirituality and, 280–281
Health, participatory, 70
Health care costs
cost shifting, 266
emergency room medicine and, 266
health care crisis and, 265–266
Health care crisis, 265–268
federal reform efforts, 266
health care costs and, 265–266
managed care role in, 268
Health care services, as community context,
9–10
Health maintenance organizations (HMOs),
267

Health proxy, 139–140
Healthy personality, in Erikson's model,
37
Hearing, effects of decline in older adults,
134
Hendrix, H., 41
Herbal remedies, 279, 281
Heroin
abuse of, 160–161
pharmacological treatment, 176
Heterosexism, defined, 118
Heterosexual, in sexual continuum, 115, *115*
Hispanic Americans, 22–23
cultural values, 22–23
historical perspective, 22
Historical hostility, in culture differences, 15
Hitting bottom, in addiction, 169–170
Holistic health movement, 276–281
Home place, in rural America, 29
Homophobia, defined, 84, 117
Homosexuality (*See also* Gay, lesbian, bisexual
or transgendered (GLBT))
prejudice and, 84–86
in sexual continuum, 115, *115*
situational, 122
Honeymoon phase, in domestic violence, 186,
188
Hospice (*See also* End-of-life care)
in-home, 142
pain management, 142
Hospitalization, involuntary, 238
Human development, 35–56
aging and, 133–136
life course model, 39–54
theories of, 35–39
Erikson's model of ego strengths, 35–37,
36t
Freudian theory of psychosexual development, 35–37, 36t
Kohlberg's model of moral development,
36t, 38
Piaget's model of cognitive development,
36t, 37–38
Human sexuality (*See* Sexuality)
Humor and laughter, in stress management,
107–108
Hypnotherapy, 279

Hypochondriasis, *vs.* somatization disorder, 247
Hypoxyphilia, 125

Ibogaine, abuse of, 163–164
Id, 35
Illness beliefs, 245
Imagery, guided, 279–280
Imago Theory of Relationships, 41
Immune system, stress and, 97
Impotence
  primary, 123
  secondary, 123–124
Impulse-Control Disorders, 166
Independent practice association (IPA), *266*
Individual belief systems, 1–2, *2*
Individualism, rugged, in rural America, 29
Infantilize, older adults and, 86–87
Infants, parenting of, 42
Ingroup, 79
Inhalants, abuse of, 164–165
Institutionalized persons, sexuality and, 121–122
Instrumental activities of daily living (IADLs), 137
Insurance
  coverage of mental disorders, 222
  health care costs and, 265–266
Integrative medicine, complementary and alternative medicine and, 277, 280–281
Interconnectedness, in family systems, 3, *4, 5*
Interdisciplinary team meeting (*See* Team approach)
Isolation
  in child sexual abuse, 211–212
  in domestic violence, 190–191, 193–196

Karma, 24
Ketamine, abuse of, 163
King, T., 83
Klismaphilia, 125
Kohlberg's model of moral development, 36t, 38
  conventional morality, 38
  postconventional morality, 38
  preconventional morality, 38

Language (*See also* Communication)
  non-heterosexual, 85
Legal issues
  in assisted suicide, 185–186276
  in domestic violence, 185–186
  reporting requirements in child maltreatment, *217,* 217–218
Lesbians (*See also* Gay, lesbian, bisexual, or transgendered (GLBT))
  LUGs (lesbians until graduation), 115
Libido, 36
Life course model of human development, 39–54
  adulthood, 50–52, *51*
  career, 52–54
  college and extended adolescence, 47–50
  couple formation, 39–42
  family as context, 39
  parenting, 42
    child birth, 42
    preschool to middle school, 42–44
    puberty and adolescence, 44, 46–47
Like-ability
  discrimination and, 79, 82
  of patient, 67–68
Listening, in communication, 63
Living will, 139–140
Long-term care, financing of, 139
Look back period, in long-term care financing, 139
LSD, abuse of, 163–164
LUGs (lesbians until graduation), 115
Lyme disease, 26–28

MADISON Scale, for pain assessment, 249
Magical thinking, in children about death, 146
Malingering, 254–255
  disability certification and, 254, 257
  drug-seeking patient and, 254–255, *255*
  in pain disorder, 249
  treatment, 254–255
  types of, 254
  vs. factitious disorders, 250
Manageability of patient, discrimination and, 67, 82
Managed care, 266–268
  bargaining power of, 267

capitation in, 267
continuum of, 266
impact on provider care, 268
role in health care crisis, 268
usage controls, 266–267
Managed care organizations (MCOs), 266, 267
Marijuana
abuse of, 160
medical uses of, 160
with PCP, 163
Marriage
sex before, 114–115
sexuality in, 114
Masturbation, attitudes about, 114
Medicaid
long-term care financing and, 139
role in health care crisis, 266
Medical history
culture differences and, 68
sexual history in, 116–120
with adolescents, 118–119
barriers to taking, 117
basic questions, 117
detailed, 118, *119*
health care provider self-awareness, 117
heterosexual bias in, 118
Medical neglect, of children, 206–207
Medical Power of Attorney, 139–140
Medicare
hospice reimbursement, 142
role in health care crisis, 266
Medicare risk contracts, role in health care crisis, 266
Meditation, 279
in stress management, 107
Menopause, 54
Mental disorders, 221–241
anxiety disorders, 234–237 (*See also* Anxiety disorders)
assessment in, 227–230
Mental Status Examination, 227, *229*
mini mental status examination, 227–228, *230*
Patient Health Questionnaire (PHQ), 229
PRIME-MD, 229

Quick PsychoDiagnostics Panel (QPD), 229
short cuts for, 228–229
borderline personality disorder, 257–260
depressive disorders, 231–234
Diagnostic and Statistical Manual of Mental Disorders (DSM-VI) for, 225–227
factitious disorders, 250–254
mood disorders (*See* Depressive disorders)
pain disorder, 248–250
prejudice and, 87
provider barriers, 224–225
societal beliefs about, 221–224
fear of disclosure, 221–222
fear of discrimination, 222–223
stigma, 221
somatoform disorders, 243–250
Mental retardation, in Diagnostic and Statistical Manual of Mental Disorders (DSM-VI), 226
Mental Status Examination, 227, 229
Mescaline, abuse of, 163–164
Midlife crisis
career and, 52–53
in women, 53
Mifepristone (Mifeprex), for abortion, 270
Mini mental status examination, 227–228, *230*
Minnesota Model, 12 step program, 174–175
Monoamine oxidase inhibitors, for depression, 238
Mood disorders, 230 (*See also* Depressive disorders)
Moral development, Kohlberg's model of, 36t, 38
Moral issues, 268–282
end-of-life issues, 274–276
reproductive issues, 268–274
Mourning, 143–145
Munchausen syndrome, 250
nonprototypical, 251
prototypical, 250–251
by proxy, 251
causation, 252–253
incidence, 251
symptoms, 252
treatment, 253

National Canter for Complementary and
    Alternative Medicine (NCCAM), 277
Native Americans, 18–21
    attitudes toward health care, 19–20
    effective communication with, 19–20
    historical perspective, 18–19
Necrophilia, 125
Neglect of a child
    elements of, 207
    incidence, 207t
    medical, 206–207
Neighborliness, in rural America, 29
Netherlands, doctor-assisted suicide in, 274, 276
Neurotoxin-mediated illnesses, vs. somato-
    form disorders, 244
Neurotoxins
    causes of, 244
    Visual Contrast Sensitivity (VCS) examina-
        tion for, 244
Neurotransmitters, in addiction, 156
Nihilism, therapeutic, 254
Non-normative life events, 39
Norepinephrine, in addiction, 156
Normative life events, 39
Norms, defined, 13
Nose rub, in non-verbal communication, 61
Nutritional therapy, 279–280

Obesity, prejudice and, 87–88
Oedipus complex, 36
Office of Alternative Medicine (OAM), 277
Old-old, defined, 134
Older adults, 134–135 (See also Aging)
    age discrimination, 86–87
    anxiety disorders in, 237
    childrenization of, 132
    crisis of care in, 136–137
    decline in five senses, 134
    dementia in, 134–135
    depressive disorders in, 232–234
    developmental tasks of, 133–136
    health care for
        assessment, 136–139
        care planning, 135–136
        communication, 135–136
        in-home care, 138
        sexuality in, 120

social losses in, 135
    transference and countertransference, 136
Openness, in end of life care, 151
Opioids
    abuse of, 160–161
    negative health effect of, 161
    pharmacological treatment for, 176
Oregon, doctor-assisted suicide in, 274,
    276
Orgasmic disorder
    female, 124
    male, 123
Orthomolecular therapy, 279
Osteopathy, 279–280
Outgroup, 79

Pain disorder, 248–250
    assessment, 248–249
    child maltreatment and, 248–249
    treatment, 249–250
    vs. somatization disorder, 247
Palliative care (See also End of life care)
    feeding issues, 141–142
    hospice, 142
    pain management in, 142
Pan-Indians, 20
Paralanguage, 61
Paraphilias, 124–125
Parental notification, regarding minor's
    abortion, 271
Parenting
    child birth
        difficulties, 42
        tasks and challenges, 42
    preschool to middle school, 42–44
    puberty and adolescence, 44, 46–47
        difficulties, 46–47
        tasks and challenges, 44, 46
Passive-aggressive, 36
Patient education, 68–69
    patient's perspective in, 68–69
    questions to answer, 69
Patient Health Questionnaire (PHQ), mental
    disorder assessment, 229
Patient history
    importance of patient's perspective, 67
    obtaining, 67–68

Patients, challenging, 243–260
  borderline personality disorder, 257–260
  factitious disorders, 250–254
  pain disorder, 248–250
  somatoform disorders, 243–250
  team approach for, 253, *253*
Patterns, in family systems, 3, *4, 5*
PCP, abuse of, 162–163
PEACE assessment, in domestic violence, 194,
  194
Pedophilia, 125
Perfectionism, in physicians, 93
Perpetrator
  in child maltreatment, 208
  in domestic violence, 186
Person perception, process of, 79, *80*
Personality
  Freudian theory of, 35–37, 36t
  stress and, 93–94, 99
  Type A, 99
Personality, type A, stress management and,
  102
Personality disorder (*See also* Borderline per-
    sonality disorder)
  in Diagnostic and Statistical Manual of
      Mental Disorders (DSM-VI), 226
Physical abuse, of children
  discipline *vs.,* 208
  elements of, *207*
  incidence, 207t
Physician aid-in-dying, 274
Physician-hospital organization (PHO), *267*
Physicians
  expectations of, 94
  stress and, 93–96
  training process for, 94–96, *103*
Piaget's model of cognitive development, 36t,
    37–38
  concrete operational stage, 38
  formal operations stage, 38
  preoperational stage, 38
  sensorimotor stage, 37
Post-formal thought, 48
Postnatal decisions, moral issues in, 273–274
Posttraumatic stress disorder (PTSD), 98
  secondary, in domestic violence, 202
  traumatic grief and, 144

Poverty
  affect on family system, 3, 4
  in rural America, 28
Practice, closure of, 74–75
Preferred provider organizations (PPOs), 266,
  267
Pregnancy, adolescents and, 269–270
Prejudice, defined, 13, 79
Prejudice and discrimination, 79–90
  age, 86–87
  counteracting, 88–89
  in health care, 80, 82
  in mental disorders, 222–223
  mental illness and, 87
  obesity and, 87–88
  racial, 82–83, *83*
  self awareness about, 80, 82, *82,* 88–89
  sexual preference and, 84–86, 117–118
  smoking and, 87
  stereotyping, 79–80
  in the workplace, 90
Premature ejaculation, 123
Prenatal screening, genetic markers and,
  272–273
Prevention of relapse, in addiction, 170,
  175–176
Preventive care, uninsured clients and, 266
Primary gain, in pain disorder, 249
PRIME-MD, mental disorder assessment,
  229
Prisons, sex in, 122
Problem solving, stress management and,
  106–108
Projection, transference and, 72
Pseudo dementia, 135
Psilocybin, abuse of, 163–164
Psychogenic pain, 248
Psychosexual development, Freudian theory
  of, 35–37, 36t
Psychosis, LSD-induced Persistent, 164
Psychosocial perspective
  community as context, 8–10
  components of, 1
  family as a system in, 3–8
  individual belief systems, 1–2, *2*
Psychosomatic disease, stress and, 97
Psychosomatic pain, 248

Psychotherapy
in addiction treatment, 175
in borderline personality disorder, 259
Puberty (*See* Adolescence)

Qi, in traditional Oriental medicine, 277
Quick PsychoDiagnostics Panel (QPD), mental disorder assessment, 229
Quitting, active, in addiction, 170

Race, defined, 13
Racial prejudice, 82–83, *83*
Rapport, in communication, 63–65
Ratey, J., 97–98
Reciprocal influences, in family systems, 3, *4, 5*
Referral, procedures for, 74–75
Reiki, 280
Reimbursement, for mental disorders, 222
Relaxation techniques, in stress management, 101–102, 107
Religion (*See also* Spirituality)
of Asian Americans and Pacific Islanders, 24
as community context, 9
Hispanic Americans and, 23
stress and, 99
Reporting requirements, in child maltreatment, *217,* 217–218
Reproductive issues, moral issues in, 268–274
abortion for minors, 270–271
difficult postnatal decisions, 273–274
eugenics, 271–273
Resilience, stress and, 99, *99*
Resistance, stress and, 96
Respiratory avoidance response, in non-verbal communication, 61
Responsiveness, in end of life care, 151
Retirement, as a developmental task, 134
Right-to-die issues, 274
Right-to-life activists, 274
Rural Americans, 26, 28
effective communication with, 29–30
rural values, 28–29
Rural health care, state of, 26, 28

Schaie, K. W., 48
Secondary gain, in pain disorder, 249

Sedatives, abuse of, 164–165
Self care, for the healer (*See* Stress management)
Self-denial, in physicians, 96
Self-diagnosis, patient education and, 68, 70
Selye, H., 96, 98
Serenity Prayer, 101, *101*
Serotonin, in addiction, 156
Serotonin selective reuptake inhibitors (SSRIs), for depression, 238
Sex education, 113
about sexual dysfunction, 126–127
about sexually transmitted infections, 114, 126
characteristics of effective, *113*
Sexual abuse
in adolescents, 120
Sexual abuse, child, 211–217
child interview, 213–216
false memories and, 215
materials for, *215*
precautions for, 215–216
defined, 208
developmental issues in, 213
documentation, 217
elements of, *207*
evaluation of severity in, 212, *212*
incidence, 207t
indicators of, 213, *214*
medical examination, 216–217
secrecy issue, 211–212
Sexual addiction, 123
Sexual attraction, range of, 114–116, *115*
Sexual aversion disorder, 123
Sexual behaviors, defined, 118
Sexual desire
hyperactive, 123
hypoactive, 122–123
Sexual dysfunction, 122–125
hyperactive sexual desire, 123
hypoactive sexual desire, 122–123
incidence, 122
in men
ejaculatory incompetence, 123
premature ejaculation, 123
primary impotence, 123

secondary impotence, 123–124
paraphilias, 124–125
  fetishism, 125
  frotteurism, 125
  hypoxyphilia, 125
  klismaphilia, 125
  necrophilia, 125
  pedophilia, 125
  referral to mental health professional, 127, *127*
  sexual masochism, 125
  sexual sadism, 125
  telephone scatologia, 125
  transvestic fetishism, 125
  treatment, 127
  voyeurism, 125
  zoophilia, 125
referral to mental health professional, 126–127, *127*
sex education about, 126–127
sexual addiction, 123
sexual aversion disorder, 123
treatment, 126–127
in women
  dyspareunia, 124
  orgasmic disorder, 124
  vaginismus, 124
Sexual history, taking, 116–120
Sexual masochism, 125
Sexual sadism, 125
Sexuality, 111–128
  adolescence and, 111, 113
  American cultural messages, 111–114
    in advertising, 112
    conservative beliefs, 111
    libertine philosophy, 112–113
    on television, 112–113
  in the chronically ill, 120–121
  denial and, 111
  in the disabled, 121
  gay, lesbian, transgendered (GLT), 115–116
    (*See also* Gay, lesbian, bisexual, or transgendered (GLBT))
  gender differences, 116
  institutionalized persons and, 121–122
  masturbation, 114
  in older adults, 120

range of, 114–116, *115*
sex education (*See* Sex education)
sexual dysfunctions (*See* Sexual dysfunction)
sexually transmitted infections (STIs) and, 113–114
taking sexual history, 116–120
Sexually transmitted infections (STIs), 113–114
  in adolescents, 113–114
  sex education about, 114, 126
  treatment, 125–126
Shaffer, Jonathan, stages of addictions, 168–170, *169*
Shaken baby syndrome, symptoms of, 210–211, *211*
Shorter, E., 44
Signs, defined, 227
Slavery, affect on African Americans, 16
Smoking
  as gateway drug, 157, 159–160
  prejudice and, 87
  as substance abuse, 159–160
Social interaction, as community context, 9
Social services, as community context, 9–10
Socioeconomic status
  career and, 51–52
  college and, 47–48
  low
    affect on family system, 3, 4
    in rural America, 28
Somatization, of mental disorders, 224–225
Somatization disorder, 245–248
  assessment, 245–246
  child maltreatment and, 246
  etiology, 245
  treatment, 247–248
Somatoform disorders, 243–250
  characteristics of, 244–245
  diagnosis, 244
  somatization disorder, 245–248
    assessment, 245–246
    etiology, 245
    treatment, 247–248
  vs. neurotoxin-mediated illnesses, 244
Spend down, in long-term care financing, 139

Spirituality (*See also* Religion)
  in belief systems, 1
  in end of life care, 151–152, *152*
  healing and, 280–281
  in stress management, 107
Splitting
  in borderline personality disorder, 258
  defined, *257*
  in factitious disorders, 253
Stereotyping, 79–80
Steroids, abuse of, 165
Stigma, of mental disorders, 221
Stimulants
  abuse of, 161–162
  medical uses of, 161
Stress, 96–101
  assessment of, barriers to, 100–101
  beliefs that produce, 98
  beliefs that reduce, 98–99
  career and, 52–53
  characteristics of, *110*
  defined, 96
  external, 97
  in the health care setting, *103*
  internal, 97
  nature *vs.* nurture, 98
  phychosomatic disease and, 97
  physiological reaction to, 96–97
  role of appraisal in, 97–100
  substance abuse and, 157
Stress management, 93–108, 280
  coping, 102–106
  culture of health care and, 94–96
  holistic approach to, 101
  personal factors related to, 93–94
  problem solving, 106–108
  relaxation techniques, 101–102
Stroke, dementia associated with, 134–135
Substance abuse, 155
  affect on family system, 5–6
  alcohol, 160
  barbiturates, 164–165
  cannabis, 160
  child maltreatment and, 209
  club drugs, 162
  of a colleague, 105–106
  as coping mechanism, 104

  dissociative drugs, 162–163
  drug-seeking patient and, 254–255, *255*
  hallucinogens, 163–164
  heroin, 160–161
  sedatives, 164–165
  steroids, 165
  stimulants, 161–162
  tobacco, 159–160
Suicide
  in adolescents, 149, 232
  depressive disorders and, 232
  doctor-assisted, 274
  grief and, 145
  rational, 274
  stigma of, 145
Superego, 35
Support groups, 12 step programs, 173–175
Support networks, stress management and, 102–104
Survivors
  in domestic violence, 198
  of sexual abuse, symptoms of, *214*
Symptoms, defined, 227
Systems approach, to family, 3–8

Tao, 24
Team approach, 253, *253*
  in anxiety disorders, 238
  in borderline personality disorder, 259
  in caring for older adults, 137
  in child maltreatment, 210
  in factitious disorders, 253
Teen Abstinence Movement, 113
Telephone scatologia, 125
Television, sexuality and, 112–113
Terminal care (*See* End of life care)
Termination, defined, 75
Termination issues, 74–75
  reasons for, 74
  referral procedures, 74–75
The Making of the Modern Family, 44
Therapeutic community, in addiction treatment, 175
Therapeutic nihilism, 254
Therapeutic touch, 280

Tobacco
  abuse of, 159–160
  as gateway drug, 157, 159–160
Tolerance, in addiction, 155
Traditionalism, in rural America, 29
Transference, 72–74, 74
  counter, 72–74
  management of, 72–73
  negative, 72
  with older adults, 136
  positive, 72
  unconscious, 72–73
Transgendered sexuality, 116 (*See also* Gay,
      lesbian, bisexual, or transgendered
      (GLBT))
Treatability
  discrimination and, 67, 82
  of patient, 67
Treatment adherence, enlistment, 70–71
Tricyclic antidepressants
  abuse of, 164
  for depression, 238
Trust
  client care and, 135, *136*
  physicians and, 94–95
TWEAK assessment, for addiction, 171
12 step programs, *173*, 173–175
  Alcoholics Anonymous, 173–174
  Minnesota Model, 174–175
  steps in, *174*

Type A Personality, 99
  stress management and, 102

Unemployment, stress and, 53
Uninsured, health care costs and, 265–266
United States
  health care crisis in, 265–268
  sexuality in, 111–114

Vaginismus, 124
Values
  defined, 13
  in individual belief systems, 2
Virtue, 37
Vision, effects of decline in older adults,
      134
Visual Contrast Sensitivity (VCS) examina-
      tion, for neurotoxins, 244
Voyeurism, 125

Wheel of Non Violence and Equality, *201*
Wheel of Power and Control, in domestic vio-
      lence, 186, *187*, 190
Wisdom, aging and, 133
Withdrawal, addiction and, 155
Workaholism, in physicians, 94

Xenophobia, in rural America, 29

Zoophilia, 125